CONNECTING WITH THE NEW HEALTHCARE CONSUMER: DEFINING YOUR STRATEGY

DAVID B. NASH, M.D., M.B.A.

MARY PAT MANFREDI, MPH

BARBARA BOZARTH, MSEd

SUSAN HOWELL, MSS

McGraw-Hill

New York   San Francisco   Washington, D.C.   Auckland   Bogotá
Caracas   Lisbon   London   Madrid   Mexico City   Milan
Montreal   New Delhi   San Juan   Singapore
Sydney   Tokyo   Toronto

McGraw-Hill

A Division of The **McGraw·Hill** *Companies*

3 4 5 6 7 8 9   BKM BKM   9 0 9 8 7 6 5 4 3 2 1 0

ISBN 007-134672-4

Printing and binding by Book-Mart Press, Inc.

Cover illustration by Steve Dininno.

This book was typeset using 11 point New Century Schoolbook.

This publication is designed to provide accurate and authoritative information in regard to the subject matter covered. It is sold with the understanding that neither the author nor the publisher is engaged in rendering legal, accounting, or other professional service. If legal advice or other expert assistance is required, the services of a competent professional person should be sought.

—From a Declaration of Principles jointly adopted by a Committee of the American Bar Association and a Committee of Publishers.

To all of our children, the real future consumers: That they may always be "connected" to the blessings of good health, peace and happiness.

Leah, Rachel, and Jacob Nash
Duke and Sara Bozarth
Nicholas Manfredi

FOREWORD

Although the history of medicine goes back thousands of years, the idea of a healthcare "consumer" is still relatively new. As the end of World War II loosed a tidal wave of pent-up consumer demand, the healthcare field awkwardly dipped a cautious toe into the murky waters of consumer communication. A community hospital or two competed politely for news coverage of a maternity wing. A health plan here or there paid a sales call on a labor union representative. A continuing medical education course counseled physicians to listen better to their patients, particularly to their female ones.

Yet signs that change would be more than incremental were already apparent. In 1946, Dr. Benjamin Spock's *Common Sense Book of Baby and Child Care* dared advise parents to trust their own instincts rather than deferring to their pediatrician for even such everyday decisions as when to feed their baby. In 1969, a collective of Boston feminists published *Our Bodies, Ourselves,* which brought the sensibilities of the Civil Rights movement to medicine. "Obedience" to the doctor was out; "dialog" was in. So were the beginnings of more aggressive "doctor shopping."

Soon, consumer and government pressure forced hospitals to adopt a "bill of rights" that acknowledged patient control in certain areas of treatment. The news media discovered that different "brands" of hospitals had different attributes: a 1973 story in the Long Island newspaper *Newsday* about local bypass surgery programs was the first to compare hospital mortality rates. A series of court decisions reinforced the new, more open climate. By the early 1970s, for example, physicians had a clear obligation to disclose to patients in simple language information about the procedures they were recommending and the likely effects, good and bad. Even more powerful, a 1975 Supreme Court ruling held that the traditional "learned professions" of law and medicine were subject to antitrust law. Professional societies could no longer prohibit advertising and other forms of competition.

The cultural, legal, and economic forces that were in place by the mid-1970s have steadily increased in power. Today, "the consumer voice has advanced from a whisper to a holler," as David B. Nash, M.D., MBA, this book's editor, puts it in his introduction. The healthcare community is paying attention. Even the American Medical Association (AMA), champion of the one-to-one doctor relationship, now has consumer-oriented Web sites. For the patient sitting in front of his or her home computer, "mouse calls" have supplanted "house calls." Just as interestingly, the financial support for the AMA sites typically comes from pharmaceutical companies, who now spend more than $1 billion annually on direct-to-consumer marketing efforts.

Indeed, healthcare "consumerism" has become trendy. Liberals love the "empowerment" of the common man, and conservatives and moderates warm to the idea that marketplace efficiency provides the best path to optimum care at minimum cost. Unfortunately, connecting with the new healthcare consumer is not as simple as creating a Web site. There are new kinds of healthcare organizations—various permutations of managed care plans and integrated delivery systems—and new kinds of healthcare consumers, including the consumer activists who make the healthcare purchasing decisions for some of the nation's largest corporations.

Connecting with the New Healthcare Consumer: Defining Your Strategy is a must-read guide to building a successful strategy in this critical area. Consumerism represents a fundamental change in how healthcare will be delivered and financed. The depth of knowledge of the authors of this book's chapters and the breadth of topics that they address make this a volume that will be pulled down from the shelf frequently for both consultation and quotation. This text is filled with interesting facts and provocative predictions, whether the topic be government involvement, online trends, or the evolution from disease treatment to health management. When the book's component parts are taken as a whole, the result is a thought-provoking examination of a phenomenon whose extraordinary impact is just starting to be widely understood.

In an influential 1988 article in the *New England Journal of Medicine,* Paul Ellwood, M.D., called for "a technology of patient experience." That focus on the patient experience is, I be-lieve, what ultimately will determine the success of the health-care consumer connection. The outreach to the patient as con-sumer must be done with the kind of thoughtfulness that this book's authors provide; the alternative is to rely only on the tools of public relations and advertising. The potential reward, however, is great: better clinical quality of care, more humane care, and more cost-effective care.

The great Albert Schweitzer, M.D., posed the challenge this way: "Each patient carries his own doctor inside him. They come to us not knowing that truth. We are at our best when we give the doctor who resides within each patient a chance to go to work."

Michael L. Millenson
Visiting Scholar, Northwestern University Institute
for Health Care Research and Policy Studies.
Author, *Demanding Medical Excellence: Doctors and
Accountability in the Information Age.*
Chicago, IL
September, 1999

PREFACE

As both an industry and a commodity, healthcare has been swept into the consumerism movement. The new generation of consumers is described as "empowered, pragmatic, narcissistic and manipulative" (Herzlinger, 1997), and the impact of this generation is nothing less than revolutionary. Managed care and roller coaster cycles of mistrust of healthcare providers and payment and delivery mechanisms have served as potent catalysts in healthcare consumers' evolution into informed, influential, and assertive players in the healthcare arena. Moreover, the rise of the Internet and World Wide Web has fostered a new class of consumers who have both an increased supply of educational resources at their disposal and greater access to these resources. In response to this new healthcare consumerism, forward-thinking leaders of health plans are asking themselves, "How can we attract and retain our members and offer the most and best we can without breaking the bank?" Physicians are asking, "How can I manage my patients' care more effectively?" Employers are competing more fiercely for employees by enticing them with even more job "perks." Health system "brand" names are appearing on billboard space, proclaiming their strengths in the marketplace, to draw future "customers."

Consumers of healthcare have made great strides away from the passive roles once played by patients of a few decades ago. As such, the phenomenon coined in healthcare business literature as "asymmetries of information" is breaking down (Kleinke, 1998; Starr, 1997)—the balance of medical information is not as heavily weighted toward healthcare professionals. In the paternalistic medical model of the past, the healthcare provider was the keeper of information. Today's healthcare consumers are aided by a plethora of resources that enable them to participate in the process of getting, receiving, and *understanding* healthcare. Consequently, patient expectations have increased.

The magnitude of consumer empowerment is being steadily uncovered. Recently, a survey by the accounting firm KPMG, with Northwestern University, found that consumerism influences "policy, strategy, operations, and investment decisions of health care organizations within all segments of the industry" (KPMG/Northwestern, 1998). The consumer portion of the survey showed clearly that consumers *are* asking employers, health plans, and providers for more information about their benefits and their healthcare treatment. Consumers *are* paying attention to medical and health news and information. A recent survey by Roper Starch, titled "Americans Talk About Science and Medical News" (Roper Starch Worldwide, Inc., 1997), demonstrates that consumers are listening and making use of their knowledge.

Why did we create this book? *Connecting with the New Healthcare Consumer: Defining Your Strategy* was the outgrowth, first, of our revelation that few industries are exempt from the consumerism movement. Companies like Wal-Mart, The Home Depot, and Nordstrom's have all devised sharp business plans around a central and winning theme: responding to consumers' needs and, within limits, desires. All three companies exemplify a movement by corporate America based on consumer-focused services that dilute competition from other companies. Consumer preferences are becoming solid marketing tools. The consumer's voice has pervaded virtually every aspect of healthcare and has advanced from a whisper to a holler. Those health plans, employers, and health systems, for example, who do not pay heed to the consumer voice and develop a business plan accordingly will fall behind others who craft their offerings based on the consumerist model.

And what does the corporate retail example have to do with healthcare? Here in the Office of Health Policy and Clinical Outcomes at Thomas Jefferson University in Philadelphia, where our mission is in large part to serve as a bridge between academia and industry, the "business of healthcare" is our invariable marketplace. Our sensitivity to so-called consumer issues, in all their forms, is not unlike anyone else's: we all aim to please our customers, who are from all walks of the delivery spectrum. Through our customers, we have heard, "What exactly does 'consumerism' mean? How can we strategize to meet our clients' needs?" (In the old days, the only client in healthcare was the patient—who remains at the center of the consumerism movement in healthcare.) Furthermore, to the best of our knowledge, there was no book or literature supporting our need to know more about the key issues and help us grasp the tools that could enable us better meet our customers' needs. We wanted a "compass" to navigate the changes that have sprung from the era of the new healthcare consumer. From these needs, this text was born.

This book, narrated by experts, walks the reader through the maze of new consumer-related developments in healthcare. Each chapter offers a unique perspective or topical angle, based on the author's area of expertise. Therein, the interests of those consumers whose voices were once unheard, if not silenced—women, the elderly, the mentally ill, among others—are highlighted.

The book has several aims: to convey the trends and developments that have shaped the consumer revolution in healthcare, to help readers better understand the impact of this revolution on the healthcare industry, and to familiarize readers with the issues germane to their own consumer markets. Success in the healthcare marketplace will increasingly be tied to how much and how *well* organizations understand and respond to the new healthcare consumer.

This text provides a solid knowledgebase and the tools to help readers form and cultivate their consumer-focused strategies. We invite this book's audience to pick those chapters most appropriate for his or her interest; each chapter is solid as a stand-alone work.

Connecting with the New Healthcare Consumer: Defining Your Strategy is for anyone trying to grasp how consumers are revolutionizing healthcare, particularly for healthcare professionals who are decision makers and leaders in their fields, as well as for those at the corporate or legislative level. It is for individuals who are proactive and willing to be introspective and reflect upon their current ideas and strategies focused on new consumers. Those who make the best use out of this book have the drive and the commitment to incorporate elements from the consumerist model into daily practice.

Now for a road map. The first chapter, "Listening to the Consumer: A Historical Review," by John Coombs, James Hereford, and Paul LePore, provides an excellent overview of the history of consumerism in healthcare, a helpful context for the remainder of the book.

Chapter 2, "The Public View of Healthcare," by Joel Miller, elaborates on American's vacillating opinions on healthcare that have been gleaned from public opinion surveys.

The self-care trend, encompassing the consumer's ability and inclination toward self-care, is illustrated by Steven Haimowitz in Chapter 3, "The Self-Care Trend and the New Healthcare Marketplace." This chapter explores the evolution of self-care and its scope in shaping modern healthcare consumers.

The power of information dissemination to today's healthcare consumer cannot be underestimated. Chapter 4, "Medical and Health Reporting in the News Media," by Ira Nash, highlights the history and trends in communicating medical and health-related information through various news media channels. Shifts in the patient–doctor–press relationship dynamic and the effect on the "power of the press" are likewise highlighted.

The Internet and World Wide Web, in particular, have been the catalyst for the explosive growth in health and medical information resources available to the lay public. Chapter 5, "The Online Community as a Healthcare Resource," by Stu Gitlow, illuminates how the Internet is changing the way we do business and the way in which we interact with one another.

An enduring theme throughout much of this book is the relationship between healthcare providers and their patients. In Chapter 6, "Relationship-Based Care: Strengthening the Patient–Physician Relationship," Mike Magee explores the intricacies of this unique human bond and offers insight and recommendations for both physicians and patients to strengthen the relationship.

In Chapter 7, "Dynamic of the Patient–Provider Relationship," Naomi Klayman offers a look at this relationship from a different perspective. This chapter offers strategies for individuals and providers in adapting to new roles created by the changing dynamics in healthcare, including those inspired by medicine's culture, health insurance, and the pharmaceutical industry.

Just as the patient–provider relationship is unique, so too are the factors motivating individual behavior. Intertwined within consumer-focused research are behavior-based, "biopsychosocial" theories, serving as conceptual bases for individual health-related behavior. These theories are explored and applied to consumers' interface with healthcare and, in particular, disease management, in Chapter 8, "Improving Consumer Health through Disease Management," by Marnie LaVigne.

A significant element of most managed care plans is their managed care drug benefit, which is examined by Tim Covington in Chapter 9, "The Drug Benefit: Design and Management." This chapter addresses selected healthcare megatrends that influence drug utilization and drug benefit design and management.

Many consumers are increasingly engaging in self-medication, thanks in large part to the switch of prescription-only medications to nonprescription status, or the Rx-to-OTC switch movement. The movement reflects the growing roles and influence of healthcare consumers and has continuing and urgent implications for major players in healthcare. Chapter 10, "The Role of Self-Care and Nonprescription Drug Therapy in Managing Illness: The Rx-to-OTC Switch Movement," by Mary Pat Manfredi and Tim Covington, explores these implications, as well as how this movement can impact strategies of managed care organizations.

The expanding body of information available to consumers, as well as the variations in healthcare quality that are omnipresent in American healthcare, command the need for organizations such as the Foundation for Accountability, or FACCT, which serves healthcare consumers by helping them make healthcare decisions based on clear and understandable quality information. Two leaders of FACCT, David Lansky and Christina Bethell, provide a look at quality performance measurement and the efforts that FACCT is undertaking to bridge gaps consumers may have with performance information in Chapter 11, "Empowering Consumers to Make Informed Choices."

Employers, long involved in healthcare, are interested in health plan comparative information when selecting health plans to offer to employees. Chapter 12 by Suzanne Mercure, "The Ascendancy of the Employer as Consumer Advocate in Healthcare," provides a historical perspective that illustrates employers' increasing role in healthcare purchasing on behalf of their employees and in promoting employees' health.

Chapter 13, "Employer Groups (Purchasers) and the New Healthcare Consumer," comes from the front lines, so to speak; it is authored by Woodrow Myers and Diane Bechel of Ford Motor Company. Myers and Bechel examine the role of employers as purchasers of healthcare, highlighting the dimensions and challenges of such a position. Specifically, the authors present a look at what Ford has done in terms of its Hospital Profiling Project and Quality Consortium.

On a different level, Marvin Bentley explores the health-related activities of state and federal government to meet the needs of new healthcare consumers in Chapter 14, "Government Connections to the New Healthcare Consumer." This chapter focuses on the current and historical initiatives of state and federal government regarding both data and programs for consumer use.

In Chapter 15, "Health System Initiatives: Responding to the New Healthcare Consumer," Philip Newbold and Diane Stover showcase health system initiatives that are exemplary for their innovation and success in reaching, and in turn helping to empower, the new healthcare consumer in the community.

The community dynamic across the country provides an exciting workshop in which to determine the reach of activities and programs designed to empower healthcare consumers. In Chapter 16, "The Healthwise Communities Project: Where Health Care Is Practiced by All," Molly Mettler of Healthwise, Inc., presents such a consumer-focused program.

In Chapter 17, "Nursing: Linking Today's Consumer to a Changing System," Linda Stutz examines key roles of nursing professionals in the current, dynamic healthcare system. This chapter explores nursing's myriad evolving roles through examination of its relationships with consumers/patients, primary care providers, the healthcare system, managed care, Medicare, employers, and the community.

The elderly population in America, growing in numbers, presents many unique healthcare challenges. In Chapter 18, "The Elderly as the New Consumer of Healthcare," Elizabeth White and Ann Danish present issues and strategies surrounding information, communication, and access, for example, in relation to the special needs of the growing elderly population.

Perhaps one of the more fascinating developments over the past few decades has been the advancement of our appreciation of women's health issues. Julianna Gonen, in Chapter 19, "Women's Health: Women as the (Not-so-New) Healthcare Consumer," looks at women's path toward making significant inroads in healthcare decision making and influence on a national level.

Felicia Gevirtz, in Chapter 20, "Consumer Advocacy and Mental Health: Public Attitudes and Private Battles," delves into the often-misunderstood world of the mentally ill and their unique role as "new" consumers of healthcare. This chapter addresses the advances and challenges inherent in rendering appropriate care for mental illness.

As a response to variations in healthcare quality and disenchantment with the traditional healthcare system, many healthcare consumers have turned to alternative medicine. John La Puma, in Chapter 21, "Examining Alternative Medicine: What Consumers Want from Physicians and What Physicians Should Tell Them," provides an interesting walk through the growth of alternative medicine and the shifts that have occurred as a result. Specifically, this chapter presents concomitant issues for healthcare professionals who may wish to familiarize themselves with the latest trends and their implication for medical practice and self-care.

Connecting with the New Healthcare Consumer: Defining Your Strategy, as a whole, will assist readers in getting their arms around the consumer movement in healthcare. In the future, the consumerism theme will certainly intensify, and professionals within wide-ranging industries can have the upper hand with knowledge and tools to understand and respond to the new healthcare consumer. Each chapter in this book provides key information, insight, and strategies for making connections with new consumers in our changing healthcare environment. We are confident this book will be your compass in guiding you toward consumer-focused strategies, programs, and services.

REFERENCES

Anderson JG. The deprofessionalization of American medicine. *Curr Res Occup Professions* 1992; 7:241–256.

Herzlinger R. Market-driven health care: who wins, who loses in the transformation of America's largest service industry. New York: Addison-Wesley, 1997.

KPMG, Northwestern University Institute for Health Services Research and Policy Studies. *Consumerism in health care: new voices,* 1998.

Mechanic D. Public trust and initiatives for new health care partnerships. *Milbank Q* 1998; 76(2):281–302.

Roper Starch Worldwide, Inc. *Americans talk about science and medical news: The National Health Council Report.* December 1997.

Starr P. Smart technology, stunted policy: developing health information networks. *Health Affairs* 1997; 16(3):91–105.

ACKNOWLEDGMENTS

Creating a multiauthored, edited book reminds me of a raucous family reunion complete with rambunctious children, doting aunts, and even tipsy cousins. Despite the din, the values of a loving family are evident in their act of coming together to celebrate their connectivity and reinforce their traditions.

Our Office of Health Policy staff, including Barbara Bozarth, Mary Pat Manfredi, and Susan Howell, all worked hard over a long time to solicit, review, revise, and reconnect seemingly disparate chapters from across the country. As the senior editor, I owe them a great collective debt of gratitude for a tough job done exceedingly well. They routinely went beyond the call of duty to help produce this first-rate book on time and on budget. It would try the patience of any "family," and they did it with exceptional grace, poise, and humor.

I am also grateful to all of our busy contributors who found the time to tackle yet another project and who had the courage to stare down another deadline. We pestered and cajoled them; we held their hands; indeed, we even sometimes offered them a shoulder to cry on just like any supportive family would. Without them, there would be no book, no tangible evidence of our own labors. We are forever "connected" to them and they to us.

Our leaders here at Jefferson provided us, and especially me, with the kind of enduring support often found only in a few lucky families. My tenth anniversary as the leader of our Office reminds me how truly lucky I am to have had the same two bosses throughout the last decade. Dean Joseph S. Gonnella of Jefferson Medical College, arguably the longest serving medical school dean in the nation, has been an enthusiastic supporter and takes great paternal pride in our accomplishments. Mr. Thomas J. Lewis, the CEO of our university hospital, has demonstrated steadfast support for our efforts in good times and bad. He is always approachable and sympathetic. Any parent has a visceral appreciation for his predicament.

Our publisher, McGraw-Hill, had confidence in our abilities to produce the first text in this new field. Mr. Tom Sharpe and then Ms. Kristine Rynne, gave us the autonomy we needed to stake out this new territory, set up the boundaries, and work the soil. We have had a bountiful harvest because of their leadership and support.

Finally, to our real families, we owe a collective debt of missed time, those precious fleeting moments of togetherness, which serve as a gold standard against which we measure all other activities in life.

CONTENTS

Chapter 7

Dynamic of the Patient–Provider Relationship   163

Chapter 8

Improving Consumer Health through Disease Management   187

Chapter 9

The Drug Benefit: Design and Management   207

Chapter 10

The Role of Self-Care and Nonprescription Drug Therapy in Managing Illness: The Rx-to-OTC Switch Movement   237

Chapter 11

Empowering Consumers to Make Informed Choices   265

Chapter 21

Examining Alternative Medicine: What Consumers Want from Physicians and What Physicians Should Tell Them   493

1

Listening to the Consumer: A Historical Review

John B. Coombs, M.D.

James Hereford

Paul C. LePore, Ph.D.

> Where once all practitioners were fairly free to decide how to manage their relations with patients, now administrators attempt to control the pacing and scheduling of work in the interest of their organization's mission which may regard the collective interests of all patients (or of investors or insurance funds) to be more important than the interests of individual practitioners and their relation with individual patients.
>
> *Eliot Friedson*

> Medicine is one of the oldest professions, but one of the youngest industries.
>
> *Michael Maccoby*

The pace of change in American medicine has never been so dramatic or pervasive as it is today. Fueled by scientific discovery and new technology, the increasing accessibility of new information, the introduction of complex health-related business arrangements, coupled with annual double-digit cost increases to the consumer, healthcare now accounts for 13.5% of the country's gross national product and 20% of the federal budget. Concern with rising costs has focused the attention of the healthcare market on four areas pertaining to care: medical

appropriateness, excellent access, patient satisfaction, and predictable, low cost. Hopes for better control over the growth and
evolution of the healthcare delivery system has now placed increasing emphasis on managed care and managed competition
among providers and payors. As might be suspected, the effect
on patients as consumers has been substantial.

As American medicine navigates these uncertain times, a
period characterized by futurist Leland Kaiser as the "white-
water period of American medicine," one principle remains clear:
choice is of central concern to the patient. With the evolution
from the doctor–patient relationship to the doctor–purchaser–
payor–patient relationship, maintaining the ability to choose
one's doctor (and insurance plan) has become a critical focus of
the American public. A study by the American Association of
Health Plans (AAHP) indicated that after cost, 50% of people
surveyed ranked the ability to choose their own physician as the
most important factor in choosing a health plan. Among health
maintenance organization (HMO) patients, Schmittdiel et al.
(1997) similarly found that on average, patient satisfaction with
the care received was 20 percentage points higher if the patient
had been initially allowed to choose his or her own physician
rather than being assigned one.

This chapter focuses on the doctor–patient bond, emphasizing how social, cultural, and macrostructural forces have altered the dynamic between doctor and client. It is hoped the
reader will be provided a historical perspective on how the patient as a *consumer* has influenced the development and evolution of the healthcare delivery system in the United States. To
achieve this objective, the focus of this chapter is twofold. First,
the transformation of American healthcare delivery over the
course of the twentieth century is examined from the perspective of the patient as a consumer, both as to the influence of the
consumer (and public opinion) on the evolution of the healthcare
delivery system in the United States, as well as the impact
brought by the consumer on those seeking and receiving medical
services. Second, with the increasing complexity of the healthcare delivery system in the United States, specific initiatives
created during the evolution of the healthcare delivery system
(which have brought to bear the consumer's influence and direct

input) are examined separately. Two examples include the measurement and use of patient satisfaction, and the incorporation of patient preference into the medical care and treatment options provided.

The aim is not to provide an exhaustive or for that matter a detailed history of medicine or of the healthcare delivery system in the United States. Space limitations imposed on this chapter alone would make this a daunting and unrealistic task. Others have already chronicled the nuanced history of modern American medicine. This book, however, intends to highlight those significant trends and events that have shaped the growth of American healthcare over the course of the twentieth century, underscoring those forces that are particularly germane to the perspective of the patient as consumer.

THE DOCTOR–PATIENT RELATIONSHIP

The doctor–patient relationship represents one of the most familiar and unique of all personal bonds. Taken at its most basic level, the doctor–patient relationship embodies the private connections between two individuals—the medical practitioner and his or her client. In its ideal form, this relationship reflects a union based on the emotions of trust, caring, confidence, and nurturance, coupled with attributes of familiarity, mutual respect, intimacy, and to a large degree, a veil of privacy.

Defined more broadly, however, the doctor–patient bond can also denote a classic intersection of interests, or perhaps more appropriately, interest groups. Doctors as members of a profession on one hand and patients as a collectivity of consumers on the other are two obvious and central groups of actors in this dynamic. Although varying in their effects on the doctor–patient bond, the interests of hospitals and hospital administration, medical schools, governments and governmental agencies, pharmaceutical and medical research companies, labor unions, the insurance industry and other third-party payors, businesses, and corporations are just a few of the many groups and collectives that also affect the relationships between caregivers and receivers.

If the changing and fluid nature of the doctor–patient bond that has historically occurred in the United States has been acknowledged, it is also important to recognize how the *combined* influences of cultural, economic, legal, ethical, and not least of which, technological trends throughout the twentieth century have shaped and, in some cases, drastically affected the relationship between the medical practitioner and the patient.

Figure 1–1 depicts the evolution of the doctor–patient relationship in a contemporary model that incorporates the purchaser and payor. Many of the thoughts expressed in this text are built upon this schematic representation.

PATIENT CARE AND PHYSICIAN PRACTICE IN EIGHTEENTH AND NINETEENTH CENTURY AMERICA

Before 1900, the healthcare delivery system in the United States might best be described as disparate and disorganized. The system strongly favored a public health approach. For most Americans, particularly the rural, the disenfranchised, and the poor, professional medicine offered patients few treatment solutions or choices. In general, only the most wealthy, urban Americans could afford to pay for or have access to private or professional medical care on a regular basis (Woods & Chi, 1986). As was the case with most aspects of eighteenth and nineteenth century life, in times of need, the sick and injured looked to family and the home for help (an aspect of the domestic economy that even today remains an integral part of the healthcare delivery system in the United States)—addressing disease and injury through a combination of improvisation, folk remedies, and "common sense" (Starr, 1979; Starr, 1982; Stevens, 1971).

Physicians practiced medicine as a "cottage" industry, working largely in isolation from one another (Hafferty & Wolinsky, 1991). With most of the population unable to pay for most doctors' services, few doctors managed to get rich providing healthcare. In fact, by the end of the nineteenth century, physicians' incomes placed them, at best, near the bottom end of the middle class. As a result, many doctors found it essential to complement their medical livelihoods through secondary employment (e.g., as farmers, dentists, midwives, pharmacists, and

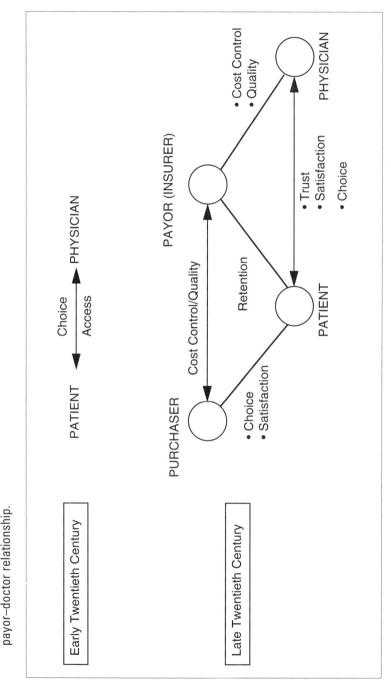

FIGURE 1-1

Schematic evolution over the course of the twentieth century of the doctor–patient relationship into the patient–purchaser–payor–doctor relationship.

even morticians) or to leave the practice of medicine altogether (Starr, 1982).

Although at odds with the contemporary status enjoyed by physicians in the United States today, the commonly held distrust toward the medical profession sustained by most eighteenth and nineteenth century healthcare consumers was, in a significant measure, warranted. Before 1900, medical training for physicians in America remained unregulated and unstandardized, and given the state of medicine and natural science, what preparation that was offered rarely provided doctors any degree of competence in curing patients' disease (Woods & Chi, 1986).

Within the medical profession itself, warring sects of practitioners also actively derided each other's work and treatment regimens (Shryock, 1966; Starr, 1979). Indeed, a number of prominent physicians would go so far as to question the validity of almost all medical therapies, suggesting that doctors had little value to add to their patients' well-being. Physicians in pre–Civil War America thus offered the healthcare consumer a muddled and disjointed view of the medical profession—a view that extended no unifying theories to explain either the causes or cures of disease or provide effective solutions for society's pressing health problems (Woods & Chi, 1986).

Governmental regulation over healthcare and medical licensure policies reflected these same levels of cynicism and skepticism. By the mid-1800s, the notion that *any* occupation (let alone physicians) should be given special and unique privileges through the formal conference of professional/expert status ran counter to widely held egalitarian and democratic ideals. The common fear that doctors would use this type of franchise and monopoly advantage to their own gains led many states and municipalities in the 1830s and 1840s to revoke earlier medical regulatory statutes and to eliminate both medical school accreditation and physician licensure altogether.

The result was a proliferation of for-profit medical schools and the largely unencumbered, and unregulated, entrance of significant numbers of medical school students, and eventually doctors, into the healthcare profession. In the early nineteenth century, virtually anyone who desired to become a doctor could do so with limited amounts of training and little personal investment (Woods & Chi, 1986). Not surprisingly, these combined deregulatory forces resulted in general declines in both health-care standards and practice and an erosion of consumer confidence in medicine more generally (Starr, 1979; Starr, 1982).

FROM COTTAGE INDUSTRY TO THE GOLDEN AGE OF MEDICINE: THE RISE OF THE PROFESSIONAL PHYSICIAN

Given this early history of American medicine, how did the diffuse, unregulated, and disorganized practices of isolated eighteenth and early nineteenth century doctors become transformed into a well-respected and politically savvy twentieth century profession of physicians and become a part of a powerful/influential healthcare industry? More important, how have these changes affected the patient as a consumer?

By the midnineteenth century, medicine had largely lost its authority and legitimacy in the eyes of many healthcare consumers. Sectarian fights within the profession had seriously undermined any confidence patients might have had in physicians, and repeals of most state and local medical licensing statutes removed any legal standing the profession and doctors once enjoyed.

However, important advances in medical technology served to quell many of the disagreements among the warring factions of physicians. For the first time, the once varying approaches to medicine could be united around a common set of interests—interests that were built upon a core of natural science and medical technology (Starr, 1982). The development of modern medicine made a quantam leap forward with William T. G. Morton of Massachusetts General Hospital's development of anesthesia in 1846; Florence Nightingale's use of improved hygiene to reduce military hospital death rates during the Crimean War of 1855; Louis Pasteur and Robert Koch's work in the 1860s and 1870s to develop a germ theory of disease and lay the foundation for a theory of protective immunization in the 1880s; Joseph Lister's principles of antisepsis in surgery published in 1867; and other notable achievements in the development of treatment and diagnostic tools.

For the healthcare consumer, the increased efficacy of treatment regimens, particularly the effectiveness of surgical practice, served to undermine traditional reliance on "self-help" medicine and to restore a sense of the legitimate complexity and scientifically based authority of the medical profession (Starr, 1979). These developments resulted in an unprecedented growth in both the volume and the types of medical surgeries and health-related procedures performed, and (not inconsequentially) offered a new source of revenue and expansion for both doctors and hospitals (Starr, 1982).

In the first 20 years of the twentieth century, hospitals began to shift their focus from serving as alms-houses and social welfare agencies to serving as medical and surgical centers. Doctors similarly reoriented their emphasis from providing in-home patient care to concentrating their practices based on clinical- and hospital-based treatment methods (Goodrick, Meindl, & Flood, 1997; Rosner, 1987). By providing hospital care in exchange for the use of hospital facilities, doctors also started to coordinate their own practice of medicine in cooperation with the work of hospitals and with other physicians.

Hospitals soon became dependent on doctors for their supply of patients; as such, the control of hospitals and other medical facilities ultimately moved from the hands of non-medical trustees to those of physicians. Equally important, doctors shifted from a reliance on individual patients as their primary referral sources to referrals from other professionals. Reasserting their *collective* claim of competence over medical authority through advances in natural science, doctors would come to view their counterparts not as competitors, but as colleagues.

THE ORGANIZATION AND CONTROL OF MEDICAL PRACTICE

Bolstered by improvements in medical technology, the common interests of physicians would become more salient to both doctors *and* their clients. Medical societies in the late nineteenth century reorganized their memberships and began to use their collective strength to exercise greater levels of political influence over the practice of medicine. Legislatures, in turn, began restoring, and later strengthening, the medical licensing laws revoked earlier in the century. The American Medical Association (AMA), for example, which was founded in 1847 and operated for the first few decades as a largely ineffective, politically weak arbitrator of internal quarrels within the profession, eventually overhauled its organization to produce a much more powerful and influential political force. By 1910, 50% of doctors claimed membership in the AMA—a fivefold increase from just 10 years earlier (Woods & Chi, 1986).

Doctors became successful in coordinating their own medical practices as profit-making ventures as well. With the increased use of surgical techniques and the movement of medical practice out of the homes of patients and into hospitals, consulting rooms, and clinics, some enterprising doctors established physician-run group practices as one means of corporately and cooperatively organizing healthcare delivery. The Mayo Clinic, for example, founded by two surgeons (brothers William and Charles Mayo) in Rochester, Minnesota, would become a model of cooperative teamwork among doctors, emulated by other groups of practitioners around the country. Beginning in 1880 as a collective among just three physicians and considered by many to be an unethical movement that supported physician employment, the practice grew tremendously as the Mayo brothers eventually invited dozens of young, well-trained diagnosticians, pathologists, interns, and technicians to join their practice. By 1929, the clinic had become an enormously successful and profitable organization with a staff of more than 350 physicians/dentists and close to 900 nurses, laboratory technicians, and other allied health workers.

At the same time, legal decisions, rendered across a number of local and state jurisdictions, set limitations on the ability of non–physician-owned corporations to provide healthcare. "Corporate medicine" was illegal according to the law. Arguing that "commercialism" in medicine reflected poor public policy, potentially compromising the best interest of patients, and that only doctors, not businesses, could be licensed to practice medicine, these decisions strengthened the growing level of autonomy and power that doctors and the AMA held within the healthcare professions and retarded the evolution of for-profit medical care enterprises. Outsiders and middlemen were what the profession and the AMA regarded as most threatening to the physicians' autonomy. Consequently, medical societies did everything possible to limit private enterprise from interfering with the doctor–patient bond.

However, the states of Washington and Oregon provide interesting counter-examples to this general trend. It is true that most courts and legislatures around the country limited the ability of profit-oriented firms to enter the field of medicine. Unique aspects of workmen's compensation laws in both Washington and Oregon actually encouraged firms in the mining, railroad, and timber industries (among others) to establish contracts for medical services with for-profit hospital associations (Starr, 1982).

These companies, few of which owned and operated hospitals, exacted strong controls over their employee physicians and placed substantive limits on their professional sovereignty. By providing medical and hospital care for a fixed cost per worker, subcontracting work to doctors in private practice, restricting medical fees paid to physicians, requiring second opinions for major medical expenses, and reviewing the length of inpatient hospital stays, the hospital associations of Washington and Oregon effectively controlled costs while at the same time antagonizing local medical societies and the AMA.

In the wake of these threats to physicians' autonomy, neither the profession nor the AMA rested idly by. Although early attempts by medical societies to limit the role that these organizations played in providing healthcare were largely ineffective, in the 1940s, Oregon doctors were able to establish their own statewide medical program—the Oregon Physicians Service—as a means to compete with hospital associations. The establishment of the Oregon Physicians Service coupled with some inventive boycotting strategies on the part of doctors proved to be highly successful. Market share in healthcare services for hospital associations dropped considerably. The once powerful hospital associations were forced to change from being direct purveyors of medical care to assume a much more limited role as third-party insurers (Starr, 1982). Once again, the power of physicians and the AMA to manage and protect the parameters of the doctor–patient bond was substantial.

PHYSICIANS' AUTONOMY OVER MEDICAL EDUCATION AND TRAINING

During this same time, medical licensing boards exerted stronger and more exacting controls over those entering the medical field. New requirements for medical education, which included more extensive and longer training periods in modern laboratory, clinical, and library facilities, were established. Hospitals would emerge as the scientific training and treatment facilities for physicians (DeSwann, 1989). Not surprisingly, these increased standards resulted in escalating costs for physician education. As a result, many smaller medical schools, particularly independent for-profit medical schools, were forced to merge with one another or to close altogether.

By the time the highly critical and much-celebrated Carnegie Foundation Report (produced in conjunction with the AMA's Council on Medical Education) on the state of medical education in the United States was published in 1910, the dye had been cast as state and local licensing bodies had already begun, independently, to strengthen standards for medical school accreditation. Medical practice was accordingly defined as a clinical profession, requiring a structured, formal curriculum based in a hospital setting. Unfortunately, many medical schools fell short of the requirements outlined in the recommendations. The result was that from 1910 to 1915, both the number of medical schools in operation and the number of medical school graduates decreased significantly (Starr, 1982). Perhaps more consequentially for the practice of professional medicine, state and local medical boards began to recognize the AMA ratings of medical schools as definitive. In effect, the AMA's Council on Medical Education had quickly become a forcible and instrumental national accrediting agency for medical schools.

Consumer protection from highly variable practices in medication availability also became a focus. With the passage of the Pure Food and Drug Act in 1906 and the establishment of the AMA's Council on Pharmacy and Chemistry, the AMA also became equally powerful in restricting the fraudulent/misleading claims of drug makers and the unregulated advertisement of prescription medication. To the detriment of patent medicine manufacturers, when doctors began to make their claims to authority based on science and technology, public opinion also started to recognize and endorse the physician's unique and singular jurisdiction over the rules for medical practice and patient care (Starr, 1982). Labor laws likewise supported the dominant ideology that provided doctors a privileged position in society—a position that warranted legal and institutional protection (Swiercz & Skipper, 1982). Indeed, the self-regulatory power of the AMA extended into all aspects of the medical profession as licensing laws were strengthened throughout the 1940s to the point at which the AMA exercised virtually complete control over not only the professional activities within organized medicine, but also the supply of healthcare workers (DeSantis, 1980; Ritchie & Sommers, 1993).

Several decades earlier, public policy and popular opinion vehemently resisted the attempts of any occupation establishing itself as a self-regulated entity; however, by the 1930s, the AMA had succeeded in firmly fixing its authority over medical practice without the need for legislation, debate, or for that matter, very much concern or fanfare (Havighurst, 1986; Starr, 1982; Swiercz & Skipper, 1982). Doctors reached the height of respectability and authority and had established for themselves "professional sovereignty" in what would come to be known as the golden age of physician-controlled medicine (Betz & O'Connell, 1983; Burnham, 1982; Hafferty & Wolinsky, 1991; Starr, 1982). By extension, physician control was publicly represented as acting in the best interest of the doctor–patient relationship.

For patients, the reforms in medical education and state licensure can be seen as a mixed blessing. Although state and local licensing boards and the efforts of the AMA Councils clearly improved the standards of medical practice, the increasing costs and regulations associated with drug manufacture, medical practice, and physician training had their downsides, particularly with regard to the labor supply of trained medical professionals. Declines in the numbers of medical schools and medical school graduates led to substantive shortages of doctors in the early decades of the twentieth century (particularly hard hit were minority communities and the rural poor). Proprietary medical schools that had traditionally provided poor cities and towns with doctors were also the schools *least* likely to conform to state and local accreditation standards and new AMA guidelines. The result was that fewer minorities and poor graduated from medical school, and fewer still provided medical care to the less fortunate (Starr, 1982).

Physicians' ability to exercise both political and economic control over healthcare affected consumer choice in a variety of ways. By specifying the training requirements for physician licensure and medical school accreditation, the profession effectively restricted the supply of doctors and, by consequence, were able to produce an affluent, tightly knit, homogeneous supply of medical practitioners—practitioners who would come to share a common ideology and approach to medical practice (Havighurst, 1986). There appeared to be little interest, or exerted success, on the part of the general public through the political process to alter these trends and direction.

Standardization and limitation of the entrance of almost all nonphysicians into medicine also meant that consumers had essentially no choice of healthcare practice and little knowledge as to what nonstandard and nonsanctioned treatment alternatives might be available. Even when doctors collectively attempted to specialize *within* the field of medicine, effectively signaling to the consumer that the skills of healthcare professionals were not all the same, it was the AMA that sponsored the creation of medical specialty boards—governing bodies that would ultimately and authoritatively describe the terms and conditions under which physicians could or could not specialize and that would limit the ability for individual practitioners or groups of practitioners to diversify and experiment within their own subspecialties. Regulating the training and certification requirements for each subdiscipline, specialty boards also carefully negotiated the boundaries between fields, effectively avoiding interdisciplinary competition and reducing interspecialty competition. This resulted in a restored sense of homogeneity within each subfield and a level of standardization, in both practice and medical training, which had always been advocated by the AMA for the profession as a whole (DeSantis, 1980; Havighurst, 1986).

COLLECTIVIZING CONSUMERS: THE PURCHASE OF HEALTHCARE IN EARLY TWENTIETH CENTURY AMERICA

The ability for turn-of-the-century physicians to collectively organize the practice of medicine around natural science led to significant gains in consumer confidence in medical technologies and substantial economic and political advantages for doctors. Unfortunately, for the patient-consumer, with the increased efficacy of surgery, prescriptive medicine, and medical treatment regimens, also came increased out-of-pocket expenses for healthcare services. Thus, while consumers' demand for physicians' services grew steadily in the early twentieth century, an equally important move to control the rising costs of medical care began as well.

THE RISE OF THE CONSUMER CLUB

Fraternal orders and benefit societies played an important role as consumers of health services in nineteenth century America. Estimates in the early parts of this century suggest that between one-quarter and one-third of all families belonged to these types of associations—groups that offered their members a wide range of services, including life/burial insurance and relief aid and sickness benefits to the diseased and disabled. Beginning in the 1890s, fraternal orders also started to contract with specific doctors (in the form of consumers' clubs) to care for their groups' members. The fees charged for these services were exceptionally low; typically between $1 and $2 per person per year (Starr, 1982).

Not surprisingly, in poor and immigrant communities, consumer plans of this type became popular. For the middle class consumer, however, healthcare services provided by fraternal societies, and the doctors who ran such practices, were met with suspicion and criticism. In short, prevailing opinion suggested that prepayment healthcare plans were a substandard form of medical practice—a healthcare option warranted only for the poor and working classes.

Among doctors, attitudes toward this type of contract practice varied as well. Some young physicians, just entering medical practice, viewed consumer clubs as a pragmatic means of covering expenses and establishing a larger, more stable practice. In fact, many consumer club doctors left contract work once their practices were more firmly incorporated. By the 1920s, however, the attitude of most other physicians, and in particular the AMA, was staunchly against *all* forms of medical "commercialism" and corporate or governmental control over physicians. Advertisement, competition among doctors, the provision of physicians' services by contract, and allowing other third parties (e.g., companies, hospitals, fraternal organizations, the state) to reap profit from physicians' labor were practices viewed to run counter to the best interests of doctors and the medical profession (Havighurst, 1986; Starr, 1982).

The AMA deemed contract services, as provided by consumer clubs in particular, to be both unethical and unfair in that they introduced an element of competition into medicine—an element of commercialism that many medical practitioners feared would ultimately bankrupt the profession. However, while state and local medical societies actively fought against this form of corporately sponsored medicine (often revoking medical society membership for doctors who practiced contract medicine), the real death knell for consumer clubs resulted not from the condemnation of other doctors or the AMA, but from the severe shortages of cheap labor; namely oversupplied and underpaid doctors. As noted earlier, the AMA's ability to control medical education and medical school accreditation led to substantive supply shortages and misdistribution of physicians. With the demand for physicians' services increasing sharply, doctors no longer needed the meagerly, although guaranteed, payment offered by fraternal societies; pay-for-fee services proved to be a far more lucrative and worthwhile venture for most practicing physicians (Starr, 1982).

THE COMPANY DOCTOR

Along with consumer clubs, some of the earliest attempts among businesses and corporations to provide healthcare to their workers, and then later regulate and control the costs of medical services, came through the establishment of "company doctors."

Becoming more common in the decades after the Civil War, railroad, mining, lumber, textile, and steel companies were the first industries to employ physicians on corporate payrolls. For most of these industries, high rates of work-related accidents and fatalities, coupled with geographic isolation and remoteness of work sites, served as prime motivating forces for becoming involved in healthcare delivery. Not surprisingly, the earliest role for the company doctor was that of emergency surgeon in the treatment of industrial accidents (Starr, 1982).

For many employers, healthcare was also used as an additional means of attracting, recruiting, and motivating workers. Thus, alongside the company store and subsidized housing, schooling, and religious programs, healthcare became an integral part of a dedicated movement among employers toward a broader policy of "corporate paternalism"—a movement that sought to bind employees through appeals to loyalty and dedication to their companies.

Employees reacted to these forms of corporate welfare with a combination of distrust and cynicism. In actuality, employees had few choices regarding healthcare matters. Whether health services were provided through a company-owned medical facility or through contracts to specific doctors and/or hospitals, the corporation nearly always controlled the choice of physician. For employees, this resulted in severe misgivings because participation in these healthcare plans was as a rule involuntary, achieved through mandatory payroll deductions. Moreover, for most healthcare consumers, it was unclear for whom the company doctor was actually working—the employee, the patient, or the owner. Because a significant role for the salaried physician was to limit employer liability and to evaluate employees' claims resulting from workplace injuries, workers naturally distrusted the company doctor. Salaried physicians were uniformly perceived as serving the interests of corporate owners before those of workers and therefore not in a position to support optimal doctor–patient relationships.

As with consumer clubs, the age of the company doctor would be short lived. Unions, which were strongly against the paternalistic policies of businesses, argued to remove all forms of corporate welfare, pressing companies to provide workers access to health services *not* through company-run medical plans but through increases in workers' pay. Changes in state and federal policy, specifically the establishment of workmen's compensation laws in the 1910s, and later the enactment of post-Depression (New Deal Era) Social Security plans, further increased employers' unwillingness to offer company-run medical services. The Depression meant that many companies could no longer afford to pay for corporately provided medical services for their workers, even if they had wanted to offer such care, and with the changes in workmen's compensation laws and Federal Social Security policies, many corporations felt that they no longer needed to afford such services. By the 1940s, the locus of and responsibility for social welfare had moved from the varying and uneven paternalistic policies of individual corporations to rest squarely on the shoulders of federal and state governments (Starr, 1982).

HEALTHCARE IN POST-WAR AMERICA

Before World War II, most governments took a "hands-off" approach to the healthcare profession, an attitude described by one observer as "benign neglect." The distribution of health resources was largely driven by market forces; as such, healthcare was perceived primarily as a "consumption good," available to individual consumers fundamentally in their private capacity (Weller, 1977).

Perhaps more important for doctors, healthcare was a service that arguably was to be furnished *solely* by physicians. Thus, although federal, state, and local governments could and often did provide limited medical care to select groups of consumers (e.g., veterans, the mentally ill, schoolchildren, tuberculosis patients, and the poor), when physicians perceived the government was becoming too entangled with the provision of medical services, the AMA responded politically. It is perhaps not surprising then that efforts in the United States to establish a national health insurance plan have been uniformly defeated since the turn of the century. However, government action in the form of legislative decisions, industrial regulation, and fiscal policy *did* help alter the balance of control over the emerging healthcare industry and affect the healthcare choices available to consumers.

THE DEVELOPMENT OF COMPREHENSIVE THIRD-PARTY INSURANCE

The failure for New Deal reformers to enact a comprehensive national health plan, coupled with increasing costs for medical care, left the door open for the rise in the cost of private health insurance (Starr, 1979). Consumers were interested in improving access to a continued shortage of physicians while covering costs that now threatened patients' ability to pay for services rendered. Hospitals were the first major players to respond, developing Blue Cross insurance plans starting in 1929. Initially advanced as a means of expanding the demand for hospital services in difficult economic times and guaranteeing the collection of medical service fees, Blue Cross plans offered a *retrospective* cost reimbursement scheme for paying hospitals—plans that effectively insulated consumers from considering costs when choosing hospitals, which greatly enhanced the pricing and spending freedom of hospitals (Havighurst, 1986; Starr, 1979).

The AMA, fearing that such insurance schemes would lead to fee-for-service controls over their own labor, blocked efforts of Blue Cross to offer a generalized plan for medical insurance. In the 1940s, medical societies, replicating the obvious successes of the Blue Cross programs, developed similarly organized insurance programs of their own under Blue Shield to cover physicians' services. The Blue Shield plans further strengthened physicians' control over medical practice, refusing to pay nonphysicians for services that physicians wanted to provide and establishing a commitment to compensate doctors or reimburse patients on the basis of "usual, customary, and reasonable" fees. In essence, Blue Shield plans allowed doctors to charge whatever fee they chose without fear of frightening away patients (Havighurst, 1986; Starr, 1979).

The "Blues" along with other third-party reimbursement plans developed during the 1930s and 1940s proved to be remarkably successful for a number of reasons. First, federal and state tax policies introduced during this period offered significant tax benefits to employers extending health insurance to their workers by providing a substantial economic incentive for companies choosing to offer health insurance benefits. Second, health insurance, for the first time, became an important employment "fringe benefit," popular among workers and their families. It also became a meaningful rallying point bargaining "chip" for increasingly powerful unions.

For "covered" employees, unlike the medical services offered from consumer clubs and company-run health plans, the insurance policies established by Blue Cross and Blue Shield (and most other third-party insurers) allowed workers a significant range of medical options and choice of physician. Moreover, even with escalating costs for healthcare, third-party payment of medical costs significantly reduced out-of-pocket expenses for workers. In fact, by 1960, third-party payors paid roughly half of the total costs of medical care. By 1980, despite substantial increases in healthcare costs, that proportion continued to increase as insurance companies, now joined by the federal government with the introduction of Medicaid and Medicare, and other third-party payors assumed payment for more than two-thirds of patients' expenses (Betz & O'Connell, 1983).

For doctors and hospitals, insurance plans effectively protected the medical profession from difficult economic times, offered more predictable rates of payment on outstanding debt, and removed competitive cost controls that threatened to reduce physician profits. Most important, these benefits were accomplished *without* limiting doctors' control and autonomy over medical practice or, for the most part, interfering with the doctor–patient relationship. However, the move in healthcare away from a "cottage industry" into a medical industrial complex was well under way.

GOVERNMENTAL FISCAL POLICY IN THE AGE OF PHYSICIAN-CONTROLLED MEDICINE: THE CREATION OF MEDICAID AND MEDICARE

Throughout the twentieth century, the spending policies of federal and state governments have had consequential effects on the healthcare delivery system in the United States, significantly shaping the healthcare choices of patients. In addition to the financing of Social Security in the mid-1930s, federal and state legislatures in the post-War era passed a series of long-term spending measures that largely underwrote the development of medical facilities, scientific technology, and investments in human capital, specifically, through the training of healthcare professionals (Havighurst, 1986; Starr, 1979). The Hill-Burton Act, passed in 1946, provided construction funding for community hospitals in poor and underserved regions. Grants to universities and medical schools by the National Science Foundation (NSF) and the National Institutes of Health (NIH) were increased and targeted to fund medical research and physician training programs (NIH funding of medical programs rose significantly from a level of about $4 million in 1947 to more than $400 million in 1960). Through changes in the Social Security Act, federal and state governments in the 1950s began to reimburse private institutions for healthcare services provided to patients receiving public assistance. Additional monies for physician training were also made available through the Health Professions Educational Assistance Act (HPEA) passed by Congress in 1963, among other spending plans (Ritzer & Walczak, 1988; Starr, 1982).

Perhaps at no time, however, was the impact of the federal government's fiscal policies felt more strongly than with the passage of Medicare and Medicaid. Enacted into law in 1965, the measures served as central platforms of Lyndon Johnson's "Great Society" domestic program and were formed to serve the healthcare needs of the elderly and the poor. In the wake of these reforms, patient demand for medical care increased substantially, and although both programs demonstrated themselves to be remarkably successful (e.g., increasing rates of doctor visits and hospital treatment among the poor and elderly), they also proved to be costly. With public expenditures for Medicaid rising from $3.5 billion in 1968 to $19 billion in 1977, by the late 1980s, more than 40% of healthcare expenditures came from public coffers—Medicaid and Medicare alone accounted for 10% of all federal spending (Anderson, 1992).

However, even with these remarkable increases in fiscal spending on medical investment, the federal government's regulatory and oversight role in the healthcare industry remained largely passive. Reimbursement plans followed by Blue Cross, Blue Shield, and other third-party insurers were emulated in the Medicare and Medicaid programs. Doctors and hospitals were similarly promised that no changes would occur in either the organization of medical practice or with the payment of healthcare expenses. In fact, Blue Cross and other third-party insurers were enlisted to serve as fiscal "go-betweens," processing claims and making claims (and taking their own profit) on behalf of Medicare and Medicaid beneficiaries (Starr, 1979).

Under these plans, healthcare was entirely self-regulated and "fattened" itself on the unfettered reimbursement policies of the government and other third-party insurers. Perhaps not surprisingly, the industry would prove to have a remarkable capacity for spending on both medical technology and human capital investment, devouring entire percentage points of the Gross National Product (GNP) after the introduction of Medicare and Medicaid (Havighurst, 1986). Doctors' incomes grew substantially during this period, as did the profit-making capacity of hospitals (Anderson, 1992). In 1950, medical expenses totaled about $12.7 billion (4.5% of GNP). By 1970, healthcare costs rose to just over 7% of GNP (at about $31 billion). Today, expenditures on medical care account for a startling 15% of GNP—a more than fivefold increase in real per capita spending on healthcare since the mid-1960s. There is little indication that this escalating trend will abate (Anderson, 1992).

IN THE AFTERMATH OF THE GREAT SOCIETY—REGULATION AND COMPETITION IN HEALTHCARE

As Anderson (1992) notes, with the dependence of organized medicine on high technologies, the lucrative success of medicine as a profit-making enterprise, and the increasing levels of healthcare consumer demand, the medical profession in the 1970s had become vulnerable to both competition from profit-seeking investors and regulatory cost control from healthcare purchasers.

Early attempts by the government and third-party payors to control cost, limit wasteful duplication, and ensure quality—through certificate-of-need (CON) and profession-sponsored professional standard review organizations (PSROs) and the subsequent professional review organizations (PROs)—proved to be

largely ineffective. These types of plans underestimated the political difficulties of making cost–benefit calculations on healthcare decisions and ignored some of the obvious conflicts of interest imposed on the doctor–patient relationship when medical
professionals are asked to regulate healthcare spending
(Havighurst, 1986).

Despite the early failures of most cost-containment strategies, court decisions in the 1970s and 1980s (specifically judgments ruling that the medical profession was not exempt from
the antitrust provisions of the Sherman Act) and enabling legislation on the part of the federal government (providing for the
formation of alternative health delivery organizations) led to significant increases in competition for the healthcare consumer's
dollar and accelerating levels of "corporatization" and bureau-
cratization of healthcare delivery (Goodrick, Meindl, & Flood,
1997). Prepayment or capitation health plans; independent
practice associations (IPAs); physician–hospital organizations
(PHOs); free-standing, profit-oriented primary care facilities
(e.g., Humana's Medfirst medical clinics and Health South's
chain of outpatient rehabilitation and surgery centers, nicknamed "McDoctor's" or "Docs-in-the-Box"); and the creation
of for-profit hospital chains (e.g., the Hospital Corporation of
America) are just a few examples that have emerged from this
increased entry of corporate actors into the provision of healthcare (Havighurst, 1986; Kassirer, 1998; Ritzer, 1999; Starr, 1982).

For-profit corporations have also established themselves
into allied health fields as well, operating alcohol- and drug-
abuse centers, nursing homes, renal dialysis programs, ambulatory surgery centers, and others. It is important to note that although prepayment plans (precursors of the later HMOs) have
been around since the 1940s (e.g., Group Health Cooperative of
Puget Sound, the Kaiser-Permanente Health Plan located in
California and Oregon, and the Health Insurance Plan of New
York), it was not until federal and state regulations over their
operation were eased in the 1970s that these plans became popular, and more important, profitable (Starr, 1982).

More recently, the government strategy has moved toward
a prospective payment system (PPS) to reimburse hospitals for
the medical costs of Medicare recipients. Known as diagnosis-

related groups (DRGs), the federal government has established the amount it is willing to pay hospitals for a given medical diagnosis, regardless of how long an individual patient is actually hospitalized. In the ideal case, DRGs provide an external control, pressing doctors and hospitals to become more efficient in their use of ancillary services and to discharge patients from care as quickly as possible (Ritzer & Walczak, 1988). In actuality, DRGs have resulted in the increasing unwillingness of many hospitals, both proprietary and voluntary, to accept uninsured or indigent patients (Anderson, 1992).

Both private and public payors have become more aggressive in purchasing medical services, negotiating directly with doctors and hospitals over the price for specific healthcare services. States like California now require hospitals to bid for the right to treat Medi-Cal program recipients. Preferred provider organizations (PPOs) have become an important means for both corporations and governments to contain spiraling healthcare costs. Indeed, although it was once perceived that healthcare costs were beyond the control of private/public purchasers, the move today appears to be one in which corporations and governments are becoming "prudent buyers" rather than passive intermediaries (Havighurst, 1986).

HEARING THE PATIENT: THE CONSUMER MOVEMENT IN MEDICINE

It was not until recently that participants in organized medicine appeared to be listening to the patients. Although the interests of doctors, hospitals, corporations, federal and state governments, and third-party payors have effectively shaped the expansion and distribution of healthcare resources in the United States, for the greatest part of the twentieth century, the voices of individual consumers have remained virtually silent. To a large extent, the exclusive authority and the importance of privacy that patients vested in their doctors contributed to this silence. Unquestioning obedience to the doctor's control was part and parcel of physicians' sovereignty. Medical decisions, particularly important ones, were viewed by patients as best handled by doctors; interestingly, the same can be said of many patients today (Friedlander, 1995).

However, physicians' regard toward their patients has proven to be an equally salient part of this dynamic. Oliver Wendell Holmes, a noted nineteenth century professor of anatomy at Harvard Medical College, captured these thoughts well, arguing to a medical audience: "Your patient has no more right to all the truth you know than he has to all the medicine in your saddle bags. ... He should get only so much as is good for him." The 1847 AMA Code of Ethics, similarly held, "The obedience of a patient to the prescriptions of his physician should be prompt and implicit. He should never permit his own crude opinions as to their fitness, to influence his attention to them. A failure in one particular may render an otherwise judicious treatment dangerous, and even fatal" (Friedlander, 1995). Even as late as the 1950s, the notion that the patient had a right to learn about alternative therapies, treatment risks, and possible complications, or should be included as an integral partner in a *shared* decision-making process, proved to be foreign to most physicians. The public, for many reasons, did not believe themselves to be in a position to question this issue.

Since that time, however, the relationship between the physician and the patient has clearly shifted. Intensified by the historical battles for equal rights waged on behalf of minorities and women, patients today are demanding their individual rights to healthcare as consumers. Whereas physicians once operated their practices based on their own notions of what was in the best interests of their patients, by the 1960s, a new movement of informed consent, in which the patient actively participated in making medical decisions, was born (Friedlander, 1995; Haug, 1986). This practice was fueling the rising concern of medical malpractice in the 1970s. The publication of a series of widely published and readily accessible how-to guides on home medical care (e.g., Benjamin Spock's *The Common Sense Book of Baby and Child Care* first published in 1946, and *Our Bodies, Ourselves: A Book by and for Women* published by the Boston Women's Heath Book Collective in 1973) helped "demystify" healthcare and loosen physicians' hegemony over medical knowledge (Haug, 1986).

Today, information provided electronically, particularly over the Internet, coupled with the general relaxing of the

Federal Drug Administration (FDA) advertisement bans on prescription drugs and medical treatment regimens, and apparent position by the AMA of tolerance for advertising by physicians has led to an explosion of medical information for the consumer. "Consumerism," in all of its forms, and the information revolution we are currently experiencing in medicine has clearly shifted the locus of decision making, at least in part, to the consumer. Only time will tell, however, whether these fundamental shifts in the doctor–patient dynamic will result in greater levels of patient satisfaction and the more efficient delivery of healthcare services, or simply information overload.

Finally, over the course of the 1990s, the increasing prevalence of managed care has introduced a wide variety of methods aimed primarily at reducing the cost of healthcare and attempting to ensure that only "appropriate care" is provided for patients. The institution by payors of case management, mandatory second opinion for specified procedures, and concurrent review of care rendered by physicians and institutions has brought ever-increasing "intrusion" by the insurance industry into the once inviolate doctor–patient relationship. The proliferation of physicians, particularly specialists, physician groups (e.g., IPAs, large multispecialty practices), and hospitals has led to managed competition and exclusive contracts that require the consumer to make often difficult choices when selecting a health plan. Medicine appears to have truly made the transition from a "cottage industry" to a medical industrial complex with no turning back.

Figure 1–2 schematically outlines many of the significant events and milestones just reviewed that have shaped the healthcare delivery system as we know it today. This schematic history is divided into four sections: (1) the transformation from cottage industry to medical industrial complex, (2) professionalism and the evolution of the doctor–patient relationship, (3) science and medicine, and (4) consumerism and its effect on medicine.

To support this change while still supporting the consumer's position in a service industry, explicit systems of enlisting consumer input and outcome have emerged. Patient satisfaction and the integration of patient preference are two means by which the

FIGURE 1-2

Schematic timeline of events shaping the evolution of American healthcare delivery

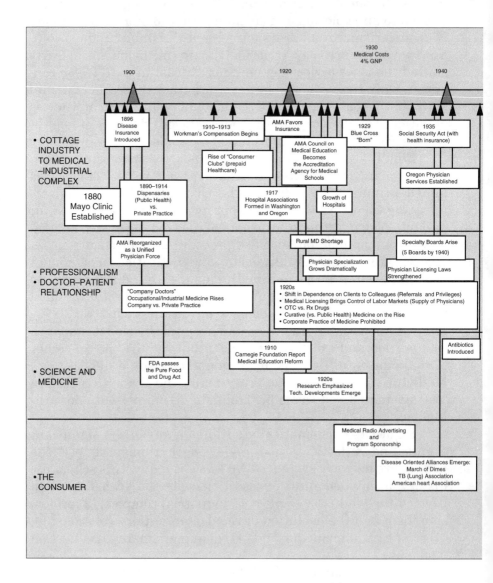

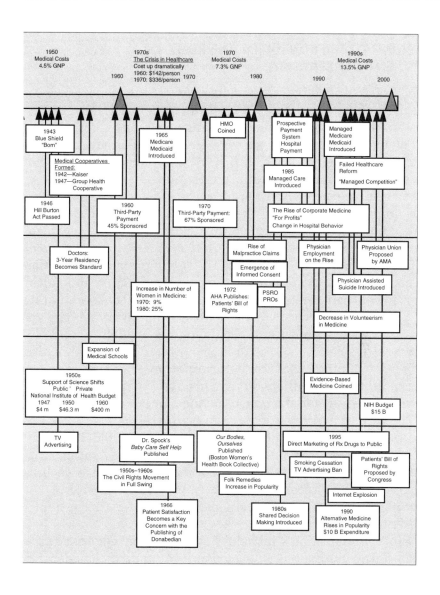

formal position of the patient may be registered, lending this essential element to the definition of optimal care.

LISTENING TO THE CONSUMER: THE ROLE OF PATIENT SATISFACTION

As the practice of delivering care has evolved into a more broadly organized endeavor, the viability of the integrated delivery systems and their ability to meet patient needs has emerged as a vital element to continued success. Healthcare provider organizations (whether they are a staff HMO, multispecialty physician group, or physician–hospital organization), like any business, have to be concerned with their ability to generate sufficient revenues to pay for the cost of the operation, make capital investments, and generate a return on the investment to the organization. They also need to ensure that services provided meet community standards for quality. The use of patient satisfaction information as one component of measuring quality in healthcare is first attributed to Donabedian (1966, 1980). Given that he described technical care within healthcare delivery as "the application of the science and technology of medicine, and the other health sciences, to the management of a personal health problem," he opined that the determination of value to the patient could be accomplished only through "achieving and producing health and satisfaction, as defined for its individual members by a particular society or subculture, as the ultimate validator of the quality of care" (Donabedian, 1966, 1980). He further concluded that information gained through patient satisfaction surveys reflects the patient's judgment of the technical care he or she received indirectly, primarily providing evidence of the practitioner's personal concern for the patient's health and welfare.

Since Donabedian's introduction of the concept that satisfaction data could serve as a measure of quality, considerable research has been done to explore its potential meaning for this purpose as well as the strengths and weaknesses of applying the results of patient satisfaction surveys to communication of quality to policy makers, regulators, and other patients. Several excellent reviews of this research and its implications are provided in the literature (Cleary & McNeil, 1988; Lochman, 1983; Pascoe, 1983; Swan & Carroll, 1980; Ware, Davies-Avery, & Stewart, 1978). Conclusions from the reviews are many, but four points are worth noting here: (1) patient satisfaction is the patient's reaction to salient aspects of his or her service experience (Pascoe, 1983); (2) characteristics of providers or organizations that result in more "personal care" are associated with higher levels of satisfaction (Cleary & McNeil, 1988); (3) good communication skills, empathy, and caring appear to be the strongest predictors of how a patient will evaluate the care received (Cleary & McNeil, 1988); and (4) patient satisfaction, with rare exception, is positively related to accessibility, availability, and convenience of care. Having a regular source of care and length of time with the same provider are positively related to satisfaction with care (Lochman, 1983; Pascoe, 1983).

One concludes from reading reviews to date that the inconsistency of methods and results does not allow for the incorporation of satisfaction assessments into evaluations of the quality of care (Cleary & McNeil, 1988). Furthermore, it is clear that the medical profession does not agree on what role patient satisfaction should play in the measurement and monitoring of quality. Little is known about what information consumers seek to help them in making decisions (Cleary & Edgman-Levitan, 1997). Hibbard and Jewett (1996) found that consumer preferences for data centered on information about preventive care and consumer satisfaction. They also noted that when receiving a health plan report card containing a variety of information, indicators that were not understood were disregarded, adding little to the consumer's overall understanding of quality within the plan (Hibbard & Jewett, 1997). Commenting on the 1994 Consumer Information Project, which surveyed senior opinions, Edgman-Levitan and Cleary (1996) noted that many elderly patients found information contained in report cards confusing and not helpful when choosing a physician. Polled seniors indicated that summary satisfaction ratings were not helpful because, as an example, they did not allow for testing another person's tolerance for waiting times for appointments. Surveyed participants overwhelmingly preferred actual explicit information on waiting time as a better measure upon which to make their own judgment. These conclusions were reinforced in a study done for the Kaiser Family Foundation, which concluded that "word of mouth information from families and friends was viewed as more trustworthy than summary satisfaction scores" (Frederick/ Schneiders, Inc., 1995).

Concern has been raised about the lack of standardized surveys used to measure patient satisfaction and other quality measures (Epstein, 1995). In 1987, the Picker Institute was established with a mission to find ways of providing medical care that would be sensitive to and address the needs and concerns of patients. Since its inception, and with a central purpose of promoting patient-centered care, Picker now provides a full spectrum of standardized survey instruments for use by healthcare providers as well as analyzing and benchmarking results over time (Cleary et al., 1992; Cleary et al., 1993). From its experience, Picker concludes that the predictor of satisfaction is directly related to the number of perceived problems encountered by patients during a given visit and that providers (e.g., institutions, physicians) can enhance satisfaction by improving the processes of care that "touch" the patient.

Until the mid-1990s, patient satisfaction played only a minor role in the decision-making process of larger organizations. There were much more important factors to consider: the reputation and prestige of the organization, largely established through the credentials and reputations of the providers who practiced there, and the availability and application of medical technology, which was a direct source for revenue growth, and hence was not identified as priority. However, the development of methods by which satisfaction could be measured was becoming an essential element given the need to measure in aggregate the doctor–patient relationship within ever-growing and complex organizations.

For individual providers and smaller organizations, patient satisfaction was almost exclusively determined by retention of patients who enjoyed the freedom of "voting with their feet" and "doctor shopping." Again, the measurement of aggregate patient satisfaction was not seen as a critical organizational need.

The lesser importance placed on measuring and using patient satisfaction was also reinforced by the relationship the patient had with the provider and the provider's attitude toward the patient. Doctors traditionally have been trained to deal with the disease. Patients' attitudes, perceptions, and needs were given far less value or were even seen as disruptive to the process of diagnosis and treatment. A number of factors in the past decade have increased the awareness of the need for using patient satisfaction data to inform the decision-making process of organizations. First, competition, for patients and payor contracts, has increased among healthcare organizations as a result of the abundance in most communities of physicians and healthcare facilities. Each individual patient has become more important because competition has made it more difficult to find new patient-consumers. This has created a heightened sense of awareness about the importance of customer loyalty. Likewise, competition among health plans or payors has intensified as new products enter the market given the history of rising investment and profitability in healthcare.

Second, the patient-consumer has changed. As other service industries have become increasingly more competitive, they have worked very hard to find new ways to satisfy the customer's needs. With each successive improvement and innovation experienced by the customer, an expectation was developed about how service should be provided and what a service organization should be able to deliver. These experiences changed the expectation the patient-consumer had for healthcare organizations.

The patient-consumer has also changed in *reaction* to the changes in the healthcare industry, as well as specifically to the changes made in the healthcare insurance industry. Cost increases were automatically passed on to the purchaser, which resulted in double-digit annual increases in healthcare spending. Annual healthcare spending became a point of focus for purchasers, who were looking for ways to control costs. As purchasers moved away from indemnity plans and toward plans that restricted patients' choices (as a cost control mechanism), many patient-consumers found that they had fewer choices and were increasingly dissatisfied with services provided by the choices they did have.

These changes have made healthcare organizations and providers increasingly aware of the importance of patient satisfaction and loyalty in determining the viability of the organization (Jones & Sasser, 1985). Patient satisfaction is commonly defined in terms of the degree of satisfaction experienced by the customer after healthcare services are rendered. Patient loyalty is indicated by their willingness to return again to receive services from the same service provider. Satisfaction, however, is not the same as loyalty. Very satisfied customers may still "defect" to other provider organizations or payors, and only those that are completely satisfied across a wide array of service and content indicators will consistently return (Jones & Sasser, 1995).

The increased focus on measuring patient satisfaction has also been reinforced by accreditation organizations. The Joint Commission on the Accreditation of Healthcare Organizations (JCAHO) and the National Committee for Quality Assurance (NCQA) have included requirements for the acquisition and use of patient-consumer satisfaction measures in their monitoring and improvement activities, understanding the increased recognition of patient satisfaction in measuring the value of both providers and payors.

This has also created momentum for the implementation of standardized surveys. The NCQA survey was put forward as data from their Health Plan Employer Data and Information Set (HEDIS) data set, a standardized tool, and was quickly followed by the Consumer Assessment of Health Plans (CAHP) survey, which has now replaced the NCQA survey, and is required by the Health Care Financing Administration (HCFA) for programs such as Medicare and Medicaid. These standardized surveys provide the basis for evaluation of healthcare organizations' provision of service quality and, perhaps most important to the patient-consumer, a means by which comparison across health plans and providers might be made.

Applying Patient Satisfaction to Improve Outcomes of Care

Once patient-consumer data has been gathered, whether through surveys, focus groups, point of service questionnaires, complaint data, or operational data, it can be applied in a variety of ways. Data marketing provides the opportunity for both use and abuse of the information gained. For example, one of the most common methods for creating the appearance of great customer satisfaction is to group a number of responses together to form the reported statistic. Although the organization may report that 90% of their members are satisfied, this result has been obtained by grouping together all of the responses on the response scale that are dissatisfied.

More appropriate uses of the data include focusing improvement efforts in areas that add value to patient care and are in need of attention. Applying data collection to quality improvement efforts often answers a critical quality question: "Did a change made result in an improvement to the overall care of the patient?"

Another application of the customer data is in the development of new products and services to meet previously unmet needs. For example, some HMOs have begun to offer open-access plans that provide some direct access to specialists without the need of a referral from a primary care provider (PCP). These plans were offered in response to customer dissatisfaction with the role of the "gatekeeper" and the referral process. Finally, collection and analysis of customer satisfaction information is becoming increasingly important in the achievement of full accreditation status by healthcare organizations.

In summary, the use of information about patient satisfaction data and its application to quality measurement in healthcare delivery is still in debate. The growing complexity of healthcare delivery and increasing competition among providers have created a strong argument for continued interest in this not yet fully understood aspect of quality measurement. The greater availability of standardized surveys that measure and compare patient satisfaction along with the integration of this information into accreditation standards for health plans and healthcare providers, ensures that greater emphasis will be placed on reporting and further understanding its meaning.

LISTENING TO THE CONSUMER—INTEGRATING PATIENT PREFERENCE INTO MEDICAL PRACTICE

In 1982, a presidential commission studying ethical problems in medicine published the report "Making Health Care Decisions: A Report on the Ethical and Legal Implications of Informed Consent in the Patient–Practitioner Relationship" (President's Commission, 1982). The report concluded that: "Clinicians should foster the informed participation of patients in medical decisions by: providing relevant information about the clinical situation, alternatives, risks and benefits; assessing the patient's understanding; and giving the patient a clear opportunity to voice a preference."

The expression of patient preference has become one means by which the corporate medicine dilemma has attempted to blend the notion of the "doctor knows best" with the "customer is always right." Today, forces at work on both sides of this issue are taking the once straightforward decisions within the doctor–patient relationship into a new world of complexity. On the "doctor knows best" side, the rising cost of healthcare has forced computerized medicine to provide only "appropriate care," whereas evidence-based medicine applies the tools of science in defining what works (and what works best) from an ever-advancing bank of knowledge. On the "customer is always right" side, autonomy, choice, and patient satisfaction all influence the dynamic. Further fueling the dilemma is the ready availability to the patient-consumer of complex and technical information (e.g., through the printed media, the Internet), coupled with the strong interests of the payors and purchasers of care. All of this calls for providers and patients to pay greater attention to the decision-making process, to expect that expression of preference is an essential element of the therapeutic process, and to anticipate that outcomes will be strongly influenced by choices that emerge from this shared process.

Shared decision making (SDM) combines physician-based decision making (best practice for a given clinical condition/informed consent) with patient-based decision making (patient preferences/risk/benefit assessment). SDM, then, creates a formal structure upon which "the doctor knows best" and "the customer is always right" can meet. Interestingly enough, when asked, not all patients gravitate toward SDM. Mazur and Hickam (1997), within a Veteran Administration setting, found that 68% of patients preferred SDM, whereas 21% preferred the physician-based, and 11% the patient-based decision-making model when deciding about an invasive medical intervention. The significance of the decision appears to influence how patients want to approach the decision-making process. Beaver et al. (1996), studying decision making for women with newly diagnosed breast cancer, found that 52% preferred the "passive" or physician-based decision, 28% the shared (SDM) approach, and 20% the patient-based approach. However, when deciding on options for care of benign breast disease, 45% preferred SDM, 24% the patient-based, and 31% the physician-based.

Other than the nature and content of the decision to be made, the fundamental interest of the patient to engage in decision making varies widely among individuals. Cassileth et al. (1980) found that age accounted for a significant part of variation in patient interest for involvement, the youngest patients expressing greatest interest as a rule: 87% (age 20 to 39 years), 62% (40 to 59 years), and 51% (60 years and older).

The physician does not always accurately predict if or how the patient wants to approach decision making. Strull, Lo, and Charles (1984) found that physicians underestimated their patients' interest in discussing therapy in 29% of cases, while overestimating it in 11% of the cases. Some patients have no interest in discussing tough questions. Murphy et al. (1994) reported that 40% of patients were not at all interested in discussing with the doctor their feelings about do not resuscitate (DNR) wishes in the event that a serious, life-threatening event might occur. A patient's trust in his or her doctor is a powerful influence on the patient's willingness and interest in discussing decisions. Kao et al. (1998) found that 69% of patients surveyed in a managed care setting believed that their doctor would put their needs above all other considerations. They further reported that patients who had the choice of their physician, a longer relationship with him or her, and a level of trust in their managed care organization were more likely to also express trust in their physician.

Braddock et al. (1997), applying six criteria reflecting the informed decision-making process to recorded doctor–patient interviews, concluded that physicians commonly describe the nature of the decision but less often discuss risk and benefits with the patient and seldom assess the patient's understanding of the final decision once made. In nearly one in five cases, however, the interview did come to some clear expression of patient preference.

Many published examples of how patient preference substantially influences or changes medically defined best practice can be found in the literature. O'Meara et al. (1994) demonstrated that despite prevailing evidence that management of deep vein thrombosis is best approached using a combination of streptokinase and heparin, rather than heparin alone, when patients were objectively presented with the risks and benefits of each approach, a strong preference for heparin alone emerged. This patient-preferred choice emerged for the simple reason that most patients are not willing to risk a threefold greater chance of bleeding and possible death associated with streptokinase while accepting the relatively common and chronic complication (90%) of postphlebitic syndrome associated with heparin alone.

Nease et al. (1995), studying the relationship between patient preference and management of coronary artery disease by disease severity classification, demonstrated the absence of predictive certainty between disease severity classification, defined best clinical management strategy, and the choices preferred by patients. Central to this finding was the observation that patients vary substantially in their willingness to tolerate the same level of functional impairment and the varying risk of death associated with different remedies.

Flood et al. (1996), studying screening for prostate cancer using the prostate-specific antigen (PSA) blood test, found that the patient who learned more about the disease and implications of testing (e.g., prostate cancer and its treatment, the frequency of false-positive test results) preferred not to be screened and, if at some time were diagnosed in an early stage of development of prostate cancer, would elect to have no active treatment for the disease.

In one last example, Murphy et al. (1994) found that patients between the ages of 60 and 99 years, when asked if they wished to receive cardiopulmonary resuscitation (CPR) in the event of cardiac arrest, answered yes 41% of the time. After the same patients reviewed evidence regarding survival after CPR, the number dropped to 22%.

Critical to the issue of allowing patients to express their preferences and to share in decision making is the creation of methods to efficiently, and in an unbiased way, provide information. Kasper, Mulley, and Wennberg (1992) describe one approach to using an interactive videodisc program to provide information about treatment options to patients diagnosed with benign prostatic hypertrophy. Using a process that combined two visits to the physician along with an intervening viewing session, 75% of the patients believed that program was balanced in its presentation, did not provide "more information than patients want," and did not interfere with the doctor–patient relationship. Use of this approach resulted in increased clinician efficiency, improved patient satisfaction, and within some managed care settings, a 40% to 66% reduction in surgical solutions with a greater number of patients electing for a "watchful waiting" approach.

What can be learned from these recorded observations? First, the expression of informed patient preference may substantially alter evidence-based defined best practice. Second, how decisions are best made between the doctor and the patient varies according to patient age and the nature and significance of the clinical question. To this point, Kassirer (1994) observed that patients should, when possible, participate in decisions affecting their well-being. He observed that those decisions that rise to the top priority in this regard are "utility-sensitive" decisions such as those where major differences in the kinds of possible outcomes (e.g., death versus disability) or when one of the choices can result in a small chance of a grave outcome.

Finally, as medicine becomes subject to the increasing availability of evidence-based approaches, managed care utilization schemes, disease management, and the like, it is clear that the need to explicitly provide for patient choice and preference will become increasingly more important to achieve optimal outcomes in patient care.

CONCLUSION AND SUMMARY

Over the course of the twentieth century, medicine has undergone profound and pervasive change. Although access, quality, breadth of what medicine has to offer, as well as cost, have all increased during this time, so has the complexity of the delivery system and the expectations of the patient-consumer.

While attempting to review this transgression from the consumer's perspective, four summarizing observations can be drawn. First, the healthcare delivery system in the United States listens to and is more responsive to the customer today than at any other time in its history. Limited access and highly variable quality in the early twentieth century, along with the privacy and relative mystery of the doctor–patient relationship, have given way to far greater access for more people, greater content and quality through scientific discovery and consumer protection measures, and increased interest and confidence of the consumer, while maintaining the importance of patient choice to patients when choosing their provider. Innovators in information technology hold promise that even though complexity and bureaucracy is the price patients have traded for this greater access and quality, in the future, improved communication and transfer of information may lessen this burden.

Second, consumers now have greater access to and are using more available information about medicine and health. This has resulted in the creation of expectations on their part that are more self-determined and explicit than ever before. Providers are now more commonly confronted with patients who are informed (often misinformed) about their healthcare needs. Armed with this information and a predetermined sense of what is right for them, patients now seek their own solutions or access to products (e.g., drugs, therapies) directly. The professional provider, especially in straightforward medical situations, runs the risk of being viewed as a barrier to the consumer's individually determined approach to his or her own health. The result has been a blurring in the eye of the consumer between medicine as a profession and medicine as a business.

Third, as increasingly complex systems of care have emerged, the increased influence of the consumer, and of consumerism, has created greater strains in the doctor–patient relationship. Frequent tales of physicians being accused of insurance fraud and abuse, conflicts created by managed care, conflicting information about cures and therapies, and continued prevalence of medical malpractice claims have tended to cast doubts on the part of the public on the trustworthiness of physicians in general. Not all of this has been without benefit. The increased awareness created by consumer interest and a generally broader interest in healthcare has brought additional attention on the part of the physician and his or her patients on items and issues that, in fact, might provide for better outcomes of care.

Finally, listening to the consumer has meant paying greater attention to patient satisfaction and the interjection of patient preference into medical decisions that used to be made through a paternalistic approach to problem solving on the part of the physician. It is becoming increasingly clear from the literature, that while attempting to directly apply to a specific disease entity or clinical problem, best practice as defined by an evidenced-based approach, an optimal patient outcome cannot be achieved if patient values and expressed preferences are ignored.

REFERENCES

Anderson JG. The deprofessionalization of American medicine. *Curr Res Occup Professions* 1992; 7:241–256.
Beaver K, et al. Treatment decision making in women newly diagnosed with breast cancer. *Cancer Nurs* 1996; 19(1):18–19.
Betz M, O'Connell L. Changing the doctor-patient relationship and the rise in concern for accountability. *Soc Prob* 1983; 13:84–95.

Braddock CH, et al. How doctors and patients discuss routine clinical decisions. *J Gen Intern Med* 1997; 12:339–345.

Burnham JC. American medicine's golden age: what happened to it? *Science* 1982; 215:1475–1478.

Cassileth B, et al. Information and participation preferences among cancer patients. *Ann Intern Med* 1980; 92:832–836.

Cleary PD, Edgman-Levitan S. Health care quality—incorporating consumer perspectives. *JAMA* 1997; 278:1608–1612.

Cleary PD, McNeil BJ. Patient satisfaction as an indicator of quality care. *Inquiry* 1988; 25:25–36.

Cleary PD, et al. The relationship between reported problems and patient summary evaluations of hospital care. *QRB* 1992; 18(2):53–59.

Cleary PD, et al. Using patient reports to improve medical care: a preliminary report from 10 hospitals. *Qual Manage Health Care* 1993; 2(1):31–38.

DeSantis G. Realms of expertise: a view from within the medical profession. *Res Soc Health Care* 1980; 1:179–236.

DeSwann A. The reluctant imperialism of the medical profession. *Soc Sci* 1989; 28:1165–1170.

Donabedian A. Evaluating the quality of medical care. *Milbank Memorial Fund Quarterly: Health and Society* 1966; 44:166.

Donabedian A. *Explorations in quality assessment and monitoring. Vol 1: The definition of quality and approaches to its assessment.* Ann Arbor, MI: Health Administration Press, 1980.

Edgman-Levitan S, Cleary PD. What information do consumers want and need. *Health Affairs* 1996; 15(4):42–56.

Epstein A. Performance reports in quality-prototypes, problems and prospects. *N Engl J Med* 1995; 333(1):57–61.

Flood AB, et al. The importance of patient preference in the decision to screen for prostate cancer. *J Gen Intern Med* 1996; 11:342–349.

Frederick/Schneiders, Inc. Analysis of focus groups concerning managed care and Medicare (Prepared for the HJ Kaiser Family Foundation). Washington: Frederick/Schneiders, Inc., 1995.

Freidlander WJ. The evolution of informed consent in American medicine. *Perspect Biol Med* 1995; 38:498–510.

Goodrick E, Meindl JR, Flood AB. Business as usual: the adoption of managerial ideology by U.S. hospitals. *Res Soc Health Care* 1997; 14:27–50.

Hafferty FW, Wolinsky FD. Conflicting characterizations of professional dominance. *Curr Res Occup Professions* 1991; 6:225–249.

Haug MR. A re-examination of the hypothesis of physicians deprofessionalization. *The Milbank Quarterly* 1986; 66:48–56.

Havighurst CC. The changing locus of decision making in the healthcare sector. *J Health Politics, Policy Law* 1986; 11:697–735.

Hibbard JH, Jewett JI. What type of quality information do consumers want in a health care report? *Med Care Res Rev* 1996; 53:28–47.

Hibbard JH, Jewett JI. Will quality report cards help consumers? *Health Affairs* 1997; 16(3):218–220.

Kao AC, et al. Patients' trust in their physicians. *J Gen Intern Med* 1998; 13(10):681–686.

Kasper JF, Mulley AG, Wennberg JE. Developing shared decision-making programs to improve the quality of health care. *QRB* 1992; 28:183–190.

Kassirer JP. Managing care—should we adopt a new ethic? *N Engl J Med* 1998; 339:397–398.

Kassirer JP. Incorporating patients' preferences into medical decisions. *N Engl J Med* 1994; 330:1895–1896.

Lochman JE. Factors related to patients' satisfaction with their medical care. *J Common Health* 1983; 9:91–109.

Mazur DJ, Hickam DH. Patients' preference for risk disclosure and role in decision making for invasive medical procedures. *J Gen Intern Med* 1997; 12:114–117.

Murphy DJ, et al. The influence of probability of survival on patient preferences regarding cardiopulmonary resuscitation. *N Engl J Med* 1994; 330:565–569.

Nease RF, et al. Variation in patient utilities for outcomes of the management of chronic stable angina. *JAMA* 1995; 273:1185–1190.

O'Meara JJ, et al. A decision analysis of streptokinase plus heparin as compared with heparin alone for deep vein thrombosis. *N Engl J Med* 1994; 330:1864–1869.

Pascoe GC. Patient satisfaction in primary health care: a literature review and analysis. *Eval Prog Plan* 1983; 6:185–210.

President's Commission for the Study of Ethical Problems in Medicine and Biomedical and Behavioral Research. *A report on the ethical and legal implications of informed consent in the doctor-patient relationship*. Washington, DC: US Government Printing Office, 1982.

Ritchie FJ, Sommers DG. Medical rationalization and professional boundary maintenance: physicians and clinical pharmacists. *Res Soc Health Care* 1993; 10:117–139.

Ritzer G. *Enchanting a disenchanted world: revolutionizing the means of consumption.* Thousand Oaks, CA: Pine Forge Press, 1999.

Ritzer G, Walczak D. Rationalization and deprofessionalization of physicians. *Social Forces* 1988; 67:1–22.

Rosner D. Heterogeneity an uniformity: Historical perspectives on the voluntary hospital. In Schmittdiel J, et al. Choice of a personal physician and patient satisfaction in a health maintenance organization. *JAMA* 1997; 278(19):1596–1599.

Shryock RH. *Medicine in America: historical essays.* Baltimore: John Hopkins Press, 1966.

Starr P. Medicine and the waning of professional sovereignty. *RI Med J* 1979; 62:179–198.

Starr P. *The social transformation of medicine.* New York: Basic Books, 1982.

Stevens R. *American medicine and the public interest.* New Haven, CT: Yale University Press, 1971.

Strull WN, Lo B, Charles G. Do patients want to participate in medical decision making? *JAMA* 1984; 252:2990–2994.

Swan JE, Carroll MG. *Patient satisfaction: an overview of research—1965 to 1978 in refining concepts and measures of consumer satisfaction and complaining behavior.* University Press, 1980.

Swiercz PM, Skipper JK Jr. Labor law and physician's privileged position: an example of structural interest influence. *Int J Health Serv* 1982; 12:249–261.

Ware J, Davies-Avery D, Stewart A. The measurement and meaning of patient satisfaction. *Health Medical Care Services Review* 1978; 1:1.

Weller GR. From "pressure group politics" to "medical-industrial complex:" The development of approaches to politics and health. *J Health Politics, Policy Law* 1977; 1:444–470.

Woods ME, Chi Peter SK. Sanitary reform in New York in 1866 and the professionalization of public health services: a case study of social reform. *Soc Focus* 1986; 19:333–347.

2
CHAPTER

The Public View of Healthcare

Joel E. Miller

Policy makers, pundits, and news audiences are bombarded every day with new polls on public opinion and by journalists' reports on the state of America's thinking. Nowhere is this truer than in healthcare surveys and polls conducted over the last 5 years.

This chapter addresses the following areas:

- Provides a brief overview of the forces impacting public perceptions on healthcare
- Presents and clarifies the various sources of public survey information (i.e., what constitutes a public view): consumer ratings, public opinion polls, patient satisfaction surveys, and focus groups
- Focuses on key themes derived from a meta-analysis of public opinion survey information.

INTRODUCTION

At a time when the economy is strong, inflation and unemployment are low, crime and drug use are down, and the public's general feelings of optimism are up, Americans now hold a dim view of the healthcare system and a pessimistic outlook for its future. This belief is prevalent despite the contradictory views found in many public opinion surveys, which show most consumers are satisfied with their own health plans and doctors. Why does this variation occur, and what does it mean for policy makers and their ability to develop solutions to pressing healthcare issues, such as the growing number of uninsured patients, rising costs, and uneven quality of care? And what do these surveys and polls mean for healthcare providers and the entire healthcare delivery system?

Americans have contradictory views on healthcare, which can be traced to a number of factors. These factors include values that have been shaped by cultural, social, political, and historical factors (e.g., the "American ethos" of a democratic society—rugged individualism and free choice) compounded by the evolution of a health insurance system that has incentivized choice and insulated all parties from fiscal responsibility.

Another force that affects our views on healthcare is technological advancement, always ingenious in finding ways to improve and extend life. And there is, most of all, the power of public demand, which has come to expect medicine to improve not only health but life in general. The public has come to see a longer and better life as not simply a benefit but as a deep and basic right.

Another force that comes into play is the media coverage of healthcare issues, specifically, coverage of managed care. One could argue whether media coverage of managed care is an accurate or distorted version of it. Media coverage is a powerful force and is linked directly to expectations that people have of the healthcare system, which is reflected in public opinion polls.

Finally, one rule that has been borne out in healthcare public opinion is the belief that controlling healthcare costs is fine for government bureaucrats and corporate financial officers, but, "Spare no expense when it comes to me or my family."

In understanding the "pulse" of the public on healthcare issues, it is first helpful to understand the variety of sources of this information.

METHODS OF OBTAINING PUBLIC OPINION

Four primary methods are used to collect information about the public's views on healthcare: (1) consumer ratings, (2) public opinion polls, (3) patient satisfaction surveys, and (4) focus groups. With the exception of focus groups, these methods rely on survey instruments/questionnaires to elicit information. The difference between consumer ratings, public opinion polls, and patient satisfaction surveys is only the means by which the information is collected (e.g., by phone, by mail survey, and electronically).

Consumer ratings measure the average experience of those who use a service. Publications such as *Consumer Reports* is an example of this kind of measurement of consumer views.

Public opinion is often driven by rare occurrences, as well as by an individual's experiences and those of their families as day-to-day consumers of healthcare. This chapter is based primarily on a review and analysis of public opinion research conducted on healthcare issues over the last 5 years. The Louis Harris and George Gallup polls referenced in this chapter are examples of this kind of public opinion research.

Patient satisfaction surveys refer broadly to interviews and surveys of patients that are conducted either at the time care is provided or later by telephone or mail. Interviews and surveys may ask patients to report on the process of care (both technical and interpersonal) and its outcome and to rate the quality of the care they received and their satisfaction. Many hospitals use this technique to ascertain patients' opinions of the medical care they received.

The focus groups typically consist of 8 to 12 individuals who are relatively homogeneous in standard demographics and lifestyles and who are unknown to each other before they are recruited for the session. During a focus group session, a trained moderator guides the discussion but allows the participants to speak freely. The importance of focus groups is displayed later in this chapter through the American Hospital Association/Picker Institute program that captures consumer experiences with the healthcare system.

Policy makers and decision makers must distinguish between general patient satisfaction surveys and surveys that ask pointed questions about the actual experiences of patients based on their interface with the healthcare system. Only by looking at the latter will focused and timely public and administrative policies evolve.

THE THREE THEMES OF THE PUBLIC'S VIEWS ON HEALTHCARE

In review of public opinion surveys conducted over the last 5 years, three major themes are found throughout:

1. Consumers believe that the problems in the healthcare system affect others but not them personally.
2. Consumers lack a basic understanding of the issues surrounding healthcare policy.
3. The public's opinions are becoming more expansive on addressing problems in the healthcare system, but there is no emerging consensus on how to fix those problems.

Furthermore, these key themes occasionally may become intertwined in reflecting the public's view of healthcare, and it is clear that public opinion will likely become more complicated to read in the future as the healthcare system continues to undergo tumultuous changes. As one commentator said, "Public perceptions in America can shift in a blink of an eye" (Moran, 1997).

The "I'm Okay, They're Not" Syndrome

To understand what is going on in the public's mind on healthcare, we first need to look at the public's overall views on the state of the nation. What one finds is that the paradox seen in healthcare surveys resides at an even deeper level throughout our society. When polled, many Americans responded that they believe the nation is in decline. However, although most Americans testify to the country's deterioration, they are equally confident that they and their families, on the whole, are thriving. The gulf between people's upbeat view of their personal lives and their downbeat judgment of the country, its public institutions, and the ability of those institutions to solve social problems helps explain much of the nation's present political paralysis on solving healthcare problems (Whitman, 1998). Many surveys show that people are satisfied with their own healthcare and its quality but believe the opposite when queried about the healthcare system as a whole. The public often believes that the growing number of those uninsured or the deterioration in the quality of care is affecting others, not them. This phenomenon is known as the "I'm okay, they're not" syndrome (Whitman, 1998).

The "I'm okay, they're not" syndrome permeates the healthcare landscape. Surveys show that 70% to 80% of the public believe that their own physicians provide quality medical care. To cut costs, most voters think it is unnecessary to place limits on their own healthcare coverage or that of the average American. A majority of the electorate believes that the rising cost of healthcare could be stemmed by cutting out profit sharing, fraud, and waste, suspected to be by other people's doctors (League of Women Voters, 1999). However, a gap exists between the public's perception and reality. Many experts point out that the aging of the population, the high costs of new medical technologies, rapidly rising pharmaceutical utilization and prices, and poor quality of care are likely the chief culprits behind high healthcare costs. The public's position is understandable, given the prevalence of everyday "horror" stories: HMOs denying medical care, Medicaid fraud, nursing home abuses, and the like.

David Whitman, who is considered by many to be one of America's best informed journalists, contends that typically the "I'm okay, they're not" attitude relieves public officials of the political pressure to address the problems. It creates a kind of self-fulfilling prophecy whereby the public's somber view of the world leads them to conclude that not much can be done about a social problem. Left unaddressed, the problem gets worse, which only confirms the public's initial cynicism about the magnitude of the problem and the futility of reform (Whitman, 1998).

The Clinton healthcare reform plan was a case in point. A 1991 Gallup poll showed that 91% of the public believed that there was a crisis in the healthcare system (*Gallup Poll*

Monthly, 1991). This kind of overwhelming majority provided much of the political impetus that helped launch the Clinton administration's healthcare reform plan. Furthermore, when the public was asked about what kind of change was needed to address the problem, a majority said that the healthcare system needed to be completely rebuilt. Initially, the electorate seemed to favor major healthcare reform because they thought the nation would be better off as a result, not because they themselves would benefit. Before long, the fact that people themselves feel "okay" overrides their sense of urgency. Ultimately, as Whitman and other commentators such as Robert Blendon conclude after viewing the events of 1992–94, the "I'm okay, they're not" syndrome helped launch the Clinton healthcare plan and then, in a bizarre twist, helped doom it (Whitman, 1998).

The high water mark of the Clinton plan occurred when the President announced the proposal in September 1993 before a joint session of Congress; nearly 60% of the electorate supported it (Yankelovich, 1995). But in the months following, surveys and focus group research tracked a dramatic reversal in public attitudes. Clinton's healthcare reform proposal failed to pass Congress for many reasons, including the lack of real public discussion of the measure. But one survey of Congress members by the Columbia Institute found that policy makers themselves believed public opinion was the single greatest determinant on the legislative debate (Columbia Institute, 1995). In response to a question on which factors mattered to the outcome of the debate, 75% of the legislators polled said that public opinion meant a "great deal" (Figure 2–1).

What spurred the shift in public opinion? According to many observers, the death knell of the Clinton plan was that consumers believed the proposal could potentially make their personal circumstances worse. By the spring of 1994, surveys showed that less than 20% of Americans believed that the President's health plan would improve their situations personally, give them more choices of physicians, or decrease the amount they paid for medical services and health insurance coverage (Blendon, Brodie, & Benson, 1995). Only 6% of the public thought that the plan provided too little government involvement. By July 1994, 9 months after the announcement, the public's favorable endorsement of the proposal had eroded from 57% to 37% (Yankelovich, 1995).

FIGURE 2–1

Sources influencing public opinion on the congressional debate on health-care reform. (Source: This information was reprinted with permission of the Henry J. Kaiser Family Foundation of Menlo Park, California. The Kaiser Family Foundation is an independent healthcare philanthropy and is not associated with Kaiser Permanente or Kaiser Industries. Conducted by the Henry J. Kaiser Family Foundation and the Columbia Institute in conjunction with the Harvard School of Public Health.)

In your opinion, did each of the following have a great deal, some, not very much, or no influence on the outcome of the congressional debate on health care reform?

	Great Deal	Some	Not Very Much	None	Don't Know
The administration	80%	13%	4%	2%	1%
Town meetings and public forums	39	38	20	0	3
The news media and broadcast print	46	39	11	0	4
Advertising by interest groups	55	36	5	0	4
Other activities by interest groups	30	45	12	0	10
Public opinion	75	16	2	4	3
PAC contributors	7	23	54	11	5
The two political parties	43	27	27	2	1
Mail and other communications from constituents	41	39	14	2	4
Radio talk shows	36	52	4	0	8

One of the noticeable incongruities during the healthcare reform debate was that 70% or more of those surveyed said they agreed with two fundamental propositions underlying the President's plan: (1) that all Americans should have health insurance coverage and (2) all employers should contribute to paying for their employees' premiums (Johnson & Broder, 1996).

In the end, the public's vague understanding of Clinton's healthcare proposal was that it would do little to help people who already had health insurance. Polls showed that voters wanted the costs of their healthcare controlled, but the typical American didn't care deeply enough about providing health insurance coverage for the uninsured, particularly if doing so might conceivably raise costs, expand government intervention, or limit their own choice of medical care. People wanted employers to pay for their health insurance. Why wouldn't they? When the follow-up question was asked, "Do you want the government to require businesses to pay for health insurance coverage if it means lower wages and fewer jobs?" the number of those supporting reforms dropped substantially (Blendon, Brodie, & Benson, 1995). The reality today as it was then is that when the electorate is asked about reform proposals, people are more concerned about the effects of reform on them personally.

In Robert Blendon's view, and that of other analysts who have tracked the voter response to Clinton's initiative, the healthcare plan died because it failed the "me first" test (Blendon, Brodie, & Benson, 1995). In a 1995 article reviewing some 28 surveys on the healthcare debate, Blendon et al. wrote that the polls disclosed that "from the outset Americans showed more concern for solving their own healthcare problems than those facing the nation as a whole. ... Americans' strong support for reform could be quickly tempered by messages implying that personal sacrifices might be required to deal with broader problems." The public's insistence that reform " ' ...do no harm' to them personally," according to Blendon, suggests that in the future, social policy initiatives that personally affect the most Americans will shrink to the least offensive common denominator (Blendon, Brodie, & Benson, 1995).

Today, we have a different target or villain and one that has directly touched the lives of many Americans in a personal way and shaped how consumers look at healthcare: consumer experiences with managed care.

The Managed Care Backlash
A reflection of the public's seemingly schizophrenic views about healthcare can be seen in recent surveys on managed care. There appear to be several parallels between the public's inconsistent views during the healthcare reform debate and

their views toward managed care. Harvard University and the Kaiser Family Foundation have been conducting surveys on the public's attitudes on managed care since 1996. Confirming the findings of a number of earlier studies, an August 1997 Kaiser/Harvard survey found that most insured Americans, regardless of whether they had managed care or traditional coverage, were satisfied with their own health insurance plan. Two-thirds (66%) of adults younger than age 65 in managed care and three-fourths (76%) of adults younger than age 65 in traditional plans gave their own health plan a letter grade of "B" or better (Kaiser/Harvard/PSRA Poll, 1997). An April 1999 Kaiser survey showed similar findings (Kaiser Family Foundation, 1999).

Although conflicting opinions were found in many surveys conducted by Kaiser/Harvard, those in late 1998 show broader worries about managed care and the healthcare system in general. In one survey, Americans reported being increasingly concerned about managed care, and support for consumer protection legislative proposals had grown significantly (Kaiser Family Foundation/Harvard University, 1998). Compared with earlier Kaiser/Harvard surveys, more Americans saw managed care plans as doing a "poor job" (36%, up from 21% the previous year) in serving consumers and worried that their insurers were more concerned about profits than about their healthcare (33% in 1998 compared with 18% in 1997) (Figure 2–2). In the April 1999 Kaiser poll, nearly 60% of Americans said they were worried that "if they became sick—their health plan will be more concerned about saving money than providing the best treatment" (Kaiser Family Foundation, 1999).

At the same time, the number of Americans supporting government regulation of health plans had risen significantly between 1997 and 1998. When presented with arguments for and against regulation, 65% said "government needs to protect consumers from being treated unfairly and not getting the care they need," versus 28% who said "additional government regulation is a bad idea and would raise the cost of health insurance." By comparison, 52% responded favorably toward government regulation when presented with this same trade-off in September 1997 (Kaiser/Harvard/PSRA Poll, 1997).

FIGURE 2–2

Percentage of Americans who say what kind of job each is doing serving healthcare consumers. (Source: Kaiser/Harvard Survey of Americans' Views on the Consumer Protection Debate, Sept. 1998; Kaiser/Harvard National Survey of Americans' Views on Managed Care, November 1997. This information was reprinted with permission of the Henry J. Kaiser Family Foundation of Menlo Park, California. The Kaiser Family Foundation is an independent healthcare philanthropy and is not associated with Kaiser Permanente or Kaiser Industries.)

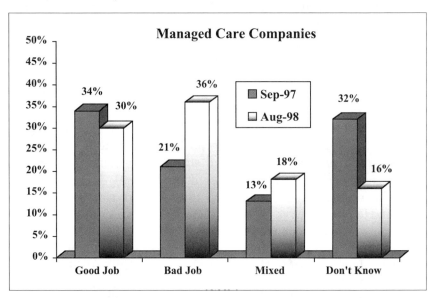

This support for regulation appears to reflect two main public concerns: (1) that managed care is hurting the quality of care available to patients and (2) that managed care is not doing as well as other means of delivering and financing healthcare. As evident in the healthcare reform debate of 1994, legislators pay attention to public opinion polls. After selected polling of the public by the GOP in July 1998 about managed care reform and patient protections, Senate Republicans decided to introduce the *Patient's Bill of Rights,* which eventually passed in July 1999 (Alverez, 1998).

However, the "I'm okay, they're not" view was still holding relatively strong even in the most recent surveys. In polls conducted in 1998, support for consumer protection in managed care dropped substantially when possible consequences were raised. For example, support for consumer protection legislation dropped from 78% to 40% when people were told that it could raise the cost of a typical family health insurance policy by $200 a year (Kaiser Family Foundation/Harvard University, 1998). Furthermore, support dropped dramatically when respondents were presented with potential problems that the "government may get too involved in the health care system, raise costs, or cause employers to drop coverage."

The April 1999 Kaiser survey also confirmed earlier findings that most Americans favored government regulation of managed care, even if it raised costs. In that survey, 74% of Americans believed that the government should protect consumers of managed care, but only 46% of that group favored such intervention if increased health insurance premiums would result (Kaiser Family Foundation, 1999).

A *Wall Street Journal/NBC News* survey conducted in June 1998 showed the contradictory views that Americans continue to have on healthcare. The poll showed that the public was angry over almost any restrictions on its healthcare. It dislikes insurance plans that require prior approval, even in nonemergencies, before paying the bill.

Large majorities complained that too many Americans lack adequate health insurance coverage and that HMOs care more about holding down costs than providing quality care. Yet, when asked about their own situation, most people were eminently satisfied with their own healthcare and coverage. Their personal experiences had been overwhelmingly positive (Hunt, 1998). However, many public opinion polls may not accurately reflect patient views because most people have no serious interrelationship with the healthcare system and many are healthy most of the time.

One example, a Louis Harris poll in 1998, showed that although most Americans believe that the healthcare system has problems, fewer believe that their own coverage and the medical care they or their families receive is less than satisfactory (Louis Harris and Associates, Inc., 1998). Of adults, 84% were satisfied with their health insurance coverage; 44% percent were very satisfied. However, 16% (a substantial minority) of insured adults were dissatisfied with their or their family's health coverage (Figure 2–3).

FIGURE 2–3

Satisfaction with healthcare coverage. (Source: Data based on Louis Harris
and Associates, Inc. *The future of health care.* 1998.)

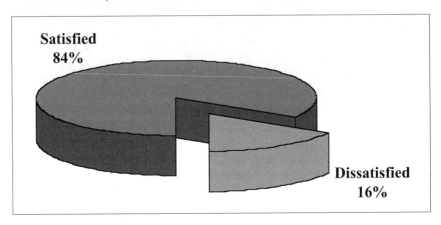

Based on these surveys, the only conclusion that can be
reached about the public's view on healthcare is to evoke an
analogy of many middle-aged characters in Woody Allen movies:
"Americans are satisfied, mixed up and worried—all at the same
time."

Three key findings from analyzing public opinion research in
the context of the "I'm okay, they're not" syndrome are as follows:

1. Consumers are alarmed about the state of healthcare.
2. The public professes to care about a national solution
   (including Medicare and the working poor and the
   uninsured), yet the public does not want to personally
   sacrifice more than they already have or give
   anything up.
3. Concern about managed care is a mile wide but an inch
   deep. Consumers are concerned about limitations and
   choices that HMOs place on the medical care they
   receive, but they are equally concerned about how
   managed care reform legislation affects them directly;
   namely, the possibility or threat of higher premium
   costs if legislation passes.

The "I'm okay, they're not" syndrome is only one aspect of
the public's view of healthcare. Another critical component in

attempting to comprehend the public's attitudes is consumer understanding of healthcare policy issues and their direct experiences with the healthcare system.

A Lack of Understanding of the Issues

Before and during the healthcare reform debate of 1993–94, there was a deep division between the way experts perceived problems in the healthcare system and the way the public did. Many experts believe this gap between public perception and reality doomed healthcare reform and has made it difficult to find solutions since 1994. For example, research conducted by the Public Agenda Foundation showed that the public believed that factors such as greed, high salaries, corruption, waste, and unnecessary care were why healthcare costs were rising so rapidly. The consensus then was that the healthcare system was not in a cost crisis but in a *profits* crisis. But experts and political leaders saw the problem of skyrocketing costs as a new problem caused by an aging population using more medical care and the explosion of new, costly medical technologies (Yankelovich & Immerwahr, 1991).

Furthermore, as the public was confronted with solutions to address the healthcare crisis, an information gap persisted. In the midst of the healthcare reform debate in February 1994, most Americans did not grasp even the most basic features of the administration's plan. Only about one in four, for example, knew that Clinton was the principal sponsor of a healthcare measure that included an *employer mandate* under which employers had to provide health insurance to full-time employees (Yankelovich & Immerwahr, 1991). By August 1994, the Harris poll was reporting that only 13% of Americans felt as if they were well informed about the healthcare plan in general, and 15% thought they had a good understanding of how the various reform proposals would affect them and their families. At the end of 1995, a slightly larger proportion of the population— about a third—actually thought that Congress had already passed healthcare reform or didn't know whether legislation had been enacted (Morin & Balz, 1996).

Ironically, members of the public, by their own admission, did not claim that their objections to Clinton's health plan were based on a well-informed understanding of it. Only a small proportion of the electorate (about 20%) said they knew a lot about what was in Clinton's plan when it was announced, and that minority actually shrank as the congressional debate wore on.

One recent survey demonstrates the confusion in the public's mind about managed care and healthcare issues (Employee Benefit Research Institute, 1998). The 1998 Health Confidence Survey of the Employee Benefit Research Institute (EBRI) found that Americans were satisfied with the healthcare they received but were confused about the type of health insurance coverage they had and about their future healthcare (Figure 2–4).

FIGURE 2–4

Managed care confusion. (Source: Employee Benefit Research Institute. Confidence in health care at what cost? *Results from the 1998 Health Confidence Survey,* July 1998.)

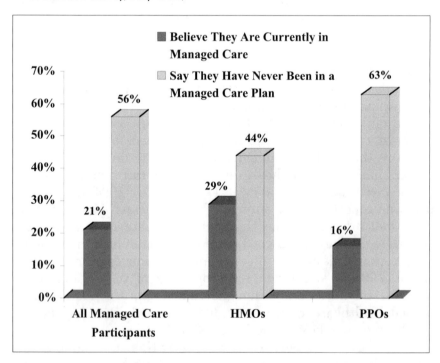

The EBRI survey showed a divergence between the magnitude of key healthcare issues and their perception of the problems. The survey showed that four of five Americans (81%) believed that the cost of healthcare had increased in the past 5 years. During this period, the rate of increase in healthcare costs and insurance premiums slowed dramatically. Although the overall rates have slowed, consumers may not have enjoyed the lower rates because of increased employee cost-sharing provisions in the form of higher premiums and deductibles. The EBRI poll also showed a gap between the public's understanding of the magnitude of the uninsured problem. Most Americans (60%) underestimate the number of uninsured in this country.

However, before any major conclusions can be made about what the public's mind-set is and what the public understands, some recent polling on Medicare reform may shed some light. A major healthcare policy debate has already begun on the best approaches to ensure the long-term financial solution of the Medicare program. In 1997, a National Bipartisan Commission on the Future of Medicare was formed and charged with developing a policy consensus on financing the program, but it was unable to achieve that consensus and disbanded without making any recommendations to Congress.

A new survey by the Kaiser Family Foundation and Harvard School of Public Health highlights the challenges for policy makers as they consider ways to shore up the Medicare Trust Fund and finance care for the growing number of seniors. Although most Americans are aware that Medicare faces fiscal problems, according to the survey conducted in October 1998, they are not ready to support changes that would produce major savings. What the survey pointed out is that generational differences and low levels of public knowledge about proposed options for reform will present more hurdles for policy makers when the debate over Medicare's future comes before Congress (Kaiser Family Foundation/Harvard School of Public Health, 1998).

Based on the National Survey on Medicare, most Americans do not believe Medicare is headed for a crisis, although they do think the program has financial problems (40% believe the problems to be major, and 26% believe the problems to be minor).

Most Americans also say they know little or nothing about the options being considered to change Medicare (50% say "only a little," and 25% say they know "nothing at all"). Even among seniors, relatively few consider themselves well informed about the options under consideration (43% "only a little," and 20% "know nothing") (Kaiser Family Foundation/Harvard School of Public Health, 1998).

The League of Women Voters in partnership with the Kaiser Family Foundation sponsored 11 focus groups in 1998 on the public's views on Medicare reform. Three major themes emerged from those focus group discussions:

1. Participants were confused about Medicare. Participants were uncertain about basic Medicare facts, such as what services are covered and who is eligible for coverage (Figure 2–5).

2. Participants' values shape their opinions about specific reform options, sometimes coming into direct conflict with one another. Participants wanted a fair and equitable Medicare system, saying things such as "Everyone needs to contribute something to pay for the system," or "It's only fair that people 65 and older who have paid into the system have access to low cost healthcare." Many also believed that it is fair for people with higher incomes and more financial resources to pay more for their coverage (on a sliding scale), but not all participants agreed with this view of fairness.

3. Participants were split on the degree of change that is needed to improve Medicare. Those who supported major change were often referring to the amount of fraud, abuse, and waste they perceived in the program, and they wanted major changes to clean up the program but not changes in other aspects of Medicare. Focus groups were concerned about the consequences of reform measures to financially strengthen the Medicare program, such as moving to a defined contribution program, raising the eligibility age to 67,

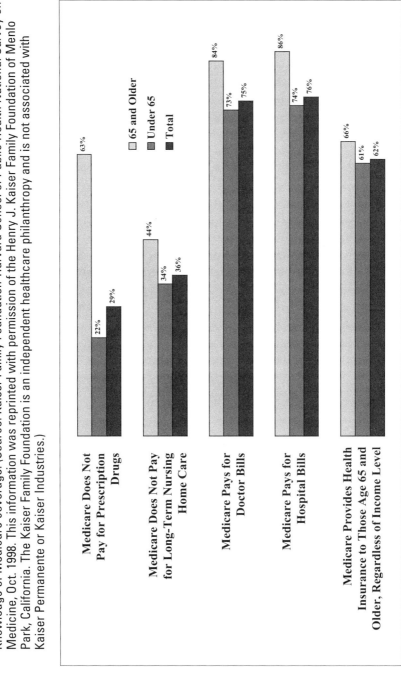

FIGURE 2-5

Knowledge of Medicare coverage. (Source: Kaiser Family Foundation-Harvard School of Public Health National Survey on Medicine, Oct. 1998. This information was reprinted with permission of the Henry J. Kaiser Family Foundation of Menlo Park, California. The Kaiser Family Foundation is an independent healthcare philanthropy and is not associated with Kaiser Permanente or Kaiser Industries.)

increasing payroll taxes, and raising contributions for all beneficiaries (League of Women Voters, 1999).

Another issue that comes into play as consumers grapple with public policy issues is their experience with accessing medical care. In this case, recent polls point out how patient satisfaction surveys can be misleading. Observers of the healthcare scene have long noted a curious phenomenon: *standard patient satisfaction surveys almost always yield high rates of satisfaction.* For example, most of the patients surveyed by the American Hospital Association (AHA) rated their care overall as "very good" (33%) or "excellent" (40%); relatively few gave marks in the "fair" (5%) or "poor" (2%) ranges (American Hospital Association, 1997). However, when patients talk or write about their experiences, they tell a different story.

Consumers who have participated in AHA/Picker Institute focus groups, regardless of their education, income, geographic location, or ethnicity, have been deeply troubled about the changes they see taking place throughout the healthcare system. Namely, they have indicated the following:

- Perception of reduced access to care and higher out-of-pocket costs
- Growing doubts about the quality of the care they were receiving and about the competence of their caregivers
- Increasing trend toward care that is cold and impersonal
- Feelings that "things" were not being done in their best interest

According to the AHA/Picker Institute survey, respondents said the healthcare "system" does not feel—or work—like a "system" (American Hospital Association, 1997).

- Few people participating in the survey perceived that there was a planned system of healthcare that operates on their behalf. Instead, they saw a confusing, expensive, unreliable, and often impersonal disassembly of medical professionals and institutions.
- If a system were in operation at all, it was seen as one designed to block access, reduce quality, and limit spending for care at the *expense* of patients. This

impression came not from sensational media accounts or the scare campaigns of special interest lobbying groups, but largely from personal experience. Patients told stories of their struggles to get past the many "gatekeepers" in the system or to get insurance or managed care approval for the care they and their doctors think they needed. They talked about how assertive they must be to get answers and the frustrations of trying to coordinate care among many different specialists (Figure 2–6). Many worried about what would happen if and when they are too sick to manage such things on their own behalf.

- They described a feeling of being abandoned when they were released from the hospital—like "jumping off into nowhere."

The issues raised in the AHA/Picker surveys highlight the frustration that many patients feel when they use the healthcare system. However, there also appears to be a basic issue that permeates the discussion on public attitudes on healthcare: a lack of understanding of healthcare issues on the public's part has complicated the ability of policy makers and decision makers to address healthcare policy on those issues.

As discussed earlier in this section, the lessons we have learned in the current Medicare reform debate in Congress are similar to those we learned about healthcare reform in 1993–94. If the public is not engaged in the policy-making process and is concerned about the ramifications of reform proposals to them personally, it will be extremely difficult to implement any significant Medicare reform measures. The implications for policy makers and others cannot be ignored. An illustrative case in this regard is the Medicare Catastrophic Health Insurance Act debacle of 1988, which resulted in the legislation being repealed a year later because of public outcry about the potential cost of the program to consumers.

There are four primary reasons why there is a lack of understanding of healthcare policy issues by the public and why it leads to distrust of the healthcare system and government:

1. There is a gap between the public's, the experts', and policy makers' perceptions of the healthcare system.

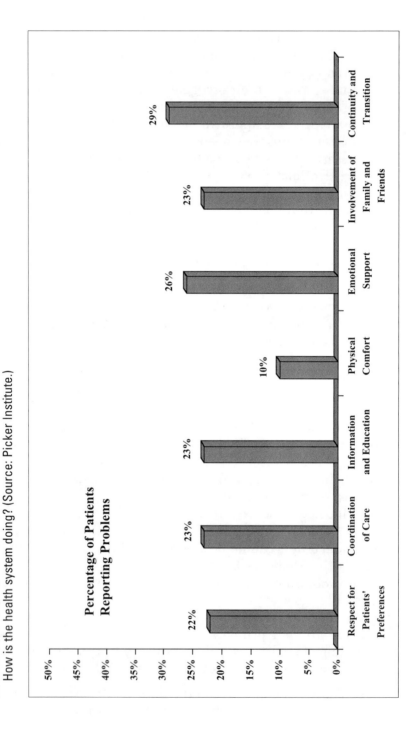

FIGURE 2-6

How is the health system doing? (Source: Picker Institute.)

2. Consumers are not able to keep track of changes in the healthcare system or legislative policies that may affect them.

3. The methods of disseminating information to the public are lacking or ineffective.

4. Consumers believe that the healthcare system is difficult to navigate.

However, as the next section shows, there are some signs that the public is becoming more attuned to the larger issues as the gap between consumer perception and reality is gradually closing (sometimes glacial-like) and we are becoming somewhat less "me" focused as we head into the next century.

Public Opinion Is Becoming More Expansive

An undercurrent throughout the recent public opinion surveys on healthcare—with their focus on the here and now—is the perception that what the medical care consumer will need in the future will not be available. This more "expansive" concern has manifested itself in recent surveys, which show a growing concern by the public with systemwide problems in healthcare and worries about how it affects them personally. This expansiveness has also been witnessed in recent actions by Congress, where several proposals have been advanced to address the uninsured problem. These measures include using the tax system and offering subsidies, and incentives to individuals and small employers to purchase affordable health insurance.

The EBRI survey points out that for all the skepticism that Americans feel about big government, the public sees a prominent role for Washington in healthcare (Employee Benefit Research Institute, 1998). Even conservative citizens insist on the government's addressing the working uninsured problem, guaranteeing more access to better healthcare, more vigorously policing managed care companies, demanding more generous coverage from employers, and ensuring that existing benefits are not pared back.

Warning signs that the public was seriously concerned about the future of healthcare came in a survey conducted in early 1997 by the National Coalition on Health Care. This survey showed a growing lack of confidence in the healthcare system. In that survey, 79% of Americans agreed with the statement "There is something seriously wrong with our healthcare system." Only 44% said they have "confidence in the healthcare system" to take care of them (National Coalition on Health Care, 1997). The survey found that 58% of Americans were not very optimistic about the future of healthcare.

A year later, the Coalition conducted a meta-analysis of public opinion surveys on healthcare and found that consumer concerns with healthcare had grown significantly since the release of the Coalition's initial survey. The study found that the public's concern had intensified from a narrow focus on managed care to broader systemwide concerns with the ability to pay for medical care, access to necessary care when health insurance coverage is lacking, and the quality of medical care delivered. These concerns were confirmed in several surveys that were released in late 1998 (Miller, 1998).

In a comprehensive survey conducted by Louis Harris and Associates in 1998, a large majority of the public believed that in the next 5 years, the problems with access to general and specialty medical care would become worse and many more Americans would be unable to afford the needed healthcare. Earlier in the decade, concerns about the cost, access, and coverage existed, but confidence in the quality of care was high. According to the survey, the public now believes the system is eroding on all fronts—in access, cost, coverage, and quality— with substantial minorities of Americans believing that the quality of their health services has declined and difficulty accessing medical care has increased in the past 5 years (Louis Harris and Associates, Inc., 1998).

The Harris poll showed that most Americans believed that minor changes to the healthcare system *will not* be enough and they were willing to vote for a candidate who would fix the healthcare system. Although a substantial minority said they would prefer that the private sector alone solve the healthcare problems, most Americans believed that the private sector alone will not be able to do so and that a joint effort of the government and private sector will be needed to ultimately fix the healthcare system. In the abstract, Americans were hesitant to trust government, but on specific issues, they thought that government has a role to play. Most people looked to government to ensure the quality of healthcare and provide healthcare coverage to those who need it. However, few were willing to spend more of their own money to sustain access to high-quality care.

Consistent with the Harris poll, a *New York Times* poll conducted in July 1998 showed that 85% of respondents believed the healthcare system needed fundamental change, barely below the 90% who said the same thing in a *New York Times / CBS News* poll in 1994 before the Clinton health plan failed (*CBS News / New York Times* Poll, 1998). But what kind of change do Americans want? Is there a public consensus emerging for solving problems in the healthcare system such as the uninsured issue?

That same *New York Times* poll continued to reflect to some degree the "I'm okay, they're not" attitude. The key finding was that although 68% of those polled said they were satisfied with the quality of their family's healthcare, 30% said they were not; that is up 19% compared with 1994. Also, the percentage dissatisfied with the cost of healthcare was almost unchanged; 46% now compared with 47% then.

In a major survey by the W.K. Kellogg Foundation's Devolution Initiative, nearly all surveyed believed that America's healthcare system needs some type of changes. Of those polled, 59% indicated that the system needs major changes (W.K. Kellogg Foundation, 1999). Almost 86% of those polled supported help for all low-income families so that the uninsured can procure health insurance for themselves and their families (Figure 2–7). Furthermore, 78% polled said that the government should pay for health insurance for children of parents/guardians who cannot afford it.

The EBRI survey showed that in response to questions about the uninsured and proposals to guarantee health insurance access, more than 77% support requiring all employers to offer health insurance to all of their employees as a means of guaranteeing access to insurance to all Americans. In fact, almost 59% indicated they would strongly favor such a proposal—another 19% would somewhat support it (Employee Benefit Research Institute, 1998).

In the EBRI survey, respondents were also asked about a series of 1% increases, in various taxes, as a means of ensuring

FIGURE 2–7

Do you believe low-income families should receive help to purchase health insurance if they are unable to afford such insurance or if their employers do not offer health insurance? (Source: Data based on W.K. Kellogg Foundation. *The national poll on welfare reform and healthcare reform.* January 13, 1999.)

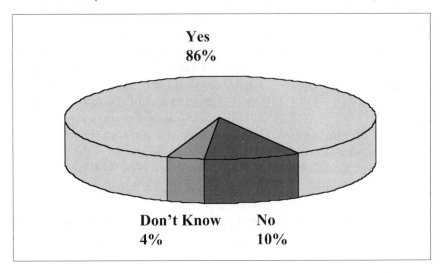

health insurance access. A majority, 57%, said they would support a 1% increase in health insurance company taxes, and 53% said they would support a 1% increase in payroll taxes for employers. Not surprisingly, the least popular tax increase was an increase in income taxes; however, 42% indicated they would support a 1% income tax increase for all to ensure access to healthcare (Employer Benefit Research Institute, 1998).

The centerpieces of the original Clinton plan, along with cost controls, were universal coverage and an employer mandate. Today, according to the *Wall Street Journal* poll, Americans (by 67% to 29%) think all employers should be required to provide health insurance for their employees. A majority of Republicans also hold that view. Support for universal coverage has actually grown in the last several years. The *Journal* poll shows strong majorities embracing initiatives to provide the same comprehensive benefits package to everyone, to charge the same for healthcare regardless of age or wealth, as well as to guarantee everyone coverage regardless of health or employment. Support is as high or higher than it was 5 years ago (Hunt, 1998).

In response to a question on the most important healthcare issue at present, the *Journal* poll showed that 37% of the public was most concerned with health insurance coverage, followed by the cost of care (29%). In addition, 23% said that quality of care was the most important problem. Only 8% of those polled in 1993 said quality of care was the most important issue. Nearly half said that cost was the most important issue in 1993 (Hunt, 1998).

A recent survey commissioned by the American Association of Health Plans (AAHP) (1999) shows that the electorate over the age of 45 is far more interested in Congress addressing the financial security of the Medicare program and that consumers have a wide range of health plan choices in Medicare and health coverage for the uninsured, rather than managed care reform (Figure 2–8).

It is becoming clearer that the public is growing increasingly concerned about the need to address the uninsured problem. In June 1999, the Health Insurance Association of America (HIAA) released a public opinion survey showing that more than four of five Americans support elements of a federal legislative proposal of targeted tax credits and tax incentives to address the uninsured problem. Of those Americans, 60% favor such proposals, even if they were required to pay an extra $100 annually in new taxes (Health Insurance Association of America, 1999).

Consistent with the AAHP and HIAA poll, a *CBS* poll (1999) conducted in late July found that the public sees healthcare as the single most pressing problem that the government should address. Of respondents, 18% said that the uninsured problem is the biggest healthcare issue, followed by the cost of medical care (8%).

However, when the public was asked to comment on the healthcare system, the *CBS* poll (1999) reflects the findings of public opinion polls in the early 1990s. When asked what type of changes should be made to the healthcare system, 86% said the current situation either requires fundamental changes or a wholesale rebuilding of the system, whereas only 12% said minor changes would suffice (Yankelovich, 1996).

Based on these recent surveys, two points can be surmised:

1. It would be a serious miscalculation for legislators, providers, and employers to underestimate the public's preference for legislative solutions to address the

FIGURE 2–8

Which one of the following healthcare issues do you think is most important for Congress to address? (Source: Reprinted with permission of Ayres, McHenry & Associates.)

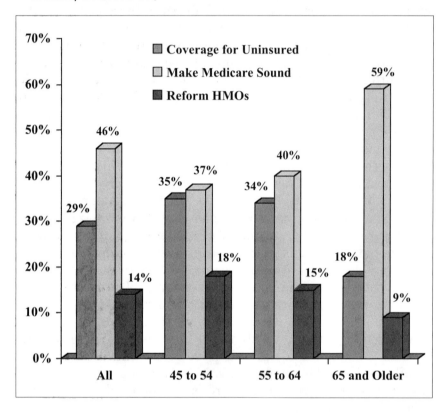

uninsured, cost, and quality problems.

2. Although the public is expressing more concern about key issues, such as the uninsured and Medicare solvency, there is no emerging public consensus on how to address these issues.

CONCLUSION

The true test of moving public opinion to support any major legislative initiative is in applying the "me-first" test. From healthcare reform to managed care reform to Medicare reform, one constant remains: the public will support initiatives that do not make their current situation worse or seem to be taking away a benefit or choice. The "I'm okay, they're not" syndrome continues to be an overarching theme in healthcare and other domestic issues, as voters continue to say "my personal situation is good," while the rest of the nation is "going bad." This view is a paradox on many fronts. Whitman's (1998) take on this construct is, "imagine how worried voters would be if the nation was in an economic recession, the arms' race were speeding ahead, violent crime were rising, and people's living standards were falling. Or if the United States was engaged in a major war."

Although there is no easy way to move public opinion to support legislative initiatives to address the major healthcare policy issues, a few key elements should be considered.

First, legislators and policy makers must recognize the public's concern, whatever that concern may be. On an issue that people have strong feelings about, most people bring with them a pet theory or preoccupation. If their preoccupation is not addressed, they will not listen to anything else the person has to say (Yankelovich & Immerwahr, 1991). In healthcare, for example, many surveys show overwhelmingly that the public believes that Medicare's problems can be fixed by eliminating waste and fraud or that managed care is limiting access to specialists. Until that concern is heard and discussed openly and broadly, the public is unlikely to be responsive to other issues or problems in healthcare.

Second, we must distinguish between the public's initial enthusiasm for new approaches and ideas for solving problems in the healthcare system and "wishful thinking," and we must begin to acknowledge the reality and trade-offs that accompany many proposals to fix the healthcare system (Yankelovich, 1996). None is a panacea that can magically solve the problem of guaranteeing high-quality medical care for everyone without bankrupting the nation.

Third, we must continue to drive home at the connections in the healthcare system (Yankelovich & Immerwahr, 1991). An outside observer might reasonably conclude that our healthcare system, even with the widespread advent of managed care, has been deliberately designed to obscure the systemwide connections and relationships between cost, coverage, and quality of care (Simmons, 1998). Our system further masks the connections between costs, demographics, and technology. The costs of high-tech medicine are mainly paid by insurance, and many workers do not pay their own health insurance premiums. The designers of Medicare deliberately structured the program to make it appear to be an actuarially sound insurance system, further obscuring the cost of medical care for seniors. Currently, many proposals have been made, ranging from providing tax credits to help pay for health insurance, to changing Medicare by providing funds directly to beneficiaries, to purchasing health insurance coverage from insurers and health plans. Such proposals should be debated not only on technical grounds but also in terms of their impact on various elements of the system.

Fourth, based on the history of reform proposals and the public's attitude to reform and change, we should not expect quick solutions. Public attitudes toward healthcare have taken a long time to evolve. Or, as Yogi Berra once said, "We're lost, but we're making good time!" In many ways, the public's views on healthcare reflect what the nation's legislative and healthcare leaders have explicitly or implicitly told them in past decades—change in deeply set values will likely come only, and very, gradually.

There are other signs of the shift in public values. There appears to be significant change in the public's willingness to forgo heroic measures designed to preserve life under all circumstances. Studies show that there has been a decline in the belief that anything and everything should be done to keep an individual alive as long as possible (Seidlitz et al., 1995).

Most of the reforms now being debated by Congress cannot succeed without a substantial level of public understanding and support. Until the public's mind-set and preoccupations are taken seriously and responded to, reform will come slowly, if at all. A good first step would be to break the "me-first," "I'm okay, they're not" syndrome that currently exists. This may be unrealistic, given our American ethos that arises from our heritage of rugged individualism and free choice.

The public also has a responsibility. Taxpayers tend to harbor unrealistic expectations of what social programs should accomplish, while simultaneously lacking faith in the government's capacity to run effective programs. In addition, the cynicism of today's voters tends to undermine the legitimacy of doing things for the commonweal. A little confidence could go a long way. Voters who trust other individuals are much more likely to have confidence in Congress, the President, and the courts than are voters who distrust others (Whitman, 1998). The former are also less likely to believe that government action hurts people.

And what about the future private sector market and the role of providers in addressing patient needs and interests? If consumers should shoulder more direct financial responsibility within the managed care paradigm, or as a direct purchasers, they will expect healthcare providers to function like any other consumer service. As direct purchasers of services, consumers will demand more information on competitive costs, quality, and expected results. They will increasingly select healthcare providers that consistently deliver convenience, responsiveness, and patient education and empowerment. To be successful, particularly in a managed care environment, providers must look beyond traditional practices and identify how to increase consumer convenience and satisfaction in providing healthcare services.

Finally, for all of those who are trying to make sense of the views of the public on healthcare, take heart from Mr. Berra's view of things: "If the world were perfect, it wouldn't be."

REFERENCES

Alverez L. After polling, G.O.P. offers a patient's bill. *The New York Times*, July 16, 1998.

American Association of Health Plans. *National survey of registered voters age 45 and older regarding healthcare issues*. Washington, DC: American Association of Health Plans, 1999.

American Hospital Association. *Eye on patients*. Chicago: American Hospital Association, 1997:2.

Blendon RJ, Brodie M, Benson J. What happened to Americans' support of the Clinton plan? *Health Affairs* 1995; 7–23.

CBS News / New York Times Poll, June 1998.

CBS Poll, July 19, 1999.

Columbia Institute. *What shapes lawmakers' views: a survey of*

members of Congress and key staff on healthcare reform. The
Henry J. Kaiser Family Foundation and the Harvard School of
Public Health, 1995.

Employee Benefit Research Institute. *The health confidence survey.*
Washington, DC: Employee Benefit Research Institute, 1998.

Gallup Poll Monthly, no. 311 (August 1991), p. 4.

Health Insurance Association of America. *Testimony before the
House Ways and Means Committee.* June 16, 1999.

Hunt, AR. Politicians risk voter backlash this autumn if they
ignore call for action. *Wall Street Journal,* June 25, 1998.

Johnson H, Broder DS. *The system—the American way of politics at the breaking point.* Boston: Little, Brown, 1996:629.

Kaiser Family Foundation. *The public, managed care, and consumer protection.* July 1999.

Kaiser Family Foundation/Harvard School of Public Health.
National survey on Medicare: the next big health policy debate?
October 20, 1998.

Kaiser Family Foundation/Harvard University. *Survey of Americans' views on consumer protection debate,* September 17, 1998.

Kaiser/Harvard/PSRA Poll, August 1997.

League of Women Voters. *How Americans talk about medicare
reform.* Washington, DC: Kaiser Family Foundation, 1999.

Louis Harris and Associates, Inc. *The future of healthcare.*
Houston, TX: Baylor College of Medicine, 1998.

Miller JE. *A reality check: the public's changing views of our
healthcare system.* Washington, DC: The National Coalition on
Health Care, 1998.

Moran, DW. Federal regulation of managed care: an impulse in
search of a theory. *Health Affairs* 1997; 7–21.

Morin R, Balz D. Americans losing trust in each other and institutions. *Washington Post,* January 28, 1996.

National Coalition on Health Care. *How Americans perceive the
health care system.* Washington, DC: National Coalition of Health
Care, 1997.

Seidlitz L, et al. Attitudes of older people toward suicide and assisted suicide: an analysis of Gallup poll findings. *J Am Ger Soc*
1995; 43(9):993–998.

Simmons HS. The forces that impact healthcare—quality and
costs. *Healthcare Forum Journal* 1998; 46–50.

W.K. Kellogg Foundation. *The national poll on welfare reform and
healthcare reform.* January 13, 1999.

Whitman D. *The optimism gap.* New York: Walker and Company, 1998.

Yankelovich D. The debate that wasn't: the public and the Clinton healthcare plan. *Health Affairs* 1995; 7–23.

Yankelovich D. The debate that wasn't: the public and the Clinton healthcare plan. In Aaron HJ (ed): *The problem that won't go away.* Washington DC: The Brookings Institution, 1996:70–91.

Yankelovich D, Immerwahr J. A perception gap. *Health Management Quarterly* 1991; 11–14.

3

CHAPTER

The Self-Care Trend and the New Healthcare Marketplace

Steven Haimowitz, M.D.

DEFINITION AND OVERVIEW OF SELF-CARE

The growing national trends referred to as "self-care" and "self-help" continue to reflect the aggressive determination of Americans to take greater command of their own health and assume greater responsibility for healthcare decisions. Accordingly, there has been an explosion in the types and scope of information sources responding to this need.

The scope of health information needs reflects the variety of healthcare decisions faced by consumers. These decisions include (1) which wellness, health promotion, and preventive health behaviors should be adopted; (2) which treatments or services should be used for specific acute and chronic illnesses; (3) which healthcare providers or facilities should be used; and (4) which health insurance options should be selected to meet consumers' needs. These decisions often involve complex interactions between family, friends, community, healthcare professionals, employers, and insurers (Sangl & Wolf, 1996).

Evidence reflecting a wide-ranging national interest in self-care is abundant. A *Wall Street Journal* survey found that 82% of respondents expressed a strong interest in self-care. Within the Baby Boomer segment (35- to 54-year-olds), 51% used vitamins or supplements, 63% always read nutritional labels, 49% restricted their red-meat intake, 78% checked their blood pressure and cholesterol during the year, and 25% regularly performed stress-reducing exercises, yoga, or meditation (Crossen & Graham, 1996).

A 1996 survey investigating the sources of healthcare information found that more households—nearly two-thirds—use print sources to read about health-related and medical information than to read about most other popular topics, including human interest stories, nature and science, or sports. More than half of all households use health-related reference books in their homes, and well over one-third use television for health-related programming (Interactive Consumers, 1996). As of July 1998, more than 17 million U.S. adults searched online for health and medical information, a number that could reach 30 million within 2 years (Miller & Reents, 1998).

These studies are consistent with multiple reports showing significant increases in consumer purchases of health-related books, videotapes, audiotapes, CD-ROMs, magazines, and newsletters, as well as an increase in the use of the Internet.

Because healthcare is a field in which millions of people have a need for sources of highly detailed information narrowly tailored to their individual situations, the proliferation of health-related sites on the Internet is not surprising (Fisher, 1996). The World Wide Web already has more than 50,000 health-related sites, hundreds of mailing lists, and Usenet newsgroups dedicated to health topics (Fitzgibbons & Lee, 1999). America Online's Better Health and Medical Network alone gets more than 1 million hits a month (Flower, 1997).

Self-care involves not only accessing information but also taking direct action, as evidenced by increased participation in fitness activities. The Health Club Industry Data Survey found a 38% increase in fitness club membership between 1987 and 1996, from 13.8 million to 19.1 million (Profiles of Success, 1996).

Factors Driving the Self-Care Movement

The self-care trend has been fueled by several important developments that reflect societal changes, economic pressures, and demographic trends. Society is placing increasing emphasis on individual responsibility for health, including behavior and lifestyle choices (e.g., diet, exercise, smoking habits), as well as on the value of applying the principles of consumerism to healthcare decisions and purchases (Sangl & Wolf, 1996). This new emphasis is responsible for new directions in corollaries of self-care, such as the increase in prescription (Rx) to over-the-counter (OTC) switches and the enormous increase in direct-to-consumer (DTC) promotional spending behind both prescription and OTC medications.

Economic pressures resulting from the increased penetration of managed care also have played a dramatic role in the self-care movement. Self-care has been identified as a "win–win" opportunity by managed care organizations. With benefits including decreased utilization of resources, increased patient satisfaction, and improved health status of enrollees, many managed care companies and employers actively promote self-care initiatives as a cost-effective means of improving both short- and long-term patient outcomes (Sangl & Wolf, 1996).

Paradoxically, consumer reaction to the *negative* aspects of managed care has also served to spur the move toward self-care. Nearly three-quarters of insured Americans—64 million people—are covered by HMOs or other managed care plans (Pear, 1997). Consumers who are unsatisfied with the restrictive nature of most managed care plans tend to view the industry as one driven by profits rather than concern for patients' health. A 1996 survey found that only 10% of consumers thought the managed care industry was credible, a number only slightly higher than that for tobacco companies (6%) (Kertesz, 1997).

Despite an expressed desire for more information, consumers are getting less face-to-face time with physicians, who must see greater numbers of patients to compensate for the decreased fees they are receiving under managed care contracts (Figure 3–1). The length of an average office visit to a family practice physician has decreased to only 12 minutes—hardly

FIGURE 3–1

Consumer Opinions of Doctors (Miller & Reents, 1998, p. 6)

PERCENTAGE OF U.S. ADULTS WHO AGREE WITH THE STATEMENT	
Doctors spend less time with patients now than 10–15 years ago.	77%
Most doctors are hurried.	65%
Not satisfied with duration of doctor's visit.	47%
Not satisfied with doctor's accessibility.	43%

Source: Yankelovich Monitor.

enough time to counsel patients at the level of detail expected by patients ("Facts About Family Practice," 1995).

This failure of healthcare professionals to satisfy patients' needs for health-related information has resulted in mutual feelings of frustration and alienation and has forced consumers to seek this information elsewhere. A survey of 85,000 consumers in 27 metropolitan areas showed that more than 25% were unsatisfied with their health plan physicians (HMO Complaints, 1997). An American Hospital postdischarge survey of 37,000 people found that one-third reported problems getting answers to important questions (Lagnado, 1997). Thus, it comes as no surprise that skeptical consumers are actively challenging both plan administrators and member physicians to ensure that they receive the best possible care, and they are turning to alternative sources for healthcare information.

The United States is also experiencing a dramatic demographic change—the aging of the Baby Boomer generation—that will have a powerful impact on the self-care movement. Currently, 27% of Americans (74.2 million people) are older than 50 years of age. By the year 2010, the over-50 group will grow to 32% of the population, according to U.S. Census Bureau projections. The 65-and-older population will grow from its current one in eight Americans, to one in six by 2020, and to one in five by 2030 (U.S. Census Bureau, 1998).

The aging of the 75 million-strong Baby Boomer generation will both increase the level of demand for health-related information and alter the nature of the information sought. The previously cited *Wall Street Journal* survey (Crossen & Graham, 1996) indicates that those currently older than age 55 have an even greater interest in health issues than do younger cohorts.

Furthermore, adults aged 55 and older now comprise 16% of health-club members, up from 7% a decade ago (Edmondson, 1997).

As the population continues to age, there is likely to be a concomitant concern in the health information marketplace about chronic health conditions (e.g., blood pressure, elevated cholesterol, osteoporosis, obesity, need for hormone replacement), age-combating strategies and cosmetic procedures, caring for ailing parents, and Medicare and other cost issues.

EVIDENCE OF THE SELF-CARE MOVEMENT

Health-Related Books

The share of consumer purchases of books in the health-related categories has significantly grown between 1991 and 1995. Data generated yearly by the Book Industry Study Group reveal that the "Health, Exercise, Grooming, Diet" category accounted for 2.1% of the total book market in 1995, representing a 10% increase from 1991. The "Love, Sex, Marriage" category experienced a 100% increase during this period, and the "Psychology, Pop Psychology" category experienced a 50% increase (Book Industry Study Group, 1996).

A review of the nonfiction, top 25 bestsellers for the years 1990 to 1996 reveals that between one and four health-related books appeared on this list each year, with a mean of 2.7 (Review of Publisher's Weekly Annual Bestseller Lists, 1990–1996). Quarterly retailing reports reveal that nine major publishers collectively increased the number of titles in this category by 32% between 1993 and 1996 (Wordstock/Titleview, 1993–1996).

Health Magazines

Health magazines have shown tremendous vitality in the last several years (Table 3–1). The most explosive growth has been experienced by Rodale's *Men's Health,* which was rated *Adweek*'s "Hottest Magazine of 1994." Since 1990, the magazine's rate base has increased 500%—from 250,000 in 1990 to

1,450,000 in 1998—making it the second top-selling monthly men's magazine in the single copy sales arena. In fact, only *Playboy* currently outsells *Men's Health* on the newsstand.

In women's publishing, magazines about healthful lifestyles, fitness, and nutrition comprise one of the fastest growing and hotly contested categories. "Nutrition and fitness are to the '90s what money was to the '80s. It's become a national obsession," states Rochelle Udell, editor-in-chief of Condé Nast Publications' *Self.*

Prevention, Cooking Light, Shape, and *Fitness* all experienced double-digit growth in advertising pages in 1996. Similar growth was seen in total circulation. *Prevention*, the category leader, has a circulation that supports two editions: a 55+ "Masters" edition (1 million circulation) and a Family edition (2.25 million circulation) (Kelly, 1996).

Health Newsletters

More than 40 health and nutrition newsletters are delivered to subscribers across the nation every month, up from five or six a decade ago. Several have circulations of 400,000 or more, larger than many metropolitan newspapers (Table 3–2). Subject matter varies from general health to nutrition, alternative medicine, women's health, mental health, and cardiovascular health. Some are sponsored by well-known medical or educational institutions such as the University of California at Berkley, Mayo Clinic, Johns Hopkins, Harvard, and Tufts. Other health newsletters represent single voices with questionable credentials.

These newsletters have built large circulations despite the fact that they are not sold on newsstands, they use minimal color or graphics, and at about $30 for 12 issues, they cost more than an average magazine (Kelly, 1996). Most health-letter subscribers are affluent, well-educated, older than age 50, and slightly more likely to be female (Kelly, 1996).

Health-Related Software

During the past 4 years, interest in "content"-based CDs has grown at an astounding pace, often as much as 64% per year (Tucker, 1996). Consumer health, medical, and nutrition

TABLE 3–1

Circulations of Top Health-Related Magazines

Prevention	3,251,555
Men's Health	1,525,000
Cooking Light	1,409,417
Self	1,141,405
Weight Watchers Magazine	1,034,082
Health	1,029,498
Shape	931,950
American Health	907,529
Men's Fitness	400,000

Source: Publishers Information Bureau, 1998.

TABLE 3–2

Circulations of Top Health Newsletters

Nutrition Action Health Letter	> 1,000,000
The Mayo Clinic Health Letter	750,000
University of California at Berkeley Wellness Letter	650,000
Health After 50, the Johns Hopkins Medical Letter	550,000
Dr. Julian Whitaker's Health and Healing	500,000
Harvard Women's Health Watch	425,000

Source: Individual Publishers Data, 1997/98.

CD-ROMs account for almost 1% of all software sales (NPD, 1996). The market for software in these categories is rapidly expanding; from 1994 to 1996, the total annual sales in these categories nearly doubled, from $11 million to $21 million (NPD, 1996).

Examples of extremely successful titles include Creative Multimedia Corporation's *Family Doctor*, which has sold more than 1 million copies since it was introduced in 1991, and Pixel Perfect's *Home Medical Advisor*, with a similar sales performance. Additional important titles now available to the public on CD-ROM include Medical Economic's *Physician's Desk Reference* and specialty family medical advisories.

From Encyclopedic to Interactive: Compliance and Prevention in Chronic Disease

In 1998, 27% of adults with children went online in search of children's health information, demonstrating the importance of the child health segment (Miller & Reents, 1998). The effectiveness of computer software in changing the health habits of individuals with, or at risk for, chronic diseases is supported by the results of an unlikely behavior modification tool: video games. Click Health, Inc., has successfully linked home video games to disease self-management to change the habits of children ages 7 to 18 in the areas of asthma, diabetes, and smoking.

Clinical trials demonstrated significant results. The diabetes-themed game reduced children's urgent care visits by 77%. Asthma sufferers showed improvements in both disease knowledge and self-care behavior after playing the asthma game (Brown et al., 1997).

For these and other disease-specific educational software products, the goal of interactivity is self-empowerment, leading to self-reliance and ultimately better long-term outcomes.

Online Health Resources

It is estimated that in the year 2002, there will be 136 million Americans, roughly half the population of the United States, accessing the Internet or World Wide Web (Fitzgibbons & Lee, 1999). Of this group, 30 million will be retrievers of health and medical information, up from just under 10 million in 1996 (Miller & Reents, 1998). The same consumer demand for health-care information (Figure 3–2) that supports the traditional publishing industries underwrites the existence of tens of thousands of health-oriented Web sites.

Online users have access to information ranging from primary medical references, once available only to medical professionals, to self-care information and disease-specific newsgroups. A recent survey found that 93% of consumer responders found the health and medical information on the Web to be "useful." Still, 53% responded that health and medical coverage on the Web needs to be increased (Medscape, 1999).

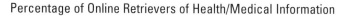

FIGURE 3–2

Percentage of Online Retrievers of Health/Medical Information

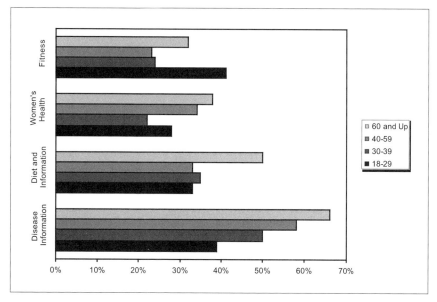

Source: Cyber Dialogue/FIND SVP.

The convergence of health and the Internet has fueled the creation of a number of major players who will be competing for the healthcare consumer over the next decade (Table 3–3). Many of these companies are collaborations between physicians, universities and/or medical centers, retailers, media companies, technology companies, and third-party payors.

Medscape is one of the more successful healthcare sites for physicians and consumers alike, offering clinical information, health-related news, and coverage of medical conventions to any registered user regardless of profession. More than 1.2 million registered users (including 180,000 physicians) view more than 6 million pages and an average of 15 million ads (banners with commercial links) each month (Medscape, 1999). In 1998, Medscape was named one of Crain's *Business New York*'s "Awesome Foursome" new media companies and was listed as one of *Fortune*'s "12 Coolest Companies in America." Medscape is

T A B L E   3–3

Major Online Players

Name	Focus
allHealth (formerly BetterHealth) allHealth.com	Content-rich forums centered around specific healthcare conditions, chat rooms, message boards, risk assessments, and other services. A subsidiary of iVillage.com, focusing primarily on women.
America's Doctor Online Americasdoctor.com	Private, real-time interactions between physicians and patients. Founded in 1997.
Empower Health Corporation Drkoop.com	Personal health information, news, e-commerce, community, and interactive services. Founded in 1997 by former U.S. Surgeon General Dr. C. Everett Koop and Dr. Nancy Snyderman.
HealthCentral.com Healthcentral.com	"Key man" strategy around Dr. Dean Edell, radio and television host, presenting health and wellness-based content including health risk assessments and personal health records. Content partnership with University of Pennsylvania. Founded in 1998.
InteliHealth InteliHealth.com	A joint venture between Aetna U.S. Healthcare and Johns Hopkins University providing personal health information, news, e-commerce, and discussion groups.
Medical Networks, Inc. healthatoz.com	Interactive health and medical site featuring the HealthAtoZ search engine, a directory of more than 50,000 medically reviewed sites and communities. Founded in 1995.
Mediconsult.com mediconsult.com	Provides clinical content, interactive communities, and health-related services, including a customized medical advisory service responding to specific clinical inquiries.
Medscape medscape.com	Customized clinical content for physicians, and controlled consumer access. More than 1.2 million members, including 180,000 physicians. Founded in 1995.
OnHealth Network Company onhealth.com	Product offerings include detailed content on specific topics and conditions, personal health tracker, and local city health guides. Content partnerships with New England Journal of Medicine and Beth Israel Deaconess Hospital.
The Health Network ahn.com	Provides consumer health information and online medical procedure video.
WebMD webmd.com	Offers both physician and consumer information and services.

Source: Individual Publishers Data, 1997/98.

just one example of the success that consumer-friendly health-care Web sites can achieve.

E-commerce, buying and selling on the Web, has been estimated at $50 billion in 1998 and is expected to soar to $919 billion in 2002 (Fitzgibbons & Lee, 1999). "Mega-sites" that serve as information hubs (e.g., Medscape and Amazon.com, online retailer) are the most heavily trafficked and the focus of continuing interest.

Across all platforms, Web advertising currently accounts for about $1.7 billion and is expected to surge to $8 billion by 2002. With the success of these and newer consumer-driven Web sites, a significant amount of revenue will be available to them to expand their reach and content (Fitzgibbons & Lee, 1999).

The explosive growth of online self-care options is not expected to slow and may in fact eclipse other sources of information, such as print. The U.S. government, as a provider of a substantial portion of consumer health information, is currently reviewing its role in the transition from paper-based information strategies to use of the full scope of existing emerging information technologies (Patrick & Koss, 1995).

It is worth noting that although the Internet is creating new opportunities to improve decision making in healthcare, it also can generate unprecedented problems. Scholarly discussion and rigorous evaluations will be important if the Internet is to meet the challenge of improving healthcare in the future (Jadad & Gagliardi, 1998).

IMPACT OF SELF-CARE TRENDS

The Pharmaceutical Industry

No other industry has been influenced more by the growing role of consumers in health decision making than the pharmaceutical industry. Most major pharmaceutical manufacturers view the self-care trend as a major opportunity and have encouraged its growth. This is best demonstrated by the increase in DTC advertising. In 1990, manufacturers spent approximately $50 million on DTC promotion. Beginning in 1995, more money was spent by pharmaceutical companies to promote prescription drugs to consumers than to doctors. In 1998, DTC spending by drug companies had escalated to an astounding $1.2 billion—44% more than was spent on physicians (CPSNet, 1999). DTC drug advertising is quickly approaching levels reached by the largest consumer brands. In 1998, manufacturer spending on advertising for Claritin eclipsed that of Coca-Cola.

Consumers are exposed to pharmaceutical advertising for prescription products within virtually every therapeutic category. The largest budgets support products for allergies, hair loss, depression, ulcers, menopause, osteoporosis, birth control, fungal infections, high cholesterol, high blood pressure, and smoking cessation. Schering-Plough's support of Claritin in 1999 represented a 300% increase over 1997 spending (CPSNet, 1999). The biggest impact on the growth of DTC expenditures came from Merck (Propecia), Eli Lilly (Evista), Zeneca (Zomig), Alcon (Patanol), Pfizer (Viagra and Aricept), McNeil Consumer Healthcare (Nicotrol), Pharmacia & Upjohn (Detrol), and Rhone-Poulenc Rorer (Nasacort) (*Managed Healthcare News,* 1999).

The figures just cited do not include promotional spending for nonprescription, OTC medications. More than 100,000 OTC medications are marketed in the United States. More than 600 OTC products use ingredients and recommended dosages available only by prescription 20 years ago (Consumer Healthcare Products Association, 1999). Since 1976, the FDA has approved 77 new and Rx-to-OTC ingredients (Consumer Healthcare Products Association, 1999).

The trend of switching prescription-only drugs to OTC status (the "Rx-to-OTC switch") is driven primarily by the desire to extend the life of products whose patents are about to expire. The shift to OTC status can lengthen marketing exclusivity and expose a new audience to the medication. Examples of recent, heavily promoted switches include Aleve, Orudis, Pepcid, Tagamet, Zantac, Axid, Rogaine, Femstat, Nicoderm, and Nicorette.

Drug manufacturers are likely to continue to support DTC advertising at current or increased levels because the payback is high. In 1987, about 18% of American patients initiated conversations with their physicians about advertised drugs. By

1995, that number had increased to 51% (Johannes, 1996). In a survey of 5,000 doctors, one-third reported that patient requests increased the likelihood of prescribing a drug not only to the patient who requested it but to other patients as well (Johannes, 1996).

Drug manufacturers are also committing significant resources to database marketing, which through the judicious use of toll-free numbers, mail-in offers, coupons, rebates, and other response devices, permits highly targeted marketing efforts. In 1996, SmithKline Beecham and Bristol Myers Squibb joined the ranks of the top 10 packaged goods database marketers, which includes consumer marketing giants such as Kraft Foods (Philip Morris) and Ralston Purina (Johannes, 1996).

Database marketing has grown almost 20 times faster among drug companies than among consumer packaged goods companies (Johannes, 1996). Today, database marketers can also take advantage of the highly targeted nature of the Internet to deliver cost-efficient, customized messages directly to prospects with the highest degree of interest.

In summary, the self-care movement has had a dramatic impact on the economics of drug marketing, fueling Rx-to-OTC switch initiatives and with it, greatly increasing DTC and prescription drug expenditures to increase awareness of these newly available treatments.

Managed Care

Managed care companies are currently involved in a number of activities that demonstrate their belief in the self-care movement. The logic behind these activities is simple: providing health information to consumers will encourage them to make healthful lifestyle decisions, reduce unnecessary visits to the doctor or emergency room, improve enrollee satisfaction ratings, and create consumer loyalty—all of which will positively affect financial bottom lines.

For example, preliminary studies demonstrate that providing consumers with online access to health information can result in cost savings. America Online's *Better Health and Medical Forum* reported the results of a survey of forum users after the first year online (Johannes, 1996). Key findings of the survey include the following:

- Of those surveyed, 5.9% avoided one or more emergency department visits.
- Twenty-six percent avoided one or more physician visits.
- Forty-three percent gained a better understanding of when to seek screening tests.
- Sixty-five percent gained an increased ability to cope with a medical problem.

The American Association of Health Plans currently lists 35 members who have established their own Web sites as resources for enrollees and potential enrollees. According to a 1995 Health Care Internet User study, 16.5% of healthcare plans are using the Internet to communicate with enrollees, and 13% have Web sites.

Managed care companies provide information to consumers through a number of other media as well. These activities include the distribution of educational books, videos, and newsletters. About 35 million Americans currently have access to phone-triage lines, up from fewer than 2 million in 1990, mostly through HMOs or doctors' group practices. These manned lines allow consumers to call and discuss their symptoms with a nurse who will help assess the condition. According to industry estimates, each dollar spent on a manned line can save the health plan as much as $2 in reduced emergency room use (Johannes, 1996).

Because self-care includes making decisions regarding choice of physician and health plan, managed care companies are also providing enrollees and potential enrollees with plan performance data, commonly called "report cards." These reports include, for example, the percentage of women between the ages of 50 and 64 who receive mammograms every 2 years, the percentage of children who receive full immunization, how many of their diabetic patients receive eye examinations, and what percentage of enrollees express satisfaction with their coverage (Johannes, 1996). Report cards encourage plans to be responsive to consumers' needs and to compete for enrollees on the basis of both cost and performance (Johannes, 1996).

Disease Management: The Patient as Case Manager

Disease management is an integral part of the managed care initiative to reduce costs. Compliance issues alone cost the healthcare system $60 to $100 billion per year. Self-care approaches, such as those online applications previously discussed, are an ideal way to control the clinical costs of chronic diseases (Fitzgibbons & Lee, 1999).

Hospitals and Health Systems

Intense competition caused by a large surplus of hospital capacity and managed care's cost focus has prompted hospitals and health systems to build a positive brand identity within the communities they serve to survive.

Many hospitals have recognized the self-care trend as a major marketing opportunity and an integral part of this brand-building process. A variety of health education, wellness, fitness, and preventive medicine programs have been initiated to fill these new needs and to achieve maximal integration of the hospital into the community.

Self-Care as a Tool for Establishing Brand Identity in a Competitive Market

Competitive pressures on hospitals today are incredibly strong. The United States has a large surplus of hospital capacity. Length of stays have decreased by about 11%, occupancy rates hover at about 58% nationwide, and once-sacrosanct academic images are eroding (Ernst & Young LLP, 1998).

These pressures have led to significant horizontal integration in which hospitals merge to form multihospital systems. With the exception of Columbia/HCA, a nationwide chain of 350 hospitals, most horizontal integration is local. This consolidation confers efficiencies in marketing the hospital system to the community and has further fueled competition among both hospital systems and independent hospitals (Dravone, 1996).

Several studies indicate that the primary determinants of survival for hospitals are consumer utilization rates and not operational efficiencies. Therefore, it becomes imperative for hospital administrators to find out why patients choose some hospitals over others, to understand consumers' perceptions of hospitals, and to mold desired perceptions by way of appropriate marketing strategies (Ugur, 1996). In fact, the most successful hospital networks have prospered mainly by establishing "brand identities" within the communities they serve.

Self-Care and Brand-Building Marketing Activities

Recognizing the self-care trend as a major marketing opportunity, hospitals have initiated health education, wellness, fitness, and preventive medicine programs within their communities. Marketers believe that maximal integration into the community will increase the likelihood that a consumer will think of their institution when healthcare concerns arise in their family (Stone, 1997). Considering that an average healthcare consumer will spend between $150,000 and $200,000 on healthcare in his or her lifetime, a program that can initiate and maintain a relationship with an individual represents a sound investment for a hospital (Thomas, 1993).

Hospital marketing departments have undertaken a number of unique self-care–related programs, demonstrating a focus on brand-building through maximal community integration. These initiatives are discussed in the following section.

Health Events

Health events, such as health fairs, are receiving increased attention as an effective tool in establishing brand preference, especially among a particular target population. In one such case study, the Cleveland Clinic reports that its Senior Health Day has proven to be a highly useful direct-marketing vehicle for increasing utilization among existing Medicare patients, as well as for attracting new patients. The event provided an opportunity for representatives from more than 50 clinical departments to promote their expertise to adults older than 60. The event was marketed through direct mail, television, radio, newspaper advertisements, and fliers, and it has grown in attendance each year (Gorbien et al., 1995).

A postevent survey revealed that 26% of attendees who were not previous patients of the Cleveland Clinic subsequently scheduled appointments as a direct result of the event. In addition, 53% said they recommended the Cleveland Clinic to family and friends. Starting in 1993, educational grants from pharmaceutical companies have covered approximately 27% of the costs of the program (Gorbien et al., 1995).

Mall Stores

More than 30 hospitals nationwide lease space in retail malls to reach out to consumers where they shop. Visitors to these mall sites can attend screenings and seminars, examine health-related books and brochures, watch videos, and interact with health educators. Seminars are usually conducted by the hospitals' own nurses and physicians. The sites provide an opportunity for a hospital to build relationships with consumers by providing them with general health information, as well as information regarding specific health concerns, in a user-friendly setting. Consumers are encouraged to call the hospital with any health-related questions so that they can receive the appropriate referrals (*Modern Healthcare,* 1996).

In Louisville, Kentucky, Jewish Hospital HealthCare Services runs four mall sites within 20 miles of its campus. Jewish Hospital, located in the city, considers the malls a major part of its strategy to penetrate the surrounding suburbs, where most of its potential consumers live. It costs the hospital about $200,000 a year to run each site (*Modern Healthcare,* 1996).

In 1995, Jewish Hospital's mall sites received 193,000 visitors, conducted 105,000 screenings, and made 15,100 physician referrals. Also that year, the hospital recorded 5,400 first-time patients who had their initial encounter in the mall (*Modern Healthcare,* 1996).

Supermarket Kiosks

The supermarket is another highly visible location where hospitals are marketing to consumers. A number of hospitals are partnering with grocery stores to offer consumers healthcare information. Carter Retail Technologies, a company that sets up and maintains hospital-sponsored kiosks in grocery stores, manages kiosks for 15 independent hospitals and 9 hospital chains in the Northeast and South. The kiosks provide healthy recipes and nutritional information and serve as a place to distribute hospital brochures and a toll-free number for the hospital's physician referral line. The supermarket advertises the kiosks on its bags and in its circulars (*Modern Healthcare,* 1996).

The University of Pennsylvania Medical Center in Philadelphia, trying to boost its following in the suburbs where it has built a network of primary care physicians, partnered with Genuardi's Supermarkets to put kiosks in 26 stores in October 1995. Carter reports that 185,000 recipes were printed by the kiosks in their first 5 months of operation. According to Will Ferniany, the hospital's Vice President for Marketing and Strategic Support, "Genuardi's stores are in markets we want to be in, that we have primary care doctors around. I've always believed every time you can get information to a person in a new setting, they see it more. Normally, you don't find hospital messages in a grocery store" (*Modern Healthcare,* 1996).

Columbia/HCA Healthcare Corporation has also invested in supermarket kiosks. Terri Reynolds Rush, a regional marketing director, points out that "With kiosks, we know the hits we're getting are in a targeted marketing area" (*Modern Healthcare,* 1996).

Fitness Centers
The explosive growth of hospital-operated fitness centers provides a powerful example of how hospitals are using the self-care trend to increase their presence in the community. Approximately 350 hospitals operated health clubs or "wellness centers" in 1997, up from 90 in 1991 and 220 in 1996 (Smith, 1996). These facilities are comparable in every way to other private athletic clubs and offer the paying public, in a nonhospital environment, everything from nutrition classes to the full array of modern exercise amenities (Stone, 1997).

Hospitals have considered a number of benefits when deciding to open a fitness center. A fitness center attracts individuals who would not normally be attracted to a hospital. Because young people tend to congregate around health and sporting events, these centers allow the hospital to integrate itself into the lives of an otherwise difficult-to-reach target audience (Hutchcraft, 1997). Furthermore, once these consumers are introduced to one service of the hospital, cross-selling other services becomes an obvious next step. The fitness center becomes a conduit to your medical staff. Delnor Community Hospital, outside of Chicago, reports that since its fitness center opened in November 1996, enrollments in its physical rehabilitation, community education, and cardiac rehabilitation programs have increased between 20% and 50% (Healthcare Wellness and Fitness Association, 1997).

By participating in the community within the context of self-care and health promotion, hospitals operating fitness centers can also establish a significant halo effect. The fitness center can position the hospital as an institution dedicated to aggressively pursuing community health goals (Healthcare Wellness and Fitness Association, 1997).

It is important to note that these fitness centers are for-profit ventures and have uniformly met or exceeded revenue, profit, and membership projections. The fitness centers have therefore demonstrated that a self-care marketing effort can contribute to profitability, independent of referral generation (Hutchcraft, 1997). The importance of diversification of a hospital's revenue stream is particularly significant in light of the American Hospital Association report that hospitals lost money on direct patient care in 1995 for the first time since 1990 (Bunda, 1996). More recently, two out of five hospitals in the Philadelphia area lost money in 1998, and losses nationwide are as high as $86 million to $200 million (Stark, 1999).

CONCLUSION

Self-care, the determination of consumers to take greater control of their own health and assume greater responsibility for healthcare decisions, is a powerful trend that has brought about tremendous change impacting every segment of the healthcare marketplace. Publishers, broadcasters, advertisers, Internet companies, managed care companies, hospitals, employers, drug manufacturers, and many other private and public companies and organizations are all vying to become providers of health information. As a result, consumers are now facing a number of challenges as self-care moves beyond a fad and becomes integrated into our healthcare system. For example, how does one deal with the barrage of health information that is increasingly available from extremely diverse sources? What sources are credible? What type of information will have the most positive impact on one's life? What action should one take based on this information? As the volume of health information increases, becoming a critical surveyor of this information will take on an importance of life-saving magnitude.

One of the most intriguing aspects of the self-care trend will be its emerging effect on the physician–patient relationship and the role of physicians in their communities. Physicians have been the traditional source of health information ("My doctor said . . ."); however, much of the self-care movement is currently fueled by sources other than practicing physicians. It remains to be seen whether physicians will emerge as "self-care leaders" and chief influencers at the local level. Clearly, self-care is a trend on an irreversible and accelerated course. The ultimate benefits of this movement, on a long-term basis, are likely to rest with the extent that physicians and other healthcare professionals take an active role to ensure that credible and actionable information is available to the public.

REFERENCES

Book Industry Study Group. Annual report. Book industry trends: 1998. New York: Book Industry Study Group, 1996.

Brown SJ, et al. Educational video game for juvenile diabetes: results of a controlled trial. *Medical Informatics* 1997; 22(1):77–89.

Bunda D. A.H.A. paints gloomier portrait of 1995's hospital performance. *Modern Healthcare*, May 20, 1996; 26(21):3.

"Consumer Demand for Online Health and Medical Information." Interactive Consumers, August 1996; 3(8):1.

Consumer Health Products Association (CHPA), "Issues." http://www.ndmainfok.org/facts/factsIndex.html. Accessed 4/10/99.

Consumer Health Products Association (CHPA), "OTC Facts & Figures." http://www.ndmainfo.org/facts/factsIndex.html. Accessed 4/10/99.

CPSNet.com. Industry News, Healthcare News Net. www.cpsnet.com/newsnet. Accessed March 1999.

Crossen C, Graham E. Lifestyles of the young, old, and in-between. *The Wall Street Journal* June 28, 1996; R4.

Dravone D. Are multihospital systems more efficient? *Health Affairs* Spring 1996; 15(1):100–104.

DTC spending eclipses 1997 total. *Managed Healthcare News* March 1999; 15(3):13.

Edmondson B. From looking good to feeling good. *American Demographic Marketing Tools*, April 1997.

Ernst & Young, LLP. Health Care Data Reference Card, February 1998.

Facts about family practice. *American Academy of Family Physicians* 1995.

Fisher L. Health on-line: doctor is in, and his disk is full. *New York Times* June 24, 1996; C1.

Fitzgibbons SM, Lee R. *The health.net industry: the convergence of healthcare & the internet.* San Francisco: Hambrecht & Quist LLC Institutional Research, January 8, 1999; 16.

Flower J. Interview with Dr. Tom Ferguson. *Wired* March 1997; 155.

Gorbien N, et al. Senior Health Day. *Journal of Health Care Marketing* Summer 1995; 15(2):8.

Health Club Industry Data Survey, Profiles of Success, 1996.

Healthcare Wellness and Fitness Association, sponsor of the Third Annual Symposium, "Hospital Fitness Programs: Improving Community Health Status," January 27–29, 1997.

HMO Complaints. *The New York Times* February 2, 1997.

Hospitals expand via mall centers. *Modern Healthcare* June 3, 1996; 26(23):50–51.

Hutchcraft C. Hospitals muscle in on fitness craze. *Chicago Tribune* February 9, 1997; Business 1.

Jadad AR, Gagliardi A. Rating health information on the Internet. *JAMA* 1998; 279:611–614.

Johannes L. Patients delve into databases to second-guess doctors. *The Wall Street Journal* February 21,1996; B1.

Kelly K. Fitness kick surges through women's titles. *Advertising Age* April 8, 1996; 32.

Kertesz L. HMO makeover. *Modern Healthcare* May 12, 1997;
37–46.

Lagnado L. Patients give hospitals poor score card. *The Wall
Street Journal* January 28, 1997; B1.

Medscape Press Release. February 1999.

Miller TE, Reents A. The health care industry in transition: the
online mandate to change. *Cyber Dialogue,* 1998; pp. 1, 6.

NPD Group's SofTrends Report, July 1996.

Patrick K, Koss S. Consumer health information. White Paper
outline, May 15, 1995. http://nii.nist.gov/pubs/chi.html. Accessed
4/10/99, p. 1.

Pear R. Congress weighs more regulation on managed care. *The
New York Times* March 10, 1997; A1.

Review of Publisher's Weekly Annual Bestseller Lists, 1990–1996.

Sangl JA, Wolf LF. Role of consumer information in today's
health care system. *Health Care Financing Review* 1996;
18(1):2.

Smith T. Hospitals are using fitness centers to improve health
status and lower costs. *Health Care Strategic Management* July
1996; 14(7):16–17.

Stark K. For teaching hospitals, a painful education. *The
Philadelphia Inquirer,* October 10, 1999, pp. E1, E15.

Stone B. Rx: thirty minutes on the stair master twice weekly.
Newsweek March 17, 1997; 46.

Thomas R. What hospitals must do. *American Demographics*
January 1993.

Tucker M. Doc-in-the-box: discs and the market for health-
oriented CD-ROMs. *CD-ROM Professional* 1996; 48–56.

U.S. Census Bureau, 1998.

Ugur Y. Competing for patients and profits. *J Health Care
Market* 1996; 16(2):30–37.

Wordstock/Titleview, Quarterly Retailing Reports, 1993–1996.

4

CHAPTER

Medical and Health Reporting in the News Media

Ira S. Nash, M.D.

The public is awash in medical and health-related information provided by the news media. Newspapers, newsmagazines, local and national television news shows, and radio news carry a large and growing number of stories about all aspects of medicine. Topics span the range from new developments in medical science to the details of the health and illness of prominent individuals. A seemingly endless stream of the latest advice from experts and the results of medical research are also presented as prescriptions for preventing illness and preserving health. The focus of this book—the new healthcare consumer—is the audience for these stories. This chapter explores the extent and nature of medical and health reporting in the news media and the factors that created it to help understand this vital influence on the public's perception of medicine. What characterizes medical health today? Why has it evolved from its current form? What are the consequences and controversies of health reporting as it exists today? What benefits accrue for the new healthcare consumer and the providers of care? What perils have been created or intensified?

TRADITIONAL ROLES OF PHYSICIANS, SCIENTISTS, AND THE NEWS MEDIA

Sir William Osler, a famous and influential physician and professor of medicine, counseled his colleagues with regard to potential interactions with the news media. In 1905, he warned the medical community to keep its distance from the news media and likened dealing with the press to a dangerous liaison:

> In the life of every successful physician there comes the temptation to toy with the Delilah of the press—daily and otherwise. There are times when she may be courted with satisfaction, but beware! Sooner or later she is sure to play the harlot, and has left many a man shorn of his strength, *viz.*, the confidence of his professional brethren (Osler, 1905).

The press, for its part, seemed oblivious to medicine despite Osler's warning. Johnson (1998), citing work by Bloom (1996a), illustrated the prior indifference of the news media to medical stories by briefly tracing news coverage of the health of presidents. In ways nearly incomprehensible to a modern audience, the press ignored Grover Cleveland's cancer, Woodrow Wilson's stroke, and Franklin Roosevelt's paralysis. Although part of this reticence stemmed from a different notion of the divide between private and public information about the nation's leaders, other factors were also at work.

Surely, one reason for the small amount of coverage of medical stories by the press in those days is that "medicine" itself had little impact on people's lives. Newspapers, alert for information that could inform or engage their readers, found little to write about. With limited understanding of the mechanisms of disease and few effective tools to treat the largely infectious scourges of the day, medical practice was a relatively unattractive subject. Likewise, in the era preceding World War II, medical research was a miniscule activity that had yielded few tangible benefits for most people. Disease and disability were seen less as opponents to be understood and vanquished and more as hardships to be endured. Compounded by a generally low rate of scientific literacy, the news media of the day—primarily newspapers—had little to say about medicine or health.

FORCES FOR CHANGE

The development of medical and health reporting in the news media is a reflection of dramatic growth in both medicine and the news industry. This growth is, in turn, both a cause and a result of comparably profound changes in the society that medicine and the media both serve.

The practice and science of medicine have been completely transformed in the second half of the twentieth century. World War II recast the United States from an inward-looking agrarian country to a global power with unprecedented industrial and technological prowess. It also vividly demonstrated the impact that science and technology could bring to bear on human society. Medical science shared in the success, and advances such as the development of effective antibiotics confirmed the ability of science to make a difference in people's lives.

The prosperity of the immediate postwar period fueled an explosive growth in medical research and the creation of a new model of healthcare delivery based on high-tech solutions applied by specialized practitioners in a hospital setting. The widespread provision of employment-based indemnity health insurance, which also grew out of the wartime economy, financed unprecedented access to the new tools of medicine. The delivery of medical services was widely perceived to be a "social good" and was supported through government sponsorship of the newly created National Institutes of Health (NIH) and the provision of tax dollars for hospitals in communities across the country. The net result was the creation of the medical research and healthcare delivery system of today—a greater than $1 trillion industry accounting for more than 13% of the economic activity of the country (http://www.hcfa.gov/stats/nhe-oact/hilites), which has a tangible impact on the life of every citizen.

It follows, then, that even if the news media had changed little over the same period, health and medicine became "bigger stories" that rightfully commanded more attention. As Bloom (1996b) points out, "Some of the most compelling political, economic, and social issues of the day are those that involve medicine and health care." Medical stories matter more to people because medicine matters more. Medical news often also has the capacity to touch people emotionally in ways that other news items cannot. For example, not everyone is drawn to a news story about a connection between toxic industrial waste and forest decline; if that same waste material were linked to a possible rise in birth defects in neighboring communities, it would become a compelling story for many people.

The growth of medical reporting is also a reflection of the dramatic transformation of the news industry over the last 30 years. One important component of that transformation has been the increase in competition in news reporting. Although big city newspapers have traditionally faced cross-town rivals, newspapers themselves were the uncontested source for news until the relatively recent rise in popularity of television newscasts. Readership of newspapers has been steadily declining, and many papers have been forced to merge or cease publishing. Those that have survived have done so, in part, by expanding their coverage of a broad range of subjects not previously considered "news." The *New York Times,* a paper of such tradition that it is nicknamed "the gray lady," now has regularly appearing sections devoted to house and home; dining in, dining out; circuits (covering the world of consumer electronics); automobiles; the arts; and since 1978, science. The science section has even spawned its own subsection on health and medicine. All this is in addition to the regular reporting of medical and science news items as part of general coverage.

Supporting this development of separate sections of papers or segments of news broadcasts devoted to health has been the growth in advertising by health-related enterprises. Health providers, such as hospitals, now spend close to $3 billion per year nationally on advertising (*Healthcare PR and Marketing News,* 1998). Direct-to-consumer advertising of prescription medication by pharmaceutical companies accounts for another $1.5 billion and is the most rapidly growing budget item for these companies (Nash, 1999). Because this advertising is often presented among health-related news stories, it has provided an important incentive to news organizations to expand such coverage (Shell, 1998).

News reporting has also changed because news reporters have changed. Newsrooms now have greater numbers of women and members of minority groups than ever before. This has occurred to the extent that "newspeople edit and write stories that affect them personally . . . the ethnic, sexual, gender and chronological composition of [the] American newsroom [has contributed to] . . . more stories—and fundamentally different kinds of stories—about medicine and health care" (Bloom, 1996b). The growth of the health reporting "beat" has also allowed news reporters to specialize in this area. This, in turn, has increased the level of expertise and sophistication among health reporters, which has also contributed to their increased access to sources of health and medical developments (de Semir, 1996). The ultimate expression of the sophisticated health reporter is the physician/reporter. "Television doctors" are now common, both at the national and local level, although their counterparts in the print media are more rare.

The diversification of news reporters has paralleled an increased openness to the public discussion of formerly taboo subjects. As was amply demonstrated by the detailed coverage of President Clinton's indiscretions, there are now almost no areas that are "off limits" to news coverage. In a news environment where the graphic details of presidential peccadilloes are the stuff of prime time television, topics ranging from breast cancer to bowel surgery no longer shock. Many observers credit part of this shift to the deliberate baring of details of their own medical problems by prominent people. Betty Ford's openness about her own experience with breast cancer heightened awareness of the disease, increased the demand for information among the lay public, and sanctioned widespread coverage of the subject in the news.

Bloom (1996b) cites a number of other changes in the news industry that have contributed to the growth of health reporting: a general rise in sensationalism (what he calls the "tabloidization" of news reporting) as a response to competition in news reporting, "personality-driven" television with its insatiable appetite for "intimate" topics for discussion, and the AIDS epidemic, which has forced medical news to the front page. These changes in medicine and the news media have contributed to the creation of a society that is now hungry for, and conditioned to, frequent stories about health-related issues in all the major news media. Indeed, the news media has become the dominant source of health information for most Americans.

Other, more general social trends have also contributed to the rise of medical reporting in the news media. A general increase in scientific literacy, as a consequence of higher levels of education, has contributed to the receptivity of the public for health news (de Semir, 1996). Although many observers still find the public level of scientific knowledge wanting (Turney, 1996), there is little doubt that there is a large segment of the population with a working knowledge of science that greatly exceeds the level of a generation ago. Closely tied to this improved facility with science is a broader social interest in scientific subjects of which medicine is just a single example. The "space race" and the environmental movement galvanized an entire generation with images of the promise and danger of technology (de Semir, 1996).

The relative affluence of the postwar United States has also contributed to a greater interest in medicine and health-related news. Only in an environment where the struggle for basic human needs is no longer dominating people's existence can interest in the relative importance of different "lifestyle" changes or the advance of medical science take hold.

Finally, there are elements of the "American character" that foster an interest in health and medicine. Americans have traditionally been optimistic and individualistic. The essence of the American dream is that strength of will and hard work will lead to great rewards. The advance of medicine can be seen as a great American success story with hard-working scientists and doctors fighting to overcome nature's obstacles and conquer disease—a kind of latter day (and more politically correct) manifest destiny. Not just the doctors and scientists are fighting this good fight. At the individual level, many believe they can each achieve a sort of personal manifest destiny, becoming the "best" person each can be. All it takes is knowledge of the latest information that science has to offer—what to eat, what to avoid, what kind of exercise to do, what vitamin supplements to take—to live "right."

MEDICAL AND HEALTH REPORTING TODAY

Coverage of medicine and health-related stories is now an established, important, and expected part of news reporting. It is also clear that the news media is the dominant source of information for most people on all subjects beyond their own work and family (Radford, 1996). News reporting in magazines, in newspapers, and in particular, on television, has become the primary source of health information for the general public (Dan, 1992). Shell (1998) reported that "Americans now rely more on the media than on their physicians" for health information. Phillips et al. (1991) reported that not only members of the general public but also health professionals (physicians and scientists) get most of their information about medical developments from the lay press. Surveys have detailed the extent of news reporting and its corresponding influence on the general public.

Wallack and Dorfman (1992) reviewed the content and perspective of a cross-section of health-related reports that they observed on television from a random sample of programming. Of a total of 105 separate news stories compiled in a single 20-hour composite "day," they found that 41% were related in some way to a health issue. These included "death or injury . . . threats of harm (lead poisoning in the workplace and radon contaminating the nation's schools), drugs (teenage drug and alcohol use . . .), and medical stories (a child's fight with cystic fibrosis and his experimental heart-lung transplant as well as various celebrity cases of heart disease)."

Although their definition of "health news" may be broad, a simple search of the Lexis-Nexis news indexing service found more than 100 references to the specific health topic of "diet and heart disease" in major U.S. newspapers in the second half of 1998 alone. The full spectrum of health stories in the same sample of newspapers numbered in the thousands.

There have been several well-documented instances of a dramatic change in public perceptions about a particular health issue after prominent news coverage. Schuchman and Wilkes

(1997) recounted the fallout from press reports in 1995 that calcium channel blockers—a class of medications widely prescribed for hypertension and some forms of coronary heart disease—had been linked by researchers with an increased risk of heart attack. A national furor ensued, with many frightened patients either anxiously calling their doctors or discontinuing the medication on their own.

Johnson (1998) reported on the "frenzy" caused by stories that appeared in newspapers and on all of the three major television news programs about preliminary results from a very small (and poorly designed) study purporting to show positive results from a new treatment for Alzheimer's disease. People from around the country responded with thousands of calls of inquiry, as well as promises for large cash payments for a treatment that was not even available.

No less remarkable is the story of the antidepressant medication Prozac (fluoxetine). Although it is now recognized as being no more effective than many other available agents (Fava et al., 1998), Prozac became a media "star" (Nelkin, 1996) and entered the popular culture of talk shows, magazines, and late night comedians through extensive reporting in the news.

CURRENT ISSUES IN HEALTH REPORTING

With the growing importance of medicine, the intense interest among the public in medical information, and the role of the press as the chief provider of medical information, a number of important issues regarding the interaction of medicine and the media need to be considered.

A fundamental question is how a particular item is deemed newsworthy. Clearly, if the news media is the most important source of health information, then the degree to which the public understands medicine is critically dependent on the decisions news reporters and their editors make regarding what to cover. In explaining how those decisions are made, Bloom (1996b) recounts the cynical (and no doubt apocryphal) anecdote about the editor of a big city newspaper. The editor orders a series of investigative reports on the deterioration of city streets only after he spills his morning coffee on his expensive suit by hitting a pothole on the way to work. The point of the story, of course, is that "news" is, by definition, whatever is important to those who report it. Johnson (1998) echoes this: "the process that leads to the official designation of information as news—meaning that it makes it into print or onto the airwaves—is far more haphazard and idiosyncratic than outsiders might ever imagine." The subject of story selection is considered more thoughtfully by de Semir (1996), who considers a number of factors that influence journalists' choices about what to report but concludes in a similar vein that ". . . in the end our intuition influences what we decide to publish. There is no defined criterion, except for the constant attempt to establish a certain complicity with our readers." He describes this ad hoc approach to defining the medical news as fundamentally "unscientific."

The great success and strength of modern medicine, however, is largely derived from its adherence to the dictates of the scientific method: hypothesis generation, experimentation, and data interpretation. Medical progress depends on the accretion of evidence to a reliable theoretical structure and the episodic reformulation of theory to account for new evidence. Consequently, physicians and medical scientists, schooled in this way of thinking, inhabit a culture quite different from the culture of news reporting (Angell & Kassirer, 1994). A number of contentious issues derive from this cultural dissonance.

One issue is the differing perspectives of journalists and physicians regarding the importance of the context of a medical news item. Because journalists are constantly striving to connect with their readers (listeners and viewers) through the presentation of "fresh and dramatic" stories (Nelkin, 1996), they often sensationalize what is, in reality, an incremental or even insignificant advance. This steady drumbeat of new advances, without a careful examination of the context in which medical research is done, has led to the seemingly endless contradictory "advice" from medical researchers, causing much confusion for the general public about what foods/activities cause/prevent which ailments. As Angell and Kassirer (1994) report:

> No sooner do they learn the results of one research study than they hear of one with the opposite message. They substitute

margarine for butter, only to learn that margarine may be worse for their arteries. They are told to eat oat bran to lower their cholesterol, but later learn that the bran they dutifully ate may be useless. They substitute low-calorie saccharin for high-calorie sugar, only to hear that some researchers find an association between saccharin and bladder cancer, while other researchers do not.

They conclude that the appropriate response to this problem is:

> ... More moderation in our response to *news of clinical research*. Every study reported in the media does not require an all-or-nothing response in our diet or lifestyle. In general, we should not embrace the conclusions of a study until other studies support them. Reserving judgement in this way, without succumbing to antiscientific nihilism, is the best protection against being whip-sawed by *media reports* of clinical research.

This is a forceful statement about the differences between medical research and medical reporting. Note in particular that they cast this as a problem with reporting about medical research, not the research itself.

Sensationalism sometimes takes other forms. For example, in 1995, a respected Spanish newspaper headlined, "The vaccine against cancer of the cervix will prevent half a million deaths a year." The story under that headline, however, merely reported that a study had demonstrated a link between a particular viral infection and cervical cancer. There was, as yet, no vaccine for the virus, and certainly no demonstration that such a vaccine, were it to be developed, could actually prevent half a million deaths (de Semir, 1996). Others have accused the media of reporting medical news as if it were a "hostage crisis," resulting in the public being "misled about the implications of [a scientific] finding" (Schuchman & Wilkes, 1997).

Closely related to the sensationalism of medical news reporting is the potential distortion brought about by the lack of follow-up stories (Schuchman & Wilkes, 1997). Dramatic advances and discoveries make for interesting headlines; later research that calls the initial findings into question does not. Schuchman and Wilkes (1997) detail several examples of this. In

1994, a study sponsored by the NIH found that a surgical procedure used to remove the fatty material in narrowed carotid arteries (carotid endarterectomy) was beneficial in lowering the risk of stroke. The initial findings were widely publicized in the lay press after an NIH-sponsored news conference. The final report in the scientific literature (Executive Committee, 1995) contained important caveats about the research findings, which made it clear that the procedure should be used selectively and performed only by highly skilled surgeons in order to derive clinical benefit. These distinctions did not receive the same level of coverage as the initial findings, leaving the public with an exaggerated sense of the value of carotid endarterectomy.

The urgent need for journalists to connect with their readers also places a premium on writing a story in such a way that the information is easily comprehended by the general public. Some medical stories, such as those reporting on the cutting edge developments in new molecular biological techniques, are difficult to explain in a way that balances accuracy and readability. A cooperative approach to this problem among researchers and reporters would benefit both: researchers who took the time to educate journalists would be more likely to see their work discussed accurately and more widely in the lay press. Journalists who are better informed could discriminate among potential stories better and obtain access to new developments more easily. Unfortunately, the cooperative spirit is often difficult to maintain in an atmosphere of mistrust (Bander, 1983) around this issue.

Finally, the nonsystematic way in which medical stories are covered by the press inevitably means that some truly seminal work never receives the attention it should. This can happen in at least two ways. The first is a general phenomenon of news reporting: the prominence of a given story is dependent on what else is competing for news at the same time. A natural disaster, plane crash, or other calamity is sure to force a medical development off the front page. A more subtle variation of this is the importance of resonance of a particular medical development with the news or popular culture of the day. This was illustrated by Ricard Guerrero, who compared the relative press interest in coincident scientific reports (de Semir, 1996). One report, which he identified as a substantial scientific achievement (the complete DNA sequencing of a bacterial species), received much less coverage than the possible discovery of viable ancient ("Jurassic") bacteria. The latter story found a public "primed" to the subject by the popular movie about dinosaurs recreated from ancient samples of DNA.

Other important issues should be considered in the present-day relationship between news reporting and the health sciences. Medical research has become increasingly dependent on public funding, and medical developments now have potentially enormous financial consequences. The NIH's budget is now well over $15 billion per year (http://www.nih.gov/welcome/nihnew. html) and growing. Fortunes are made on Wall Street on the news of a favorable clinical trial that may lead to approval of a new medical device or on the release of a drug expected to "do well." This was amply illustrated recently with the success of Pfizer based on the anticipated sales of its new medication Viagra. In such an environment, medical researchers have a powerful vested interest in seeing to it that their work receives prominent and *favorable* news coverage. This puts medical journalists in a relatively new and challenging position. Whereas they previously concentrated on accurately conveying the medical or scientific developments in a way that people could understand, they must now, in addition, assess the validity and accuracy of information being actively promoted by their medical sources. Medical researchers, formerly rather suspicious of the press, now may also see news coverage as a way to enhance the prominence of their work, with attendant increases in their prestige and funding.

In discussing the difficulty journalists may have in sorting out true medical advances from promotional "hype," Wilkie (1996) detailed the tremendous volume of unsolicited information that he, as a newspaper reporter, received regarding "medical news" in a 4-day period in 1995. He counted a total of 158 items, including 3 books, 30 invitations to press conferences, 103 press releases, and 24 journals. Medical journals, the source from which journalists often derive their stories, have contributed to this by preparing news releases and even "prewritten" articles and video clips about papers in their latest issues (Shell, 1998). Many medical journalists have become inured to this information onslaught (Johnson, 1998), which has, paradoxically, made journalists more suspicious, not better informed.

This sea of medical information, proffered or not, along with the rapid growth and diversity of medical research has raised important questions about the qualifications that journalists ought to have to cover their "beat." One would not expect a newspaper's business reporter to be adept at writing about baseball, nor would they expect the restaurant reviewer to be capable of a trenchant analysis of geopolitics. Sophisticated subject matter requires sophisticated writers. Given the range of medical subjects, what skills are required? Johnson (1998) offers the following:

> . . . good medical-news reporting requires . . . very specific skills in the understanding of biostatistics and epidemiology. . . . I think it is virtually impossible to do a good job of analyzing and reporting [medical advances] without a basic grounding in knowledge of such matters as the strengths and weaknesses of descriptive studies . . . and analytical studies, the evaluation of association . . . and potential cause and effect . . . and the critical difference between relative and absolute risk.

Although he is a physician/journalist, he felt compelled to get formal training in these subjects himself. He also proposed that others interested in health reporting obtain some "basic knowledge" of the relevant subjects. Furthermore, he suggested that health reporters be certified as qualified by "the fraternity of medical journalists" in much the same way that television weather reporters are required to be meteorologists. Others have concentrated less on the credentials of health reporters and have instead suggested a "code of practice" (Medicine and the media, 1981) for health reporting that could minimize some of the potential misunderstandings and tensions just detailed.

These issues of trust, timeliness of information, reliability of medical sources, and the qualifications of medical journalists are all manifest in the practice of premier medical journals of refusing to print scholarly reports that contain information previously "published . . . elsewhere, including the lay press" (Relman,

1981). This "news embargo," called the *Ingelfinger Rule* (named after a prior editor of the prestigious *New England Journal of Medicine*) prohibits authors of accepted manuscripts and journalists from discussing a particular paper before the actual appearance of the journal issue containing it. It also results in the rejection of manuscripts that contain previously publicized findings. The result is that these journals have considerable influence over what medical advances are shared with the public and when that information becomes available.

Lawrence Altman, a physician/journalist highly critical of the rule, sees it as an unjustified interference with the free flow of information that is important to, and often funded by, the public. He explains the way in which this may occur (Altman, 1996):

> Because the rule restricts what authors may disclose long before publication in a journal, it [the Ingelfinger Rule] helps determine not only what scientific information is disseminated but also how soon important information related to clinical care and public health is publicly disclosed . . . [researchers] have chosen not to present [their findings] at meetings where the data may become available to reporters . . . Because journals are a primary source of information on new therapies and advances in medicine, the rule ultimately influences the care given to millions of patients.

The Rule's proponents see the prohibition against early dissemination of information as a way to preserve the peer review process of medical research, whereby manuscripts describing new research findings are evaluated by qualified medical scientists before they are published (Relman, 1981). Whichever interpretation is more valid, no disagreement exists regarding the importance of the rule and the pervasive influence it has on the dissemination of health news to the general public.

CONCLUSION

Medicine and the news media are now inextricably linked. Both have profound influence on modern society, and each has learned to use its relationship with the other to its advantage.

To the medical world, the news media, once a "harlot," is now an important partner in educating the public and securing support for research. To the news media, medical research is a deep well of material to plumb for stories that engage the public in the way that few subjects do. Ultimately, the successful partnership between these different enterprises benefits the understanding and health of the public.

REFERENCES

Angell M, Kassirer JP. Clinical research—what should the public believe? *N Engl J Med* 1994; 331:189–190.

Altman LK. The Ingelfinger rule, embargoes, and journal peer review—part 1. *Lancet* 1996; 347:1382–1386.

Bander MS. The scientist and the news media. *N Engl J Med* 1983; 308:1170–1173.

Bloom SG. Health legacies from Franklin Roosevelt to Robert Dole, or how medical and healthcare issues took over the nation's news. *J Health Commun* 1996a; 1:83–97.

Bloom SG. The legend of potholes: newsroom changes increase medical and healthcare news. *The Pharos* 1996b; Summer:2–7.

Dan BB. TV or not TV: communicating health information to the public. *JAMA* 1992; 268:1026–1027.

de Semir V. What is newsworthy? *Lancet* 1996; 347:1063–1066.

Executive Committee for the Asymptomatic Carotid Atherosclerosis Study. Endarterectomy for asymptomatic carotid artery stenosis. *JAMA* 1995; 273:1421–1428.

Fava M, et al. A double-blind study of paroxetine, fluoxetine, and placebo in outpatients with major depression. *Ann Clin Psychiatry* 1998; 10(4):145–150. http://www.hcfa.gov/stats/nhe-oact/hilites.htm

Healthcare PR and Marketing News November 12, 1998.

Johnson T. Shattuck lecture—medicine and the media. *N Engl J Med* 1998; 339(2):87–92.

Medicine and the media. Summary of a consensus conference. *Br Med J* 1981; 282:1947–1948.

Nash BR. Personal communication, 1999.

Nelkin D. An uneasy relationship: the tension between medicine and the media. *Lancet* 1996; 347(9015):1600–1603.

Osler W. *Aequanimitas, with other addresses: internal medicine as a vocation*. Philadelphia: P. Blackstone Son & Co, 1905.

Phillips DP, et al. Importance of the lay press in the transmission of medical knowledge to the scientific community. *N Engl J Med* 1991; 325:1180–1183.

Radford T. Influence and power of the media. *Lancet* 1996; 347:1533–1535.

Relman AS. The Ingelfinger rule. *N Engl J Med* 1981; 305:824–826.

Schuchman M, Wilkes MS. Medical scientists and health news reporting: a case of miscommunication. *Ann Intern Med* 1997; 126:976–982.

Shell ER. The Hippocratic wars. *New York Times Magazine* 1998; June 28:34–38.

Turney J. Public understanding of science. *Lancet* 1996; 347:1087–1090.

Wallack L, Dorfman L. Television news, hegemony, and health. *Am J Public Health* 1992; 82:125–126.

Wilkie T. Sources in science: who can we trust? *Lancet* 1996; 347:1308–1311.

5

C H A P T E R

The Online Community as a Healthcare Resource

Stuart Gitlow, M.D., M.P.H.

INTRODUCTION

Online capabilities have revolutionized the healthcare consumer's ability to participate in a global dialog with both healthcare professionals and peers. The ability to rapidly access information is rapidly altering the patient–physician dynamic (Green, 1998). This chapter aims to help the professional healthcare reader better understand the online world of the healthcare consumer. It is designed to allow healthcare providers and professionals to target their audience, promote their sites, determine information about their competition, and account for the international aspects of publishing information in the online environment. Specifically, this chapter presents the following:

1. An overview of the online resources available to consumers
2. An overview of methods of online participation
3. An overview of ways in which consumers receive healthcare information

4. Case studies comparing and contrasting the different information sources
5. Examination of the important role of online demographics for the healthcare professional
6. A focus on some of the legal issues attendant with the dissemination of healthcare information within the online environment, including privacy and confidentiality, as well as professional licensure and liability

America Online's (AOL) Health Channel is highlighted as an example throughout this chapter because AOL is the online environment of choice for most healthcare consumers (America Online, keyword "OLP"). AOL's Health Channel has nearly three times as many monthly visitors as the second most visited health-related site. The author recognizes that although most academic centers are tied directly into the Internet, the consumer typically does not have the benefit of such access and therefore uses an Internet Service Provider. It is also of interest to note that despite AOL's acceptance by the consumer market, the coverage of the online healthcare industry has to a great extent ignored AOL's Health Channel entirely (Raths, 1998). A portion of this chapter is used to describe the pertinent differences between the Internet and AOL.

Just as the laser printer provides the public with the power of the printing press, the online medium provides the power to both distribute and access information. The potential value of this networking ability is tied to an individual's specific needs. For any consumer, those needs may involve gathering information, distributing information, or participating in a dialog with others about a topic of interest. In only a few years, the information distribution market has changed. Development, production, and distribution of text, audio, and video is no longer limited to a small minority but is within the grasp of anyone with time, computer access, and comparatively few financial resources.

The "robustness" of the information distributed and accessed online is subject to debate. By February 1999, more than 2 million individuals were visiting the leading online health-related site each month (America Online, keyword "OLP"). Is the information they find accurate, current, or peer-reviewed? Who is responsible for the presented information? To whom can the reader go to obtain additional support should the material reviewed not answer all questions? Which responsibilities are held by the information provider; which are held by the recipient? As the healthcare consumer seizes the power of the online community, these questions become increasingly important.

BACKGROUND

What Is Online?

The online world is divided into two major subsets. One subset, the portion of the Internet known as the World Wide Web, is the equivalent of public access television. It represents an anarchic realm within which falls content ranging from the nadir to the zenith of any topic's base of knowledge. The second subset consists of the proprietary networks. Proprietary networks, owned by a single company such as General Electric or AT&T, are at this time those that present a value in addition to that available on the Internet. For example, on AOL, one can access information not available on the Web by using AOL's proprietary software. These networks, available long before the Web, started to come into public view with The Source, CompuServe, and GEnie. Several such networks have come and gone, each providing a constrained set of information selected by the service, much as a magazine selects content. These services also create rules designed to govern or mediate the content posted by the community. At this time, AOL represents the largest such proprietary network. The lines between these two subsets have gradually blurred. One may access the Web directly from AOL. One may also access e-mail and a portion of AOL's information directly from the Internet. As of this writing, there remains a substantial portion of AOL's content that is not available other than through AOL's proprietary software.

Doctors Online

The online world is a reflection of the real world. There are locations to visit, products to purchase, ideas to share, and people to meet. Healthcare information is distributed and accessed differently online than within other contexts. This impacts the healthcare professional and the consumer most importantly, but as a result, it also impacts the hospital, the managed care organization, the community mental health center, the emergency hot-line, and all other health-related organizations. In 1997, the American Medical Association (AMA) conducted a survey of physicians to determine their patterns and habits in online use (http://www.ama-assn.org/sci-pubs/journals/archive/jama/vol_277/no_15/ed7016x.htm). Of all the physicians polled, only 20% indicated that they used the Web. Fifty-eight percent said they didn't even use computers. Of those going online, however, 89% reported using the Web at least once per week. Thirty-seven percent accessed the online world via AOL. Younger physicians, those younger than 40, were more likely than older doctors to access online services. Physicians in a group or academic setting were more likely to use online services than those in a solo practice. Medline access was of particular interest to physicians searching for healthcare-related information. By early 1999, according to a Healtheon Corporation survey, an estimated 85% of physicians in the United States were on the Internet. Of doctors surveyed, 63% use e-mail daily, with fully one-third using it to communicate with patients. One-fifth of doctors were dissatisfied with the lack of network content and services. Although apparently somewhat late to the online gathering, physicians have rapidly been making their appearance as the 1990s draw to a close. What physicians and other healthcare professionals do with that presence will determine in part whether the professional–patient relationship within an online environment can be rebuilt.

ONLINE HEALTHCARE FORMATS

Health-related information on the Web is available from a variety of sources. Medical organizations, individual healthcare professionals, commercial for-profit information providers, pharmaceutical companies, and not-for-profit support and advocacy groups have all posted material on the Internet and on other online services. Pharmaceutical company sites are often divided into two sections: one targeting the healthcare professional, and the other targeting the consumer. Because the Web sites are available worldwide, pharmaceutical companies generally take care to post appropriate disclaimers and to indicate the brand name in each country (it is unusual that brand names are consistent worldwide). Many academic and medical centers have set up sites containing articles written by their professional staff. Several media companies focus on the distribution of health-related information and have a variety of affiliations, allowing them to bring a great deal of content to the consumer. The AMA, state and county medical societies, specialty societies, and publishers of medical literature also have Web sites targeting the healthcare consumer directly. Managed care organizations, private practitioners, individual patients, and lobbying organizations have sites addressing the general consumer. Government agency guidelines are freely available to both clinician and patient. This torrent of information represents a windfall for both consumer and healthcare professional alike, who just a few years ago were unable to access most of this knowledge without consulting a medical library. Unfortunately, the ability to distinguish between accurate and inaccurate or biased and unbiased information does not come easily. Even to the trained eye, it is often difficult to determine the origin of information found online.

Online health-related material may be divided into three groups: health content, health communities, and health provision. The health information areas deal in one-way communication, much as magazines do. At these sites, the consumer can access information but cannot share his or her own ideas or beliefs with others accessing the site. Health communities are locations that provide interactive features such as message boards and chat rooms for individuals to discuss a given topic with one another. Provision of healthcare includes one-to-one contact between healthcare professionals and consumers, prescription of medications, and as broadband speeds come into play, full audio and video contacts between professionals and patients.

Health Content

Two media, print publications and television, can be used as metaphors to describe and define the online experience of obtaining health content. Consumers expect a broad range and depth of content comparable to that found in a newspaper to be available online. They also expect the timeliness of television news broadcasts. Because the audience for online information is international, information available at 3 AM elsewhere must be as timely and complete as the information available at noon local time. Within the print medium, the consumer is aware that the information received was current at the time of printing but may have become outdated since. Consumers expect information online to be the equivalent of a newspaper taken to the limit in which it is published and distributed seconds before being read, updated the moment new information becomes available, and corrected as soon as incorrect information is discovered.

For a moment, this sounds like television news. But we must recognize that within the television metaphor, there is but one story available at any given moment on any specific channel. Finding a story of interest often involves waiting for that story to be broadcast. Consumers expect information online to be the equivalent of an infinite number of television channels available simultaneously, with all information equally timely and with the depth and breadth of information similar to that found in a newspaper.

Health Communities

The aspect of health communities completes the online experience. If content is represented metaphorically by the grocery store bulletin board, communities are represented by the town meeting. The online user who regularly accesses a site becomes more than simply a user or a member but starts to perceive himself or herself as an occupant or citizen of the community. The reasons for accessing an online community are diverse. Just as in any population, some participants spend most of their time observing. Some are more vocal, perhaps finding it important that others consider the opinion they express. Any one participant might become a community leader, while most will prefer to simply participate. Whereas some participants may visit only occasionally, others will come daily as part of their normal routine. In the case of healthcare sites, clinical leadership may be drawn from participants but more often must be recruited and trained.

Here, we illustrate an example of a community from birth to death. In 1994, a small online service called eWorld was opened. The service had been constructed by Apple Computer and designed to support users of Macintosh computers. When a user first signed on to eWorld, he or she was welcomed with a screen that looked like a physical place (http://hotel.cprost.sfu.ca/eworld/). Although this was not the first time a graphic interface was used for an online service (AppleLink, MacNET, and AOL all preceded it), this was the first time the graphic interface emulated the appearance of an actual village. In early 1996, at the time the service was shut down, it had grown from a nonexistent village to a city of 147,000 participants (http://www.axon.net.au/eworld/). Imagine an area with a population of nearly 150,000 where all occupants are being told they must leave and never return. As the closing of the service loomed, many subscribers began to write messages of sadness, even despondence, over the loss of what they saw as their home (http://hotel.cprost.sfu.ca/eworld/index3.html). An area of AOL was set up for the displaced eWorld denizens to seek out upon their arrival on this other service that would be taking over the accounts. Although that location is also gone now, areas of the Web have since been set up to emulate the original village (http://hotel.cprost.sfu.ca/eworld/index3.html). One former eWorld user wrote, "Many, many people imprinted their hearts into this service. . . . That an electronic service has come to take on a quality personality and become a true community, is . . . the leadership precedent for an Internet to come . . . , that will not be 'just so much stuff' but rather a new medium for expanding the shared human experience" (http://hotel.cprost.sfu.ca/eworld/index3.html).

Health Provision

Health provision is represented by direct contact between the consumer, or patient rather, and healthcare professional or healthcare team. The professional might be a physician, pharmacist, or other clinician. The contact may be a simple one-time contact in which the consumer poses a question (e.g., What is the difference between a heart attack and an MI?), and the professional responds with, in this case, a definition of the abbreviation MI and a needed clarification. The contact may be between a patient and physician in which a relationship has already been established in a traditional setting. More provocatively, the contact could be group therapy in which a clinician regularly runs a chat group in which multiple individuals participate on a recurring basis. A pharmacy could sell prescription medications from their Web site. A radiology group could provide consultations from their online area by reading "films" submitted electronically to their site. The number of theoretical possibilities is limitless. At the close of this chapter, there is a review of some of the potential pitfalls currently present.

ONLINE PRESENTATION

Within an online environment, conventions of presentation refers to the graphic aesthetics as well as to the potentially intuitive nature of the human interface characteristics. Those distributing information often do not have a background in communications, journalism, or production and therefore may or may not be aware of interface standards generally in use by professional online production companies. To the general public approaching an online area, there is no immediate method of determining the level of expertise or professionalism present in the development of that area. Television and motion picture viewers are familiar with the convention of a scene blurring to indicate the start of a dream sequence. They are used to an echo being added to a voice to indicate that we are hearing the actor's or actress's thoughts. Readers of newspapers are used to seeing thin lines distinguishing the content from advertising. Advertisements that are formatted to look similar to the standard content often have the wording "Paid Advertisement" appended by the newspaper staff.

Presentation conventions are not universal within online services. The differentiation of editorial from advertising is often nonspecific. Amazon.com has been praised for its "thoughtful editorial voice and its staff of editors" (*New York Times,* 1999).

Amazon accepts payments from publishers that will lead to "complete . . . editorial review treatment" (*New York Times,* 1999). Only after an uproar from Amazon's community did Amazon quickly agree to distinguish between reviews chosen by the editors and paid reviews.

The separation of editorial from advertising is typically unclear. For example, the InteliHealth forum does not indicate whether advertising matter is solicited by Aetna U.S. Healthcare or Johns Hopkins, the companies that have jointly formed InteliHealth (George, 1999). There is often no disclaimer on private practitioner or medical center sites indicating whether grant income is derived from pharmaceutical companies whose products are featured within the provided content. Who are the professionals answering questions? Are they board certified? Why were they selected to participate in the forum? Are they paid, and if so, by whom? Perhaps these are unimportant questions, but educated consumers often are interested in this information.

INTERACTIVE VERSUS READ-ONLY SITES

Forums and Web sites can be set up as interactive or read-only areas. The Addiction & Recovery Forum on AOL (http://ng.net-gate.net/~bobber/eworld.html) is an interactive forum that provides opportunities for the community to discuss topics of concern with one another, with the forum staff, with the forum clinicians, and with special guests. Pfizer's Web site (http://mac-world.zdnet.com/daily/daily.15.html) represents an example of a read-only area, presenting information of value to those interested in Pfizer's products. The Pfizer Web site requires production, editorial, and design staff. These staff members are responsible for the look and feel of the site as well as for the content. In addition, interactive sites such as the Addiction & Recovery Forum require staff members to interact with the community. These staff members must be trained in forum management techniques so that the message bases and chat rooms are run smoothly. A clinical staff is also necessary if medical questions will be addressed. Clinical and community staff members require training similar to that provided by AOL's Community

Leaders' College. That college is responsible for training all Community Leaders in the skills and knowledge required for volunteer positions within AOL forums.

Online Participation Modalities

Several tools are used to provide interaction capabilities among participants in an online forum. The techniques described here are typical.

E-mail can be used for the community to address issues with the producer or editor of a given online area, but only if a method of contact is provided. Some areas, particularly those without the staff to handle many messages each day, do not provide an e-mail contact. Others provide one-way suggestion boxes in which the incoming messages are read and acted upon but not answered. Community members can also use e-mail to contact other community members who have posted public messages within the forum. This type of discussion takes place "behind the scenes" and is not observed directly by the forum publisher. Yet these discussions represent a significant and remarkable portion of the community activity.

Public message bases can be incorporated into the area. These are comparable to a public bulletin board. A message is posted by a single individual and can be read by all who access the message base. After time, each message base will contain several ongoing message threads, essentially a series of simultaneous conversations taking place at one time. The message areas allow community members to post messages that all other community participants can read or respond to. These messaging areas hold a varied number of messages depending on the area. Typically, old messages are logged and made available in another format for community participants to use as a resource. Message bases are monitored on AOL to be certain that AOL's Terms of Service are met. They are sometimes monitored on the World Wide Web, depending on the desires of those operating the site.

Chat areas allow live discussion among a limited number of community members, the number of which depends on the software being used. These chat rooms are often used when a special guest is making a presentation but can also be used for scheduled group discussions. Certain rules have become traditional in which participants type "?" if they have a question, "!" if they have a comment, and a staff member keeps a queue, calling on people in turn. Unmonitored chats are also possible, although they begin to become difficult to follow once there are more than 7 to 10 people in the discussion area.

Information Maintenance

Keeping content current is requisite for any site. According to a 1996 *JAMA* Editorial (http://www.psycom.net/depression. central.expert.html), the Internet is starting to offer medical content of high quality and utility for both physicians and patients. A 1997 editorial in the same publication (http://www. priory.com/pharmol/gingko.htm) indicates that there should be concern about medical information on the Web because "the Internet too often resembles a cocktail conversation rather than a tool for effective healthcare communication and decision-making." This concept is comparable to stating that a bookstore contains too many magazines about home repair and an insufficient number about fine literature. Both the interactive and the read-only sections of the forum require ongoing maintenance.

Maintaining the read-only sections requires that any item posted for reading by community participants have a "drop date" applied to it. On that date, the item is reviewed by forum staff to determine whether the item (1) requires an update or follow-up, (2) should be deleted, or (3) may be left posted as is. In any case, a new drop date is then applied to the item for future review.

Describing the maintenance of an interactive forum demands an example. Imagine an online area that supports the use of insulin pumps for diabetic patients. One part of the forum is a messaging area where people discuss how to use the pump. One member of the community posts a message in which he vociferously decries the fact that his medical insurer will not pay for an insulin pump; he goes on to call for legislation in his state such that this would not be the case in the future. Finally, he refers to his own insurer using an impolitic descriptive term.

Several people respond to the message by describing their own healthcare coverage. The message area, to which people come for discussion about insulin pumps, now provides discussion about healthcare coverage. The community will expect this to be fixed quickly. They will expect the provider of the site to set up another folder for discussion of healthcare coverage and to move the applicable messages to the new folder. Should the forum provider not attend to this matter expeditiously, the messaging area will quickly degrade and become minimally useful. Of note, when the producer moves the messages to a new message folder, the authors of the messages may become irate, accusing the producer of censorship before they realize their messages have simply been moved. This will be more likely to take place if the producer decides not to have any discussion on healthcare coverage and simply deletes the messages.

SEARCHING FOR INFORMATION

Searching through a beach's sands for sea glass is analogous to searching the online environment for a useful treasure. There is much to look through that is not germane to the area of interest. Even upon finding the information sought, its timeliness, its accuracy, and its relevance must be confirmed (Morrissey, 1998). There are several incompletely developed instruments to evaluate health information on the Internet. Their value is not believed to be high (Jadad & Gagliardi, 1998).

The availability of information regarding depressive disorders was previously explored. Consumers might conduct such a search by simply entering the term *depression* in a search engine such as Yahoo. They might also search for something more specific such as *St. John's Wort* or *psychiatry and depression.* The search engine used and the exact search phrase entered will both impact which sites are revealed to the consumer. During our perusal of the Web for information on the broad topic of depression, we noted that no fewer than five pharmaceutical companies, each manufacturing contemporary antidepressants, have extensive Web sites for the discussion of depressive disorder. A few of the sites mentioned generic names of competitive products, but each site focused on the trade name of the product manufactured by the company running the site. While in search of less biased educational sites, we found one that collects content on depression and combines it with a community area that includes both chat and message board capabilities. This site led us to a page set up by a private psychiatrist in New York. It instructed us as to how expert a psychopharmacologist is, based on a series of four questions. This page suggested that one's psychopharmacologist is less than expert if not occasionally combining monoamine oxidase inhibitors (MAOIs) with tricyclic antidepressants (TCAs), or using lamotrigine or gabapentin to treat depression. Links that advised on the use of Ginkgo biloba extract for antidepressant induced sexual dysfunction were quickly located.

Continuing our search for information about depression, we were led through a variety of links from a search engine to the InteliHealth site (http://www.intelihealth.com). At the time we searched, this area featured an article on depression written in the style of a news weekly's health column. The article's sidebar featured information allowing readers to determine their level of depression by checking through a symptom list. No advertising was present on the page with the article, but the remainder of the site had promotions for a variety of health-related books and products. A search of the site revealed several hundred articles covering the topic of depression, most of them rather brief and provided by Johns Hopkins to address specific issues. AOL's Depression Information Forum and Online Psych Forum both address topics of depression. Both areas provide quizzes to allow the consumer to determine whether professional help should be sought. Neither area has sponsorship from companies that might lead to editorial bias. One area is owned by AOL and is operated by an outside contractor (http://www.prozac.com). The other area is owned and operated by a partner of AOL.

During our search for depression-specific information, we found that almost all of the online areas allow the user to interact with either the developer of the forum or with a healthcare professional participating in programming within the area. AOL's two areas and InteliHealth each provide message boards, chat rooms, and other ways for participants to interact with one another and with the forum staff. Online staff members often speak to participants in a generic manner, referring them to their own clinician for psychiatric difficulties, but some staff members were willing to become more involved. All of the areas in which public message boards were present had occasional messages from participants in which suicide is threatened. There were often fearful responses to these messages posted by other participants. Staff members at AOL's Depression Forum often receive private e-mail from concerned members of the community about the potential suicidality of other members. The ramifications of this type of discourse have not been studied. Policies concerning action that staff members take in such instances vary but usually relate to the provision of helpful but generic emergency resources to which the anguished community member might refer.

DEMOGRAPHICS OF ONLINE HEALTH AREA PARTICIPANTS

During the development of Lifescape.com, the editorial staff discussed at great length the issues of expected audience demographics. As content was being written, graphics were being designed, and chat guests were being contacted, the staff kept in mind the expected number of consumers who would be using the site, as well as their demographic details. After the first week of launch, if it was determined that the actual demographics of visitors differed from the expected, new articles would be written, graphics redesigned, and different chat guests contacted. Such is the life of a Web editorial team. Demographic assessment, whether conducted on your own or using available online marketing companies, involves not only knowing the details of an area's audience, but the overall size of that audience. This is often difficult to assess. Nearly all the companies we contacted for the purposes of researching this chapter refused to share demographic information for public distribution. Some online areas depict a "counter" on their homepage. Unfortunately, they rarely indicate either what is being counted or the time period involved for the overall count. We do have information regarding several health-related areas of AOL. This information is presented to allow a general concept regarding the overall number of people who access a specific health information area. In considering these numbers, keep in mind the number of patient visits a single healthcare professional, a community health center, or a hospital emergency room might have per month.

Family members sometimes use a single online account. One individual often has several accounts, perhaps one at work and one for home use. Individual accounts on AOL can have up to five "screen-names," all of which might be used by a single person using each name for different purposes. People might visit a site, then browse other areas, then return to the initial location. Does this count as one visit or two? An individual might enter a site, then browse three additional pages within the site, then leave. This might be counted as four page views or one visit. Depending on how any one site measures visits or defines terminology, the demographic data may or may not be comparable to information from another online area.

In February 1999, Media Matrix indicated that the AOL Health Channel draws 2.1 million unique visitors to their forums each month. InteliHealth, they reported, draws 666,000 each month. DrKoop.com draws 255,000 per month. Cyber Dialogue reported in December 1998 that interest in health content is growing, that women tend to use these areas more than men, and that disease information, diet and nutrition information, and pharmaceutical information is of greatest concern (America Online, keyword "OLP").

Case Analysis of Two Popular Online Forums

Comparing online areas, even those that exist on the same proprietary service, is rife with difficulty. A specific online area may not be as easily found as others via conventional search engines. Promotional opportunities such as available links to one forum from another might be more readily available to certain areas that have formed strong rapport with other online areas. Even within AOL, some forums are featured on the Welcome screen and on Channel screens with greater frequency than other forums.

In the chart on page 128, we review the demographics for two forums within the AOL Health Channel. These two forums

were both launched within several months of one another several years prior to the dates of these demographic reports.

Forum/Date	Total Visits	Unique Visitors	Hours of Use
Addiction & Recovery/ Feb. 1999	348,140	61,920	29,122
Addiction & Recovery/ June 1999	377,820	85,240	30,318
Alternative Medicine/ Feb. 1999	401,300	114,280	18,805
Alternative Medicine/ June 1999	709,180	235,400	43,000

Within the Addiction and Recovery forum, almost 13,000 of
the total February hours were exclusively in the chat rooms,
which themselves were visited by one-sixth of the overall
number of users. It can be quickly observed that a small fraction
of users generate a large portion of the overall forum's hourly
use. This core group, if tracked, is seen to return to the forum on
a daily or near-daily basis.

Addiction and Recovery—Selected Demographic Data
- 85% male
- 80% married
- 50% have children in household
- 45% visit forum 5–6 days per week
- Majority use forum between 6 PM and midnight local time
- Majority are between the ages of 36 and 45
- Majority have at least a college education

Alternative Medicine Forum—Selected Demographic Data

- 83% male
- 80% married
- 54% have children in household
- 98% visit forum 1–2 days per week
- Majority use forum between 6 PM and 10 PM local time
- Majority are between the ages of 36 and 45
- Majority have at least a college education

If the likely incorrect assumption is made that both forums just reviewed have an equal promotional status and that all users of AOL are therefore equally aware of both forums, it is seen that the Alternative Medicine forum is more popular but the Addiction forum generates greater retention and increased attention. This is likely a direct result of the community interaction, which applies more to a forum designated to a specific illness than it does to a forum designated for a general topic. Again, this is mere speculation on my part. There is yet to be any significant research regarding this topic. Figures here are also likely to be significantly different than they would be for identical areas built on the Web because of differences in promotion, competition, and the demographic differences of the Web audience from the AOL audience. Of note, we see a large change in the audience size for the Alternative Medicine area within only 4 months. This may reflect the increasing level of interest in this field or a new form of promotion being used at AOL for this particular forum.

The AMA (http://www.ama-assn.org) revealed some demographics of their Web site (America Online, keyword "DIF") in their 1998 Annual Report. They noted that an average of 220,000 pages at the site are viewed each day. They estimate that each visitor views 10 pages per visit. At 22,000 visits per day, February would have brought 616,000 visits. The AMA estimates that they have a 50% repeat visitor rate, a low number compared with the AOL forums described, but not surprising because the AMA site focuses on information distribution rather than community building. One can tune an online information source to be "sticky," industry jargon, indicating that the site draws people back for additional visits after their first. Depending on the goals of the production, this may or may not be of interest.

TOPICS OF PRESENT IMPORT

As cable modems and digital subscriber line access become generally available, both physicians and patients will have the ability to receive complex audio and video via the Internet. This is comparable to the predecessor of this type of service, the AT&T PicturePhone shown at the 1964 World's Fair. With fast access becoming the norm, the world is becoming wired for immediate communications that will alter how and when we travel, who we speak with, and the breadth of our individual communities. Privacy and confidentiality, liability, and professional licensure issues are critically important in addressing scenarios that might arise within a high-speed communications system.

If a physician in Alabama uses a computer to talk with a patient located in Iowa, is the contact taking place in Alabama? Or is it in Iowa? Which laws apply? Which medical board has jurisdiction? Must the physician be licensed in both states or just one, and if so, which one? Under a federal licensure system, health professionals would be issued one license based on federally established standards. Perhaps administered at a state level, this system would ease the regulatory burden on clinicians (http://206.189.190.101/public/pai/ed6013x.htm). It would be similar to the federal licenses issued to aircraft pilots. Alternatively, the current system used for automobile drivers could be adopted for use by healthcare professionals. In this case, each state would offer reciprocity such that a license in a specific state allows performance of function within any state. Some states have enacted guidelines requiring out-of-state physicians to obtain full unrestricted licenses before consulting with patients in the state via electronic communications. At least one state, Mississippi, declares that out-of-state physicians do not require a state license to consult via telemedicine with state residents (http://206.189.190.101/public/pai/ed6013x.htm).

One wonders what state the patient is in if the patient is accessing electronic communications from the seatback phone available in an airborne commercial airliner.

A series of questions then arise. If an individual posts a question on a health information site and a doctor responds, has a relationship been formed? Does the doctor have a duty to that individual? Can the doctor bill for services rendered in this way? What liability issues are present? Must a chart be opened? Where would such a chart be kept? How is privacy maintained? Have patients been abandoned if an online healthcare forum closes without referring customers to other locations? Are clinic licenses required for online healthcare forums? What criteria would be used to inspect and certify online locations? Each of these questions is now being examined. It is rather distressing that it has taken the medical profession so long to recognize the need to develop standards, long after the marketplace raced ahead to quickly ease the ability of consumers to reach health-care professionals. Nevertheless, organized medicine is now willing to review these questions directly (*Psychiatric News,* 1999).

What about e-mail between a healthcare professional and patient? Is this a formal communication that must be saved just as one would append a certified letter into the patient's chart? Or is it an informal communication, comparable to a telephone call in which the professional would summarize important aspects of the communication in the medical record? Telephone calls are not recorded and appended to the chart, yet current American Medical Informatics Association (AMIA) e-mail guidelines (Kane & Sands, 1998) suggest that patient e-mails and physician responses should be kept as part of the record. Would this apply to messages posted to public message boards as well as personal e-mail?

Outside the range of topics for this chapter are issues of prescribing and pharmaceutical sales within an online environment. Here again, as technology becomes even more capable of emulating live contact between two individuals, the issue of technology will lessen. For now, however, consumers must be provided with safe healthcare professional contact without allowing excitement for accessibility to skew judgment as to what constitutes reasonable and safe provision of healthcare.

Any online health forum must consider each of these questions before launch, determine what policies they will apply to their area, and educate their employees and volunteers as to what these policies are. Consumers visiting an online health area should be informed as to these policies as well. It would be inappropriate, for example, for all personal e-mail to be permanently appended to a medical record opened for each visitor unless that visitor knew both that a record was being opened for them and that all their outgoing e-mail to forum staff was being kept within that record.

CONCLUSION

During the first half of the twentieth century, the world shrank through the use of transportation. The world moved from steam locomotive to car, airplane, and finally jet transportation. Since the mid-1960s, continued compression of the world took place via enhanced communications, which had changed little in the decades before. In 1965, for example, the black desk telephone was little changed from that which was present two generations earlier. Now, as the twentieth century ends, a 1960s car or jet goes no slower than the latest models but the rotary telephone has long been left behind. The distance between any two points on the planet, given the proper technology now readily available, is no longer germane. We can effectively "be" anywhere—anytime. A clinician who was once tied to his or her office can now see patients anywhere, perhaps from the comfort of a home office. While the public awaits the rather slow legal system to catch up to technology and for input from ethicists and medical organizations as to appropriate standards to be used, the consumers are turning to whomever is available to them using their newly discovered empowerment. Healthcare providers and professionals must strive to push forward in as rapid a manner as possible to provide quality healthcare services within the constraints of the online communications environment, a communication technology growing more rapidly than any which came before it.

REFERENCES

A benchmark study on physicians' use of the World Wide Web. American Medical Association, 1998.

America Online, Keyword "DIF."

America Online, Keyword "OLP."

George J. Providing health info means healthy returns. *Philadelphia Business Journal*, February, 5, 1999.

Green H. A Cyber revolt in health care. *Business Week,* October 19, 1998.

http://206.189.190.101/public/pai/ed6013x.htm

http://hotel.cprost.sfu.ca/eworld/

http://hotel.cprost.sfu.ca/eworld/index3.html

http://macworld.zdnet.com/daily/daily.15.html

http://ng.netgate.net/~bobber/eworld.html

http://www.ama-assn.org

http://www.ama-assn.org/sci-pubs/journals/archive/jama/vol_277/no_15/ed7016x.htm

http://www.axon.net.au/eworld/

http://www.celexa.com

http://www.intelihealth.com

http://www.priory.com/pharmol/gingko.htm

http://www.prozac.com

http://www.psycom.net/depression.central.expert.html

http://www.remeron.com

Jadad AR, Gagliardi A. Rating health information on the internet, *JAMA* 1998; 279(8):611–614.

Kane B, Sands DZ. Guidelines for the clinical use of electronic mail with patients. *J Am Med Informatics Assn* 1998; 5(1):104–111.

Media Matrix. The Industry Standard, April 5, 1999, p. 38.

Morrissey J. Medical facts online. *Modern Healthcare*, March 2, 1998.

New York Times. For sale: on-line bookstore's recommendations. February 8, 1999; p. A1.

Psychiatric issues figure prominently at AMA House of Delegates meeting. *Psychiatric News,* July 16, 1999.

Raths D. Working the Web: inside the online consumer health boom. *Healthcare Business*, October–November, 1998.

Telemedicine Report to the Congress, US Department of Commerce, January 31, 1997.

6

C H A P T E R

Relationship-Based Care: Strengthening the Patient–Physician Relationship

Mike Magee, M.D.

INTRODUCTION

It takes about as long to develop a new doctor as it does a new discovery—approximately 10 to 15 years. For the physician, the dream can begin in the junior year of high school as a young woman discusses the idea with family and friends. At about the same time, we are screening millions of compounds to come up with some 5,000 promising new chemical entities worthy of further investment and exploration. As the years progress, the doctor-to-be becomes a mature woman, focuses on her undergraduate studies, takes the MCATs, is accepted to medical school, spends 4 years studying and learning and passing boards, and chooses a specialty and residency. During those same years, most of the 5,000 possibilities drift away for lack of specificity or unacceptable toxicity, leaving few to survive Phase I, II, and III clinical FDA studies. At the end of the day, and some $500 million later, only 1 of the 5,000 survives.

The night before that single survivor is approved by the FDA, our doctor completes her residency. The following morning, she writes her first independent prescription for the new discovery and the two collide. At that point, whether the discovery ever reaches its full potential to benefit mankind has little to do with the company that birthed it, and everything to do with that doctor, her patients, their relationship, and the health system within which they are engaged. So whether one is a medical educator attempting to create physicians for the future rather than the past, or a pharmaceutical company attempting to realize a new discovery's full potential, a thorough understanding of the dynamic patient–physician relationship is essential.

A HISTORICAL PERSPECTIVE

The patient–physician relationship is at once constant and dynamic. Nearly a decade and a half ago, I described this interaction as a "covenant of caring—one individual with a need and the willingness to trust and another with knowledge and the desire to respond" (Magee, 1997). The AMA has called it a moral enterprise grounded in a "covenant of trust" (American Medical Association, 1995). Yet at the same time, this relationship must accommodate changing needs, perceptions, and expectations. Today, the patient–physician relationship is as much involved with advanced technology, innovative medical treatments, and high-tech diagnostic tools as it is the delicate interaction of two human beings.

Over thousands of years, this relationship has been known to involve varying blends of science and humanity, a complex interaction with many facets. John D. Stoeckle, M.D., Professor of Medicine, Emeritus, Harvard Medical School, said, "the communicative, educational, persuasive, supportive, and caring behaviors of the physician are central to the provision of care. The relationship is a partnership based on the care of the patient. It is care that technology, by its nature, cannot provide" (*Pfizer Journal,* 1998a). Lewis Thomas (1984) remembered it this way: "The close up, reassuring, warm touch of the physician, the comfort and concern, the long leisurely discussions in which everything including the dog can be worked into the conversation. . . . It has roots that go back to the beginnings of medicine's history."

This relationship has transcended time; place; and ethnic, social, and political origin; but changed it has and change it must as a human living entity (Kirsner, 1992). The explosion of science and technology, appearance of a health consumer movement, issues of financing, emergence of the Internet, and globalization of healthcare are simply a few of the modern forces at work. Yet faced with such change, there is evidence of a coalescence of physicians, patients, and legislators around a desire to preserve and enhance relationship-based care. Yank D. Coble, Jr., M.D., Trustee, AMA, recently noted, "physicians are returning their attention to the fundamentals—our patient-based ethical traditions, our caring tradition and our science tradition. The strength of this (patient–physician) relationship is fundamental and critical to all future healthcare reform" (*Pfizer Journal,* 1998a).

THE HUMAN ELEMENT OF CARING

Although science and technology are clearly identified by the American public as a source of American medicine's success, they are secondary when it comes to defining the modern patient–physician relationship (Magee & Dole, 1998). In a study conducted by Yankelovich Associates in 1998 of 1,600 patients and 400 physicians nationwide, there was consensus on this issue among physicians and patients. More than 96% of physicians and patients surveyed defined today's patient–physician relationship as three things: (1) compassion, (2) understanding, and (3) partnership. What is involved in consummating such a human partnership? When one considers that two very different human beings are uniting in the midst of an array of sensitive issues, the simple answer is "quite a lot." Stanley J. Reiser, M.D., Ph.D., Griff T. Ross Professor of Humanities and Technology in Health Care at the University of Texas Health Science Center, said, "There are many ethical issues that bear upon the patient–physician relationship but the central one is trust. The essential decision every patient makes is to put his/her life in the hands of a stranger and allow that stranger or multiple strangers to do things no one else is allowed to do. . . . The coin that allows trust to happen is the view that the physician will treat me according to my interests and not according to the physicians' interests" (*Pfizer Journal,* 1998a). It is clear as well that no two doctors or patients are interchangeable (Cassel, 1982). Different personalities, cultures, finances, dreams, fears, and responsibilities are a reality. Thus, overcoming the gap— whether ethnic, cultural, economic, or social—and overcoming it quickly is a necessity. This is facilitated through the initial and ensuing encounters that, in full, constitute the "covenant of trust."

INGREDIENTS OF THE PATIENT–PHYSICIAN ENCOUNTER

The result of a successful encounter would be defined by sociologists as the accumulation of social capital, that being the value that accrues between two individuals who share a relationship marked by commitment, trust, and a willingness to give at a higher level (Putnam, 1995). How important is this relationship to society overall? A recent study suggests more important than we give it credit (Omnibus Study, 1999). In fact, second only to family relationships, the patient–physician relationship is viewed as extremely or very important by 67% of those surveyed, exceeding relationships with spiritual advisors (52%), pharmacists (45%), co-workers (44%), and financial advisors (36%) (Omnibus Study, 1999). Efficient and useful patient–physician relationships, as with other societal relationships such as marriage and employee relations, evolve and expand over time as the parties gain and apply their knowledge of each other. Thus, healthcare systems that constantly rechannel patients to new physicians inadvertently relinquish valuable imbedded social capital and ensure a less efficient and more cumbersome form of care. Once a relationship is established, everything possible should be done to preserve it.

Although the relationship is central to societal well-being, the dance remains a delicate one. According to Stanley Reiser M.D., Ph.D., "Actions are taken when there is consensus. Two independent judgements have to be made, but the suggestion for action usually comes from the professional. The patient or the patient's surrogate must agree that this intervention is one they accept. As we become more sophisticated and educated as a society, I think we can be optimistic that these relational changes will evolve into beneficial changes in the partnership" (*Pfizer Journal,* 1998a).

Accomplishing this anticipated goal requires a rethinking of the standard equation for healthcare value: $Q/C = V$. Where Q represents measurable quality as reflected in outcomes measurement and captured proactively in clinical protocols; C represents cost as reflected in financial and human capital; and V represents value. This equation has been a guidepost for health policy theorists and practitioners for well over a decade. Yet despite the progress in measurable quality and success in managing cost, the end product today lacks strong public support. Why? Perhaps the answer may be found in the definition of this relationship. The patient–physician relationship = compassion + understanding + partnership. Each of these elements requires active participation of both parties with (at a minimum) focused bidirectional communication, touch, and education.

It is not that the original elements in the value equation were either inaccurate or unimportant. To the contrary, they require renewed attention and study, which is impossible without public support. Rather, the problem with the original equation is what is left out: human participation of both parties, which is time dependent and vulnerable to compromise by bureaucracy, complex processes, and inadequate preparation or education of the participants. A more accurate equation for healthcare value would therefore become the following: $Q/C + P = V$, where P represents participation by both physician and patient. Implicit in this approach is that enlightened health policy experts and health managers, doctors, and patients consider equally the impact of their proposals, actions, and directives, on all three elements of this equation and their interplay with each other. Such a reasoned approach might ensure that our efforts in reform will actually create approaches that are ultimately viewed by the public as valuable and worthy of support.

Participation is at the heart of human caring. But is there equality? The Yankelovich study clearly indicated that we are headed in the right direction. Keep in mind that when I began practice in 1978, most physicians (including myself) believed that the best patient was the one who said "whatever you say, doc. You're the boss." The health consumer movement was not yet on the radar screen. Now, a short two decades later, the study revealed quite a different reality, with more than 90% of physicians defining the best patient as an educated patient. Both doctors (77%) and patients (44%) identified a mutual 50/50 partnership as the dominant form of patient–physician relationship today, and more than 95% of healthcare providers and patients recognized the mutual partnership as the ideal relationship (Magee & Dole, 1998). Both parties saw paternalistic authoritarian care as a minority approach, with physicians recognizing its presence at lower rates (8%) than did patients (17%). Still, when doctors and patients were asked to predict what the near future would hold, only 4% (the margin of error in this study) of doctors and patients saw the existence of paternalistic care as an option for the future. Rather, some 95% envisioned mutual partnerships and mutual *team* partnerships orchestrating smoothly oiled clinical and educational community-based teams, with the physician at the helm, advancing harmonious and collaborative continuums as the preferred new reality (Magee & Dole, 1998). Mutual partnership implies a 50/50 partnership between patient and physician, with shared decision making. Mutual team partnership maintains patient–physician equality but also presumes the development and effective physician management of both clinical and educational continuums.

WHO IS IN CHARGE?

As the patient–physician relationship evolves toward mutual partnerships and mutual team partnerships, the question of who is in charge becomes central. Recent studies indicated that if one or the other is forced to take the lead, 89% of doctors and 90% of patients say that the patient has the ultimate responsibility for himself or herself (Magee & Dole, 1998). Similarly, it is clear that although the patient is increasingly comfortable with the concept of mutual team partnership that spans both clinical care and health educational objectives, the physician is expected to manage the clinical continuum and oversee the educational team's products and research to ensure their accuracy and relevance (Magee & Dole, 1998).

THE NECESSITY OF EDUCATIONAL TEAM CONTINUUMS

Clear evidence exists that patients' expectations are rising for this relationship, which they believe can and should deliver clinical care as well as educational support for informed disease prevention and health economic decision making (Magee & Dole, 1998). To accomplish these goals, the physician must embrace and coordinate all of the available human resources. These resources include not only traditionally skilled personnel, such as medical specialists, nurse practitioners, physician assistants, and pharmacists, but an array of engaged community-based citizens, such as medical librarians, elder care specialists, Alzheimer Day Centers, hospice, visiting nurse associations, voluntary health associations, hospital business departments, Internet Web site managers, and more. Just as physicians have developed comfort and expertise in constructing teams of specialists that are accessible and responsive, so now they must also construct personal educational team continuums. For example, the physician treating a patient with diabetes should have a reliable team continuum to support diabetes general education, nutritional counseling, instruction in self-treatment, self-help groups for emotional support, ongoing consumer research, and financial planning. Without such well-planned and integrated resources, it is likely that the physician's limited time for engagement in relationship building will continue to be compromised and that the patient's legitimate expectations for physician leadership will not be met.

ARE *YOU* MY DOCTOR?

In the clinical arena, most patients now interface with multiple physicians simultaneously, unlike in the past. For the patient, discerning just who is his or her physician can be a knotty problem when dealing with primary versus specialty, teacher versus student—ever the case today. In some ways, we are in the process of completing an evolutionary loop, defined by Stanley Reiser: "One can explain the development of 20th Century Medicine by focusing on the central issue: how can the generalist who dominated medicine until about 1910 be recreated as a group of people" (*Pfizer Journal,* 1998a).

Mutual Role Identification: Setting the Context

If physician identity is clear, the amount of responsibility a specific patient is willing to assume often varies. Some physicians recommend a direct approach, asking the patient how much autonomy he or she prefers. One cancer survivor and healthcare manager recently noted, "As a patient this is a delicate balance between how empowered I want to be and how much I want the physician to be in charge. As a cancer survivor, I have learned there is no magic right answer about a particular treatment regimen. Even though I want the final decision left with me, it is often confusing and difficult to make the right decision because of different, often conflicting, advice from physicians" (*Pfizer Journal,* 1998a).

In the process of searching for the proper role balance and an instructive analogy, some are looking backwards as well as forward. Dr. Jing-Bao Nie, an expert on Eastern and Western Medicine, likens today's physicians as both "kings of old" and generals, the imperative being to strike a balance among the complementary virtues of the two. He states, ". . . Wisdom, sincerity, humanity, courage and strictness constitute the five cardinal virtues of the general. In the Chinese analogy of the physician as general, patients do not relate to the doctor as a soldier but rather as a king. The general is chosen to coordinate the forces against disease. The good healer—like the good general—must know the limitations of the art, remain alert to constant changes, cultivate virtues, and fight with humility. Being a general—just as being a physician—is not easy; it requires great wisdom. As the good general sometimes needs to act independent of the opinions of the king, a good king—as a good patient—sometimes accepts the knowledge and the wisdom of the general acknowledging experience in battle" (*Pfizer Journal,* 1998a).

A second area of concern for the physician is the loss of intimacy and commitment in the name of autonomy. Physicians who descend to the role of dispassionate advisor and patients who seek "just the facts" without availing themselves of the physician's experience or wise counsel, in essence accept a partial service, product, or relationship. In effect, they have accepted a virtual relationship, one that could be easily replicated on the Internet, absent touch, warmth, full individualization, and targeted interchange leading to consensus. The challenge then is not so much who is in charge, but rather, how will we communicate with each other in a modern day world?

COMMUNICATION: THE CORNERSTONE OF PARTNERSHIP

Compassion, understanding, and partnership—the cornerstones of the patient–physician relationship—each require communication. Traditionally, face-to-face encounters between an individual physician and patient have dominated. Increasingly, information is being front-loaded before the office visit. This is as much the result of changes in information technology as it is a rethinking of health philosophy and the increasing pace of modern society. Key health information sources used by patients include books (72%), family and friends (69%), television (60%), and the Internet (18% and rising). But when asked where they turn to ensure that the information they have received is accurate, 89% turn to their physicians (Magee & Dole, 1998).

If health information is flowing outside the physician's office, is health treatment (i.e., "self-care") as well? The growth in self-treatment, homeopathy, and Internet prescribing based on cursory health questionnaires and prescriptions by invisible doctors with fulfillment by invisible pharmacists would suggest it is. Although such an approach may save time and even money short term, it short circuits the systems that allow comprehensive patient histories, physical examinations, accurate diagnostics, and compliant treatment, let alone the establishment of a fully committed relationship, marked by compassion, understanding, and trust. For communication to continue to prevail, physicians and their clinical and educational partners will need to focus on the creation of environments and experiences that are highly individualized, time-efficient, information-rich, courteous, compassionate, and enduring, and patients will need to recognize the value of these human encounters. In short, people will invest the time and energy in a relationship only if it is worth it.

THE MEDICAL INTERVIEW: THE KEY ENTRY EXPERIENCE

Medical educators have increasingly focused on the medical interview as the key entry experience. There are 734.5 million visits in the United States each year, or 2.8 visits for every man, woman, and child in the country (Woodwell, 1997). Of the U.S. population, 75% visit a doctor in any given year and 90% do so in any given 3-year period (Lipkin, 1996). The patient history is part of a ritual of words and touch, including "probing, palpating, penetrating and percussing, which is a systematic, reassuring, and comforting encounter that meets a human need for personal attention to the body" (Nie, 1996; Stoeckle, 1987). The medical history is seen as the time to elicit individualized histories, social demographics, and personal concerns, while at the same time establishing trust and educating the patient about health and disease processes, all within a compressed time framework (Lipkin, Quill, & Napodano, 1984). Mack Lipkin, Jr., M.D., Founding President of the American Academy on the Physician and Patient, notes that "each patient–doctor relationship is individualized and unique but many patients fall into groups about which some general information is available to help the physician communicate" (*Pfizer Journal,* 1998a). Studies show that 25% of the time, physicians are dissatisfied with their own ability to communicate with patients (Pendleton, Brouwer, & Jaspers, 1983). Yet interviewing is integral to a physician's life and professional success. Considering the fact that a 40-year career as an oncologist will include some 200,000 medical interviews (Fallowfeld, 1995), one can appreciate why medical educators are increasingly focusing on this skill in the medical curriculum (Stoeckle, 1987).

Studies have shown that a variety of medical interviewing communication patterns can be distinguished (Roter et al., 1997), including the following:

- Biomedical, in which the visit does not extend beyond medical issues (32% of the total), or expanded biomedical, in which most issues are medical (33%). For example, "I think I have strep throat and I need a prescription."
- Biopsychosocial, in which the visit deals with both medical and personal issues (22% of visits). For example, "This is my fourth strep throat this year, and I cannot miss any more time at work."
- Psychosocial, in which it focuses on personal issues, with very little medical discussion (8%). For example,

"I need to see you because I am really worried about all the changes going on in my life."
- Consumerist, in which all topics discussed are introduced by the patient (8%). For example, "I found this on the Internet, and I want you to tell me if it might work for me."

Surprisingly, the aforementioned research indicated that physicians preferred consumerist-style visits, perhaps because the physician burden was less with the patient in charge (Roter et al., 1997). This is consistent with our research, which indicated that more than 90% of physicians agree that the "best patient" is an "educated patient" (Magee & Dole, 1998).

Increasingly, medical schools are providing students earlier access to perhaps the most important medical school communications education resource—the patient. Real-life encounters are now supported with a rich array of educational techniques, from interactive CD-ROMs to "professional patients" able to accurately role-play patients with a wide range of disease processes. All of this curricular growth simply reflects an emerging reality: patients are increasingly driving the evolution of the American healthcare system, expressing themselves, providing active feedback, and raising the expectations. The health consumer movement has brought a change in the status quo in medicine.

BARRIERS TO COMMUNICATION

Beyond these skills and individual encounters, America, in its diversity, has created a challenging environment for communication. Physicians in the United States encounter more than 120 different languages among their patients. Dr. Lipkin notes that "The diversity of language is becoming an important challenge to patient–physician relationships in this country—to have an effective relationship, you have to communicate deeply felt emotions. Dealing with a patient who has a different language changes the complexity" (*Pfizer Journal*, 1998a). Translations may be inaccurate or incomplete, and they sometimes impede free communication. Furthermore, racial, ethnic, social, and economic barriers are common and variably appreciated by physicians and patients alike. Our desire to unite physicians and patients with common life experiences and cultures remains particularly challenging for health educators and medical school admissions departments. In addition, geriatric patients, patients with chronic diseases, and patients with mental health disorders offer special communication challenges that are attracting interest and educational initiatives.

The Crisis in Health Literacy

One final area that is just beginning to attract the attention it deserves is health literacy. The 1993 National Adult Literacy Survey estimated that more than 40 million people in the United States could not read instructions on a prescription label, notes from a teacher, or directions on a map. An additional 50 million Americans are marginally literate (Kirsh et al., 1993). Nearly 9% of patients receiving Medicaid cannot read at all, and the mean reading level for Medicaid participants is grade 5.6 (Weiss et al., 1994). A 1995 health literacy study of 265 adults in Los Angeles and Atlanta set off additional alarm bells (Williams et al., 1995). Many patients were unable to understand directions for taking medications on an empty stomach. Of the patients, 26% could not interpret their own next appointment slip. More than a third of the Spanish-speaking patients could not understand instructions for x-rays written in Spanish on a fourth grade level. The experts concluded that the status of health literacy in America is "staggering" (Parker, 1997) and "a recipe for disaster" (Baker, 1997).

Finally, what makes the issue of health literacy such a barrier to patient–physician communications is the fact that most physicians are unaware of their patients' illiteracy because many patients have managed elaborate schemes to avoid detection of their illiteracy. In fact, there are well-documented cases where illiteracy has been effectively hidden from a spouse. The good news is that the issue of health literacy has come out of the closet and is beginning to attract early intervention and the attention of researchers (Parker et al., 1996), industry (*Pfizer Journal,* 1998b), government (US Department of Education,

1997), and medical organizations (American Academy of Pediatrics, 1997).

ACCESS: A TWO-WAY STREET

It is impossible to have a strong relationship without bidirectional access. This is as true for the patient–physician relationship as it is for a relationship with a spouse, spiritual advisor, financial consultant, or co-worker. It has been seen in the last decade how low a tolerance both physicians and patients have for systems that impede live encounters. Whether it be recorded telephone access trees, health insurance forms, prior approval programs, physician disappearance from approved provider panels, or busy understaffed medical offices, the inability to consummate the relationship generates militancy on the part of those who deliver and those who receive care. Thus, the foundation of the current patient rights movement, which has effectively linked patients, physicians, and legislators, has been access and is the culmination of the first wave of development of the health consumer movement.

What these constituencies have begun to realize, as we enter the second wave of the relationship-based care movement, is that accomplishing physical access to each other can be a hollow victory. This is because ensuring face-to-face patient–physician encounters on a schedule that both parties agree is responsive and independent of perceived or real third-party interference means very little, save for the availability of modern diagnostics and therapeutics. Such a state simply reproduces 1950s medicine and forces the relationship to exist inside a medical demilitarized zone absent modern weapons to fight disease. For the relationship-based care movement to be meaningful in terms of positive impact on the relationship, patients and physicians must not only access each other but access the full range of modern science and technology.

Studies have shown that America's physicians and patients have taken such access for granted (Magee & Dole, 1998). Both groups see science and technology as the primary determinant of success of American medicine over the past two decades. Although they identify their relationship as compassion, understanding, and partnership, they identify the healthcare product as all of the above, plus quick and effective diagnosis, and counseling on how to accomplish payment. Access must be informed and responsible, but it must also be complete. Clearly, the health insurers primary concern, in light of extreme competition to protect market shares annually, employer pressures, limited ability to perform accurate and timely cost/benefit analysis, continued reliance on component rather than disease management, and a major assault seemingly from all political corners is to survive rather than evolve.

The reality, however, is immutable. First, patients and physicians highly value their relationship with each other, second only to marriage (Omnibus Study, 1999). Second, the emergence of the health consumer movement and the presence and growth of the Internet over the past two decades have elevated and firmed up patient expectations. Third, individual patients and their organizations are increasingly organized and have tasted success in their political alignment with physicians and legislators. Fourth, there will be more discoveries of greater scientific significance in the next 10 years than in the past 100 (*Pfizer Journal,* 1997). Fifth, and most important, there is clear and growing evidence that accessing and leveraging these new discoveries to their full benefit would have a transforming effect on our healthcare system, moving us from intervention to prevention and wellness (BHARC, 1991).

EARLIER ACCESS: PREVENTION

By virtue of a new discovery's ability to transmit hope, it encourages an individual to explore what is possible and to enter the healthcare system earlier in a disease state than would otherwise be the case. A good example worth noting is the discovery of Viagra (sildenafil) for erectile dysfunction. The presence of a simple, safe, and effective pill for this condition moved the percentage of men with the condition seeking treatment in the United States from approximately 7% to 13% (Pfizer Inc., 1999). Most of those additional men seeking treatment were age 40 to 70, a group traditionally resistant to use the healthcare system. The Massachusetts Male Aging study demonstrated that a standard office visit of 1 million men in this population would uncover 30,000 cases of untreated diabetes; 50,000 cases of untreated heart disease; and 140,000 cases of untreated hypertension (Feldman et al., 1994). Thus, the presence of a simple treatment that engendered hope and eliminated the fear of needles and clumsy contraptions was a sufficient magnet to do exactly what managed care had early envisioned—move us away (in the case of diabetes-induced erectile dysfunction) from costly emergency visits (devascularized limbs), surgical procedures (amputations), and hospitalizations (hyperosmolar coma) to prevention (diagnosis of diabetes by blood glucose) in the course of a standard workup for erectile dysfunction in a patient seeking Viagra.

HEALTH INSURANCE: WHO WILL PAY, WHY THE RELUCTANCE TO PAY, AND HOW ACCESS IS AFFECTED

If access to new discoveries is supportive of the patient–physician relationship and consistent with the ultimate goals of enlightened health policy, why then was there such resistance to insurance coverage? The case of Viagra points to several explanations. The first is the presence of faulty cost analysis, leading to wildly exaggerated cost estimates. For example, estimates of annual cost for covering Viagra to Kaiser (150 million) (California Department of Corporations, 1998), State Medicaid (100 million) (Associated Press Release, 1998), and the Veteran's Administration (235 million) (US Department of Veterans Affairs, 1998) have proven to be at least 10-fold inaccurate (Pfizer Inc., 1999c, 1999d). How was this possible? Analytic mistakes included presuming 100% of men with erectile dysfunction would seek treatment (rather than 13%), failing to exclude men younger than 20 (25%), failing to exclude men taking nitrates or those choosing other treatments (15%), failing to exclude men for whom Viagra is ineffective (30%), and overestimating unit cost (up to 30%) and monthly use (up to 50%). The net effect of these analytic mistakes was to limit the insurers' options.

Health industry leaders had no choice but to assume that the financial impact would be catastrophic. As a result, they left themselves no choice but to negatively impact on access, continue to cover more expensive and invasive treatments they had already approved for the disease, and exclude themselves from the financial benefit of early diagnosis and treatment of underlying conditions. This latter impact was especially felt in state Medicaid programs, which cover disproportionate numbers of African-Americans, who carry a higher disease burden of erectile dysfunction's underlying conditions, including diabetes, hypertension, heart disease, and carcinoma of the prostate.

Interestingly, with public outcry and a refocus on the numbers, as well as a validating look at actual prescription experience, strongly held public positions against coverage of Viagra by Kaiser and by 35 of the 50 state Medicaid programs were quietly reversed (California Department of Corporations, 1998b; Pfizer Inc., 1999b). But the reality is that two forces remain that will likely continue to encourage knee-jerk restrictions on access. The first is a continued reliance on component management, which seeks to manage healthcare costs by line item and is measurable in annual budget terms, versus disease management, whose savings play out in years. The second is bureaucratic structures that often silo elements of the health economic continuum from each other, such as pharmaceutical expenditures, emergency visits, hospitalization, surgery, rehabilitation, and long-term care. This not only makes it difficult to identify and connect expenditures in one component with savings in another, but also prevents effective organizational reengineering and workforce transformation that could deliver improvements in measurable quality, cost, and face-to-face participation.

The reality is that access will continue to be the leading edge of the growing relationship-based healthcare movement. Battles will likely be fought one case at a time, with access to a new transforming discovery uniting those doctors, patients, and legislators, with the discoverers most intimately involved. Careful analysis will increasingly become indisputable, and market forces will eventually align with ethical ones in support of a fully armed patient–physician relationship.

THE CONTRACT: MUTUAL RESPONSIBILITIES

In 1997, the AMA declared that "The creation of the physician–patient relationship is contractual in nature" (*Code of Medical Ethics*, 1997). Recently, there has been heavy emphasis on physician responsibilities and patient rights (Eraker, Kirscht, & Becker, 1984). However, in light of the movement toward mutual partnerships, it is essential that we recognize that although patients have rights, they also have responsibilities in a fully consummated relationship (*Pfizer Journal*, 1998a). In 1998, as part of the Pfizer Medical Humanities Initiative, a group of medical and health consumer experts on the patient–physician relationship were convened in Boston, Massachusetts, and asked to identify the responsibilities of patients and physicians in light of their rapidly evolving relationship. Their conclusions follow:

For the patient:

1. *Be truthful.* Do not hide facts or exaggerate symptoms. The relationship is based on the free flow of confidentially held sensitive information. Inaccuracy threatens your health and the relationship. Respect the confidentiality of your communications with your doctor.

2. *Give the relationship time.* As with all complex human encounters, this relationship needs time to mature and develop. Get to know each other. Be open to a partnership in decision making.

3. *Take responsibility for learning.* Your body is complex. Commit to understanding how it functions and how to keep it healthy.

4. *Take responsibility for your health.* Know thyself means more than just knowing what diseases you have and what medications you are taking. It also means having a well-defined health philosophy for you and your family. They are partners in this relationship as well.

5. *Raise issues of concern.* Hidden issues, left unsurfaced, will ultimately compromise even a stellar relationship. If something is bothering you—the doctor is rushing, the staff is rude, the room is cold, whatever—speak up.

For the physician:

1. *Act with the highest professional competency.* Trust requires a high level of physician competency and the

ability to culturally connect and communicate clearly one-on-one.

2. *Master the skills of communication.* Part of creating a good match is the ability to communicate complex science in layman's terms and in a neighborly way. Help patients understand and absorb medical developments. Always honor confidentiality.

3. *Allow patients to share ideas and help formulate priorities.* In an environment where time is a limited commodity, priority setting needs to be collaborative and ideas that are urgent to the patient must be permitted to surface.

4. *Acknowledge the fullness of your patient.* Wellness and illness are highly individualistic. They must be interpreted within the context of family, job, finances, and mental and spiritual health.

5. *Respect your fellow professionals.* Patients expect their doctors to work well with each other and with other caregivers. Turf battles are a nightmare for the patient. Open disagreement and rude interprofessional behavior cause patients to question their physician's credibility and capability.

SELECTING AND TRAINING BALANCED HEALTHCARE PROVIDERS

One cannot cure with great curriculum what has been created with poor selection. If the wrong people are selected for a career in medicine, their personality defects are most often lasting. Certain people have dispositions uniquely suited for human interaction; they are capable of being mentors and caregivers to their patients. This has been recognized for some time. Tinsley Harrison, M.D., one the fathers of Internal Medicine, said, "the misanthrope may become a smart diagnostician of organic diseases but he can scarcely hope to succeed as a physician. The true physician has a Shakespearean breadth of interest in the wise and the foolish, the proud and the humble. The stoic hero and the whining rogue. He cares for people" (Fauci et al., 1998).

This quote is displayed under the bust of Dr. Harrison at the University of Alabama School of Medicine in Birmingham. Not two blocks away is another statue of a beloved Methodist minister, Brother Bryan, a man of great local fame. It was constructed in 1934, well before he died, to express the town's love and respect for his caring contributions. The words on this statue read:

Fervent in Prayer
Consecrated in Life
Sympathetic in Counsel
Friend of the Friendless, the Sorrowful, the Poor, and the Rich
He went about doing good.

The striking compatibility of these two messages highlights that although scientific acumen is certainly expected, even presumed in our selection and training processes, it is the caring capacity that is the critical determinant of success. One approach to creating balanced physicians then would be to work on the front end of the continuum to encourage more students with humanistic strengths to envision medicine as a career path. The Pfizer Medical Humanities Initiative has established a Web site, http://www.positiveprofiles.com, to address this objective. The site includes hot links to all 143 U.S. medical schools, a collection of real-life physician role models, inspirational patient care stories, and advice on applying to medical school. In addition, the Initiative maintains close working relationships with the Association of American Medical Colleges, Alpha Epsilon Delta, the pre-med honor society, and pre-med advisers nationwide.

A reexamination is under way of both cognitive and noncognitive factors in medical school selection (Wear, 1997). It is possible to identify those noncognitive traits that define role model physicians (Hojat et al., 1999; Magee & Hojat, 1998). Some of these personality traits include conscientiousness, achievement, striving, activity, competence, dutifulness, trust, assertiveness, and altruism. Whether similar instruments that are practical in the selection process can be constructed remains to be seen. What appears intuitive is that careful selection of Admission Committee members to ensure high humanistic content makes selection of balanced medical students more likely. This is the result of the natural tendency for individuals to select others in their own image. Equally clear is that diversity of all types on the committee and in the entry pool fosters a broad and balanced medical education through exposure to varied cultures and experiences.

Presuming that the right individuals, women and men who possess a balance of science and humanity, are selected, they still face a daunting and often dehumanizing environment. Competitive pressures, personal stress, dislocation from family and friends, fatigue, and exposure to needy and dying people are realities. Some medical students describe the experience as entering a tunnel only to surface many years later scientifically equipped but with a narrower and less carefree view of the world. To counteract this dehumanizing tunnel effect, a number of strategies are being attempted:

1. *Curricular changes:* A wide variety of new experiences stressing appreciation for the social, environmental, and ethical context of caring have been instituted in U.S. medical schools. These take a patient-centered approach and present the patient within the context of family, community, and societal forces.

2. *Community service:* Various strategies to expand community service opportunities have been instituted, the idea being that exposure to other human beings in need and the capacity to respond will have a humanizing effect. Many of these programs have been the brain children of faculty. With the belief that medical students are fully formed adults who are solely responsible for maintaining their own sense of humanity, the Pfizer Medical Humanities Initiative has established a Medical Student Community Ventures Fund. Managed by the American Association of Medical Colleges (AAMC), the Fund provides seed grants to medical student–conceived and medical student–driven community service activities.

3. *Mission identification:* There has been a renewed focus on professional ethics and the physician's oath of service beginning the first day of medical school. The

Arnold P. Gold Foundation initiated the practice of a White Coat Ceremony in 1993. The popularity of the Ceremony is evident; in 1998, 85% of medical schools held one (The Arnold P. Gold Foundation, 1999). In these ceremonies, first-year students receive their white coats in a formal ceremony in front of family and friends, recite the Hippocratic Oath, and listen to an address on Medical Humanism from a faculty role model. The theme of one's ethical responsibilities is now interwoven in many schools' 4-year curricula reinforcing the Oath along the way.

4. *Role modeling:* Increasing emphasis is being placed on identifying and promoting humanistic role models in the faculty. These are human "best-in-class" embodiments of the desired result or product of medical education. The feeling is that if students can "see it, feel it, and touch it," they will more likely replicate it. A secondary benefit of this approach is to focus on an institution's values. To identify one's "heroes" requires that one define the characteristics he or she seeks in an individual and explore the obstacles he or she has overcome in accomplishing these goals. Thus, role modeling requires defining the meaning of success. Once again, placed in the hands of students, this can be a powerful tool. The Pfizer Medical Humanities Initiative has established the AAMC Medical Humanism Award. Each year, the AAMC's Organization of Student Representatives selects a single faculty member nationwide who best embodies the following qualities: positive mentoring skills, compassion, collaboration, tolerance, sensitivity, community service, and professional ethics (AAMC, 1999). In addition, national search programs in 1996 and 1999 have yielded two published collections of American physicians worthy of American Medicine's high ideals (Magee, 1996; Magee & D'Antonio, 1999).

5. *Individualized clinical training:* Considerable progress has been made in teaching medical interviews and

reinforcing interpersonal skills in medical school (Novach et al., 1993). Courses use role-playing, videotape feedback, and professional patients. The goal of these experiences is to understand one patient and his or her story at a time. The story is the entry point, the beginning of the relationship, and has a humanizing power all its own. Increasingly, medical students are exposed to patients early in their first year. This has had the effect of returning teaching to the bedside. Students, who are exposed to faculty in action and to patients with the full array of human emotions, can learn to simultaneously motivate, educate, counsel, and support (Kroenke et al., 1997).

Expectations have been raised for faculty as well. They are the relationship builders for students and need to treat the students as they hope students will treat their patients. This growing self-awareness of their role, not only as a source of information but also as a model of caring virtues, is encouraging.

Our medical education system is in a formative period from which will hopefully emerge successful approaches. Whether it be Harvard's "Patient–Doctor Relationship" (Branch et al., 1991), Northwestern's "The Patient, Physician, and Society" (Makoul & Curry, 1998), Dartmouth's "A Life in Medicine" (Moore-West, Testa, & O'Donnell, 1998), or AAMC's report on diversity and cultural competency (*Pfizer Journal*, 1998a), each and every effort has a contribution to make. What is obvious is that the issue of humanistic–scientific balance is a real issue that needs to be addressed.

SUMMARY

The patient–physician relationship is, has been, and must always remain at the heart of American healthcare. This relationship has changed substantially over the past two decades as a result of the market pressures of managed care, the emergence of health consumerism, the growth of new information technologies, and the changing demographics in America. In general, the changes have been for the better, with the relationship moving away from physician-centered paternalism toward mutual partnerships grounded in patient education and scientific progress (Magee & Dole, 1998). The good news is that patients remain highly supportive of their physicians, with 81% involved in relationships lasting more than 7 years, and only 10% expressing dissatisfaction (Magee & Dole, 1998). The bad news is that although doctors and patients still like each other, they increasingly do not have time for each other. Physicians' time constraints flow from intrusive bureaucracy, partially compatible health information systems, continuing expansion of new knowledge and discoveries, and rising patient expectations.

What might be done to reinforce and strengthen the already strong foundation of this essential societal relationship? The Pfizer 1998 Consensus Panel had the following recommendations:

1. Relieve some of the physician's pressures for time. Of physicians, 41% have reduced the time spent with each patient in the past 3 years (Collins, Schoen, & Sondman, 1998).

2. Encourage the physician's role as patient advocate. Although the physician may continue to have to act as a double agent, providing care while conserving resources, he or she should never have to act as a secret agent (Angell, 1993).

3. Encourage integrated comprehensive care. Aligning the continuum of care is essential. Physician leadership must extend beyond clinical continuums to educational continuums. Enlightened managed care must abandon component management once and for all and embrace disease management and the transformational potential of new discoveries and new approaches.

4. Expand access. If real estate is location, location, location, relationship-based care is access, access, access. This includes defining unique strategies to bring patients into the system, reinforcing face-to-face interaction and ensuring that when patients and physicians encounter each other, they have unimpeded access to modern diagnostics and therapeutics.

5. The movement toward measurable quality, critical pathways, and cost-efficient decision making has begun to address unacceptable variability in clinical decision making and cost. That said, some level of practice variation must be preserved if physicians are to continue to engage patients as individuals with unique features. Overcategorizing patients runs the risk of disengaging the physician from the patient–physician relationship.

6. Support process improvements that expand respect for patients. Compassion, understanding, and partnership are often expressed by little gestures that denote respect for patients. Temperature, touch, eye contact, timeliness, tone, and dress all have meaning to patients. At the very least, students should be taught to be sensitive to these messages.

America is witnessing a resurgence of interest in relationship-based care. This movement has now burst into the public arena, uniting patient advocates, physician organizations, enlightened healthcare organizations, public servants, and information specialists. What remains to be seen is in what direction and to what end all of this energy will be focused. What is undeniable is that it is now within the reach of all interested parties to positively transform this vital human service, increasingly setting the tone for a modern caring society. What is equally clear is that true success can be achieved only through steps that advantage our society's great scientific progress while simultaneously reinforcing, rather than degrading, opportunities for live human contact.

REFERENCES

AAMC. *Wanted: doctors with a heart: call for nominations.* Washington, DC: AAMC Publication, 1999.
American Academy of Pediatrics. *Statement on prescription for reading* (press statement). Washington, DC: American Academy of Pediatrics, 1997.

American Medical Association. The patient-physician covenant. *JAMA* 1995; 273:1153.

Angell M. The doctor as double agent. *Kennedy Institute of Ethics Journal* 1993; 3:279–286.

Associated Press Release. *Viagra decision represents unfunded mandate—NGA opposes hasty decision that increases state costs and limits flexibility.* Washington, DC: Associated Press, 1998.

Baker DW. *What is health care literacy?* Presented at Health Literacy: A National Conference. Washington, DC: 1997.

Battelle Medical Technology Assessment and Policy Research Center. *The value of pharmaceuticals: an assessment of future costs for selected conditions.* BHARC-013/90/025, 1991.

Branch WT, et al. Teaching medicine as a human experience: a patient-doctor relationship course for faculty and first year medical students. *Ann Intern Med* 1991; 114:482–489.

California Department of Corporations. Public testimony. San Francisco: 1998a.

California Department of Corporations. *State closes investigation of Kaiser's prescription practices* (press release). Sacramento: State of California, Business, Transportation, and Housing Agency, 1998b.

Cassel EJ. The nature of suffering and the goals of medicine. *N Engl J Med* 1982; 306:639–645.

Code of Medical Ethics. Chicago: American Medical Association, 1997.

Collins KS, Schoen C, Sondman DR. The commonwealth fund survey of physician experiences with managed care. Available at http://www.omwf.org/health_care/physrvy.html. Accessed August 1998.

Eraker SA, Kirscht JP, Becker MH. Understanding and improving patient compliance. *Ann Intern Med* 1984; 100:258–268.

Fallowfeld LJ. Communication skills of oncologists. *Trends Exp Med* 1995; 5:99–103.

Fauci S, et al. The practice of medicine. In Fauci S, et al (eds): *Harrison's principles of internal medicine,* 14th ed. New York: McGraw-Hill, 1998:1–6.

Feldman HA, et al. Impotence and its medical and psychosocial correlates: results of the Massachusetts male aging study. *J Urol* 1994; 151:54–61.

Hojat M, et al. A comparison of personality profiles of internal medicine, residents, physician role models, and the general population. *Acad Med* 1999 (in press).

Kirsh IS, et al. *Adult literacy in America: a first look at the results of the national adult literacy survey.* Washington, DC: US Department of Education, 1993.

Kirsner JB. Living with Hippocrates in a changing medical world, with particular reference to the patient-physician relationship (commentary). *Arch Intern Med* 1992; 152: 2184–2188.

Kroenke K, et al. Bedside teaching. *South Med J* 1997; 90:1069–1074.

Lipkin M Jr. Patient education and counseling in the context of modern patient-physician-family communication. *Patient Education Counseling* 1996; 27:5–11.

Lipkin M Jr, Quill TE, Napodano RJ. The medical interview: a core curriculum for residencies in internal medicine. *Ann Intern Med* 1984; 100:277–284.

Magee M. Ethics of advocacy. *Massachusetts Medicine* April 1997; 2:7.

Magee M. *The fifty most positive doctors in America.* New York: Spencer, 1996.

Magee M, D'Antonio M. *The best medicine.* New York: St. Martin's, 1999.

Magee M, Dole R. *What industry and society expect of their medical educators.* New Orleans: AAMC Group on Student Affairs. 1998.

Magee M, Hojat M. Personality profiles of male and female positive role models in medicine. *Psycho Rep* 1998; 82:547–559.

Makoul G, Curry RH. Patient, physician, and society: Northwestern University Medical School. *Acad Med* 1998; 73:14–24.

Moore-West M, Testa RM, O'Donnell JF. A life in medicine: stories from a Dartmouth Medical School elective. *Acad Med* 1998; 73:153–159.

Nie JB. The physician as general. *JAMA* 1996; 276:1099.

Novach DH, et al. Medical interviewing and interpersonal skills teaching in U.S. medical schools. *JAMA* 1993; 269:2101–2105.

Omnibus Study. Claremont, CA: Yankelovich Partners, 1999.

Parker RM. *What is health care literacy?* Presented at Health Literacy: A National Conference. Washington, DC: 1997.

Parker RM, et al. Literacy and contraception: exploring the link. *Obstet Gynecol* 1996; 88:725–775.

Pendleton DA, Brouwer H, Jaspers J. Communications difficulties: the physicians perspective. *J Lang Soc Psych* 1983; 2:17–36.

Pfizer Inc. Internal communication. *U.S. sales of Viagra.* New York: Pfizer, Inc., 1999a.

Pfizer Inc. Internal communication. *Medicaid coverage of Viagra by state: status update.* New York: Pfizer Inc., 1999b.

Pfizer Inc. Internal communication. *Medicaid sales and rebate report by state for Viagra.* New York: Pfizer Inc., 1999c.

Pfizer Inc. Internal communication. *Viagra sales to Kaiser.* New York: Pfizer Inc., 1999d.

Putnam RD. Bowling alone: America's declining social capital. *J Democracy* 1995; 6(1):65–78.

Responding to the challenge of health literacy. *Pfizer Journal* 1998b; 2(1):1–37.

Roter DL, et al. Communication patterns of primary care physicians. *JAMA* 1997; 22:277, 350–356.

Stoeckle JD. Introduction. In Stoeckle JD (ed): *Encounters between patients and doctors: an anthology.* Cambridge, MA: MIT Press. 1987:1–129.

The Arnold P. Gold Foundation Web site, http://www.humanism-in-medicine.org. 1999.

The evolving patient-physician relationship: maintaining a humanistic and scientific balance. *Pfizer Journal* 1998a; 2(3):1–37.

The pharmaceutical industry at the start of a new century. *Pfizer Journal* 1997; 1(1):1–37.

Thomas L. *The youngest science: notes of a medicine watcher.* New York: Bantam, 1984.

US Department of Education. *Early literacy activities in the home.* National Center for Educational Statistics. The Condition of Education 1997. Indicator 2. Available at http://nces.ed.gov/pubs/ce/c9702a01.html. Accessed December 1997.

US Department of Veterans Affairs. *VA reaches decision on Viagra* (press release). Washington, DC: US Department of Veterans Affairs, 1998.

Wear D. Professional development of medical students: problems and promises. *Acad Med* 1997; 72:1056–1062.

Weiss BD, et al. Illiteracy among Medicaid recipients and its relationship to health care costs. *J Health Care Poor Underserved* 1994; 5:99–111.

Williams MV, et al. Inadequate functional health literacy among patients at two public hospitals. *JAMA* 1995; 274:1677–1682.
Woodwell DA. National ambulatory medical care survey: 1996 summary. *NCHS Advance Data* (No. 29) December 17, 1997:1.

7

CHAPTER

Dynamic of the Patient–Provider Relationship

Naomi R. Klayman, Ph.D.

INTRODUCTION

The process of delivering and receiving healthcare services and products is changing for both healthcare providers and patients. The questions that arise from this process are how it is changing and what impact it will have on these relationships. How these relationships might change *for the better* is a more difficult issue to address. The fact that this chapter references a "provider" rather than a "physician" is in itself a sign of the times. Who is the provider? Is it a physician, a hospital administrator, a pharmaceutical benefit management company, a managed care organization, the federal or state government, an employer, or any of a host of others in the healthcare industry? One might as easily ask, who is the patient? A recipient of services can also have the role of client, subscriber (to an insurance plan), or consumer. Is it the person with the medical condition, the employer/insurance plan that dictates what services will or will not be covered, or the family who must support the patient in providing care and who may be involved in making discretionary medical decisions?

These "roles" are interconnected; no one professional and no one "individual" patient acts alone in the delivery or consumption of healthcare. The task of describing the dynamic at the intersection of these two groups is enormous and probably deserves its own book to be addressed adequately. Therefore, the goals of this chapter are to identify some of the dynamics and forces for change that are ongoing, to examine their impact on relationships, to offer some suggestions for making sense of these challenges, and to indicate what might be strategies for responding to them. There are two crucial things to bear in mind throughout this discussion. The first is that our current state of affairs is the result of a long process of change along many lines and is not the outcome of one group having taken a "wrong turn." The other is that to appreciate the *dynamics* of these relationships, one must look at the *interactions* that occur *between* each of the aforementioned groups, not just the actions taken within groups.

THE PATIENT–PROVIDER RELATIONSHIP AND THE CULTURE OF MEDICINE

It probably is no surprise that Americans are not happy with the healthcare system in the United States. In a survey of 10 nations, Americans were the least satisfied with their healthcare and the only country that would consider adopting a healthcare system in use by another country (Blendon et al., 1990). The good news for healthcare providers, as another article reports, is that although confidence in medicine collectively has plummeted, Americans remain confident in their personal physicians (Mechanic & Schlesinger, 1996).

Beisecker and Beisecker (1993) suggest two metaphors for describing the most commonly mentioned ways the patient–provider relationship can be organized. The more historical role, they suggest, is a "paternalistic" one in which "the role of the doctor was to direct and prescribe; the role of the patient was to obey and cooperate." This is typically described as a parent–child relationship (Parsons, 1951; Parsons & Fox, 1952). In this dynamic, the patient is cast as an unknowing, dependent seeker of care, encouraged to play the "sick role." In contrast, the physician is cast as the all-knowing, benevolent provider of care.

However, as early as the 1970s, sociologists began questioning the nature of this relationship and called attention to medicine as an institution of social control (Friedson, 1975; Zola, 1972). The concern was that physicians were "medicalizing" normal, daily life and that the public's acceptance of them as unquestioned experts was resulting in unnecessary and potentially harmful use of medical services and goods. These articulated concerns, combined with the growing presence of managed care, encouraged patients to take more responsibility for knowing about their health, question therapeutic recommendations, and explore medical alternatives, including the possibility that no medical care was required. Beisecker and Beisecker (1993) refer to this second kind of relationship as "consumeristic" and describe the consumer as listening "to the thoughts of the provider, or of several providers, but ultimately [making] his or her own decisions." Rather than being the voice of authority, the provider is recast as one of a number of resources for information and advice. In this model, it is the consumer who has the final responsibility for demanding or rejecting "care." At worst, the provider is self-serving, seeking to provide "care" when none was required, out of a motive of personal gain.

At either of these two ends of the spectrum, one of the participants in the dyad is cast as "the bad guy." Either the patient is pathetic for acting like a dependent child, or the provider is untrustworthy and suspect of having dubious motives. In response to this lack of viable alternatives, further efforts have been made to create a third alternative, one that is respectful both of the provider's professionalism and the patient's right to make informed decisions. Brody (1980) suggests a model of mutual participation that considers the provider's unique skill and training and also includes the patient's perspective in formulating the medical decision. He borrows from Szaz and Hollender (1956), who formulate the relationship in terms of degree of control, and he suggests that individual healthcare providers and patients will seek different levels of involvement.

He claims that the first step is to create a medical relationship in which patients are encouraged to participate, knowing that the physician reserves the right to refuse interventions believed to result in more harm than good.

The process of including the patient in medical decision making is not simple. It requires a number of skills that are not necessarily acquired during medical training. For example, in Beckman and Frankel (1984), it was found that after asking patients to state their reason for the medical visit, physicians interrupted the patient after an average time of only 18 seconds. In a study designed to revisit this issue, Marvel et al. (1999) found that physicians interrupted the patient's opening statement after a mean of just 23 seconds. Yet, the patient's opening statement may be one of the most important aspects of the medical visit. It helps the provider to assess the true nature of the complaint. By allowing the patient this initial time to speak freely, the provider communicates a sense of caring and personal concern to the patient. Although the following four suggestions are not always implemented, they suggest how physicians and patients might obtain higher levels of satisfaction with the medical encounter:

1. Physicians are encouraged to solicit the patient's agenda early in the medical encounter and to include the patient's goals and health beliefs in the discussion of the findings and therapeutic recommendations (Cohen-Cole, 1991).

2. Patients are encouraged to arrive at the medical visit with a list of questions and concerns. In light of the potential level of anxiety and "flood" of information that results from receiving medical information, patients often forget to raise the concerns they had before the visit. However, it is important to remember that in the recent past, a syndrome called *le mal du petit papier* was assigned to patients who arrived with just such lists of symptoms and concerns. Patients' lists are not always appreciated by physicians, and some take it as suggesting this might be a "problem" patient.

3. Physicians are encouraged to spend ample time giving patients information and informing them of the findings and their significance. Research suggests that physicians vastly overestimate the amount of information they provide and vastly underestimate the amount of information patients want to receive.

4. Therapeutic plans need to be chosen in conjunction with patient preferences and patient suggestions for enhancing adherence. The patient's life situation and personal goals must be a part of the treatment objectives. Physicians need to recognize that the patient's goals are not always congruent with traditional medical goals, and some kind of bridge or compromise needs to be created.

In summary, it is recommended that the medical relationship be formed as the participation of two equal but different parties, each with different skills and knowledge and each participating in different ways to achieve increased health for the patient. However, this is no small task and asks for nothing less than a cultural shift in the process of medical education that "produces" the way physicians treat patients. At least one suggestion is that medical residents be treated with the same respect that we would like them to show to patients (Frankel, 1996).

PROVIDERS AND MEDICAL TRAINING

With increasing frequency, physicians are beginning to engage their patients in conversations that address the patient's perspective of illness. However, when this skill is lacking, we need to recognize that this may pertain more to the nature of medical education than to the personal style of any one physician. Traditionally, medical education has focused on inpatient care and on illnesses that are diagnosed with laboratory values, x-ray studies, and other tests. Historically, medical education has not taught healthcare providers to listen to patients and to respectfully explore the patient's beliefs about the nature of illness, personal medical goals, and preferred paths for healing.

For programs in the United States that do include interpersonal communication training, there is great variation in the quality and intensity of courses offered (Novack et al., 1993; Schwenk et al., 1987). If medical students have a preceptor with superior interpersonal skills, they learn informally through patterning. But traditionally, little formal training has been provided in conducting the medical interview. Several benchmark papers that heralded an interest in the patient as a social being are Engel (1977) and Korsch, Gozzi, and Francis (1968). Medical providers must consider patients' personal world experiences and cultures when developing a diagnosis, when recommending therapy, and when educating for patient adherence (Kleinman et al., 1978, 1980, 1988).

To say that physicians would like to spend more time with patients but are restricted by managed care can be misleading. In fact, some physicians are rather *uncomfortable* talking with patients. In my extensive research with physicians, I have found that the syndromes that are not diagnosable with laboratory tests, such as migraine and depression, and those for which there is no "cure" but require ongoing behavioral change and medical care, such as diabetes and lupus, are the ones that may be least gratifying for the clinician. Perhaps this is because they are difficult to diagnose or manage except through extensive conversation with patients and a deep appreciation of the patient's life.

Published research suggests that medical students may actually "lose" some of their patient contact skills as they progress through medical training (Kauss et al., 1980; McKegney, 1989). In my experience teaching the medical interview, medical residents have commented numerous times that "who" they were becoming did not match the vision they had when they entered medicine. A number of them stated that they were "toeing the line" to get positive reviews from their attendings but were anxious to complete their medical residency so that they could practice medicine according to their initial vision. They also commented that they hoped they would not forget how to "talk to patients" by the time they completed training.

Providers already in practice are no less disillusioned with how they have been "forced" to change the way they care for patients. Managed care has introduced an enormous amount of paperwork into medical practices, often necessitating the hiring of one or more persons simply to attend to this task. Managed care limits the range of drugs and procedures that can be prescribed for its subscribers. At the extreme end, physicians need to ask what kind of insurance a patient has before they can obtain a urine sample. As one physician explained, "I have to know what your insurance is so I know which cup to give you to urinate in." At that point, she opened a supply cabinet to display the extensive inventory she was required to keep in the office to satisfy the "container needs" of all the managed care plans represented by her patients.

Although much of this discontent is blamed on the advent of managed care, I am not convinced that it is solely responsible. Rather, managed care can be a convenient scapegoat for the frustration that emerges from the lack of training on how to interact with patients in the ambulatory care setting. Some physicians find that their medical training and the traditional model of allopathic medicine failed to prepare them adequately to respond to the sociocultural aspects of health and illness represented in clinical practice. For example, O'Conner (1995) provides an excellent discussion of how people from different cultures blend their traditional systems of healing with Western, allopathic care and emphasizes the need for providers to be aware of *all* the steps their patients take to recover from illness. She also discusses how important it is for providers to recommend therapeutic steps that can be integrated with patients' cultural values. This has not typically been part of medical training.

Illness and health are interwoven with the patients' way of life, including family constellation and dynamics, sexual identity and orientation, death and loss of a loved one, poverty, personal violence and sexual abuse, cultural food and health traditions, illiteracy, inability to converse in English or hearing impairment (requiring interpreters), and mental and emotional disturbances. Surprisingly, the medical establishment is poorly equipped to accommodate people who are socially or physically constrained. Some providers may complain about the lack of time to talk to their patients, but it is likely that a number of clinicians would experience extreme discomfort if they were *required* to talk with patients for extended periods. The rigors of medical training often leave the medical professional with little time for personal growth and the development of self-awareness. If a provider has not had the opportunity to resolve personal emotional conflicts, it is unlikely that he or she will be able to address them with patients.

PATIENTS AND THE PATIENT–PROVIDER RELATIONSHIP

Patients view physicians from a range of perspectives, from that of "beneficent caregiver" having no personal bias to that of "profit-driven withholder of access to care." These stereotypes are easily remembered because they stand out in our thinking. However, the most prominent sentiment for the vast number of patients is probably that of anxiety and fear. As a result, much of what occurs during the medical encounter is not remembered by the patient and has the potential to become distorted when the patient recounts the visit to family and friends. For this reason, providers are encouraged to write out diagnostic findings and directions for therapeutic regimens. Patients may view the physician as having significantly more power and can become intimidated, forgetting to ask questions and voice concerns that were clear before the visit. The physician may take the patient's silence as acquiescence to the recommended procedures, when in fact, the patient is simply overwhelmed and confused.

Providers need to make efforts to determine the patient's underlying agendas. For example, they need to consider whether the patient is more interested in alleviating pain or obtaining reassurance that the illness is not terminal rather than obtaining a "cure." Therapeutic plans need to consider the agendas of all who are involved in the medical relationship, including those who will be providing daily care for the patient. Often, this is not an easy task.

THE PATIENT–PROVIDER RELATIONSHIP WITH REGARD TO PATIENT GENDER

Women may be suspicious of the care they receive from the medical establishment, and ample research supports this lack of complete trust. Research demonstrates that for the same presentation of symptoms, women are more likely to be told their complaint is "psychiatric" in nature and are more likely than men to be given antianxiolytic medications. Women are less likely to have their complaints taken seriously and are less likely to receive pain medication when recovering from surgery (Calderone, 1990; Wilcox, 1995). Women have received too much "care" and too little care. Some studies suggest that hysterectomies and cesarean sections have been performed at a higher rate than would be suggested by women's health needs (Laurence & Weinhouse, 1994). On the other hand, most pharmaceutical drugs historically have been tested exclusively in men and lack information on optimal dosing and potential side effects in women (Herman, 1994). Until recently, heart disease was cast as a "man's" disease; today, we know that heart disease is the "number one" killer of women, far and beyond the frequency of breast cancer. Reviewing death statistics for women by disease, Laurence and Weinhouse (1994) point out that in 1993, 478,000 women died from cardiovascular disease compared with 237,000 from all forms of cancer. Comparing death statistics between women and men, according to 1992 statistics, 46% of all deaths among women resulted from cardiovascular disease compared with 40% of all deaths among men. Yet, physicians continue to have less success in diagnosing heart disease in women. When a woman is diagnosed with heart disease, she is likely to receive less interventive care, and cardiac surgery is less likely to have a positive outcome (Laurence & Weinhouse, 1994).

Women and men are likely to have different agendas with regard to the patient–provider relationship (Klayman, 1997). Women more typically approach the encounter from a relationship perspective. The primary goal may be to form an ongoing partnership with the caregiver, even though the stated goal may be to effect a particular outcome. If "healing" does not occur within a specified time frame, women are more likely to "stick it out" and hope that, given another chance, the provider will accomplish the desired outcome. The need to change physicians is described as a deeply distressing transaction. At the same time, women are more likely to claim that the provider simply does not understand her true concerns. Male physicians may especially believe that a medical visit has proceeded well, only to hear later that their female patients are significantly dissatisfied.

In contrast, men appear more likely to approach the encounter from a "transaction" perspective, seeking remediation of symptoms within a particular time frame. If the present "contract" is not successful, they appear to have few qualms about moving on to another provider. They are less likely to be apologetic about switching providers and less often mention that the physician does not "understand" them.

Providers need to take patient gender into account during medical interactions. Not only does the command "take everything off, down to your waist" have a very different significance for women than it does for men, the entire understanding of the relationship and strategies for maintaining that relationship are likely to be different as well.

THE PATIENT–PROVIDER RELATIONSHIP WITH REGARD TO SEXUAL ORIENTATION

The importance of addressing sexual behavior and sexual orientation with patients encompasses far more than whether the patient's behavior places him or her at risk for sexually transmitted diseases. Sexuality includes more of a person's life than what he or she "does in bed." Appreciating whom one loves and with whom one lives is crucial to understanding who the person is. To provide care that is inclusive of all patients, providers need to be able to elicit information about whether a patient identifies as gay, lesbian, bisexual, or transgendered. If a provider is not comfortable doing this, he or she should be able to refer the patient to someone who is. Fear that one's sexuality may incur judgment from the provider inhibits lesbians from receiving adequate preventive care. This reluctance puts them at higher risk for breast and cervical cancer. This fear also prevents gay men from receiving adequate care. Once a physician learns a male patient is gay, there is a risk that HIV/AIDS will preclude the discussion of other potential illnesses. Rankow (1995) speaks to the importance of cultural competence with regard to patient sexuality, and the *Mautner Center for Lesbians with Cancer* in

Washington, DC, has begun a provider education program to address these issues.

Providers also experience discrimination and often find they must hide their sexual orientation. Oriel et al. (1996) point out that in a 1982 survey of 1,009 San Diego physicians, "30% would not admit a homosexual applicant to medical school and almost 40% would discourage homosexual physicians from training in pediatrics or psychiatry." In 1994 Oriel et al. conducted a national survey of family practice residency directors to assess the influence of homosexuality on a candidate's consideration for admittance to a residency program. Of the 291 who completed the survey, "25% admitted they might rank such an applicant lower." As discussed earlier, the process of medical education has a profound effect on how medicine is practiced. If providers are to be accepting of sexual diversity among patients, then medical students and residents need to learn medicine in institutions that are equally accepting of sexual diversity among their constituencies.

PATIENTS AND PROVIDERS AND MANAGED CARE

The United States seems to have had a cultural need to divorce discussions of money with the delivery of healthcare. Traditionally, physicians recommended medical care and patients accepted it as benevolent advice. The cost of care was not typically part of medical discussions, and any financial questions were referred to office administrators. The advent of managed care introduced the presence of a "contract" into this relationship, and both patients and physicians were forced to acknowledge that money was, in fact, a part of the healthcare transaction (Friedson, 1975).

Managed care also began requiring second opinions for some medical procedures, and it became part of the patient's responsibility to question whether the recommended care was the *only* option. To a degree, this has had a positive effect on patients, encouraging them to question medical advice, to become empowered through understanding their medical conditions, and to become an active participant in choosing therapeutic options. However, it has also served to engender mistrust in the medical profession, not all of it deserved. Malpractice cases "sell" news programs, and the disproportionate reporting of negative managed care outcomes can alarm patients inappropriately. The potential for litigation has also engendered "defensive medicine." Understandably, some medical recommendations may now be driven more from a concern for "how this might look in court" rather than whether it is in the patient's best interests. For better or worse, managed care and litigation are now a part of the dynamic of the patient–provider relationship.

AMERICAN CULTURE AND HEALTH INSURANCE

In the United States, there seems to be a cultural belief that healthcare is a right but that there is no system in place to provide this idealized, unlimited access of care to all people. Hence, an inadvertent system of rationing based on income has been developed: those able to work full-time, at some salary threshold, in certain kinds of jobs, are able to participate in private, third-party payor insurance, albeit a diminishing benefit of employment. Those who are less fortunate must rely on federally funded programs. The least fortunate are those who earn "too much" to be eligible for Medicaid but work in jobs that do not include medical care as a benefit. These individuals and their families have neither the insurance nor the income to cover the out-of-pocket costs of healthcare. Working parents may be able to obtain federally funded health insurance for their children but may not personally be eligible for coverage; this is a problem that has a particular impact on working, single mothers. These are growing problems as individuals are increasingly expelled from the ranks of welfare to obtain minimum wage jobs and become the working poor. These economic hardships also impact on the relationship between patients and their healthcare providers. These are people who are unable to "stay home from work to elevate the leg" or to afford necessary medications at the minimum dosages required for a therapeutic effect. Cost is a barrier to accessing healthcare and to patient satisfaction.

However, even those with private insurance are not uniformly satisfied with the current system. In a multinational study in 1988 that included Americans, Canadians, and Britons, Americans were the most *dissatisfied* with their health system (Blendon et al., 1990). Perhaps even more remarkable are the data from a follow-up study in 1990, reported in the same article, that included seven additional countries. Americans continued to be the least satisfied with their current healthcare system despite having the highest per capita spending rate of the 10 countries ($2,051 versus $758 for United Kingdom, the lowest of the 10 countries), while Canada, at $1,483, has the highest reported level of satisfaction. The authors conclude the following:

> American dissatisfaction arises from the interaction between our sharply rising healthcare costs and the inadequate financial protection provided by our health insurance system . . . [there is] little guarantee of continuing health insurance coverage to almost any individual . . . A 1989 survey [revealed that] in a twenty-eight month period, more than one American in four (28%) reported they were without health insurance coverage for some period of time.
>
> Similarly, Americans have no guarantee that their employer will not decide to reduce the breadth of their health insurance benefits when they may be most needed.
>
> Lastly, Americans, in comparison to citizens of the other nations surveyed, appear to pay more out-of-pocket at the time they are ill. Surveys show that Americans, on average, pay 26% of their healthcare bills out of pocket, and one in six (19%) report paying more than 40% of these cost directly (p. 191).

Although this and other studies (e.g., DiMatteo et al., 1995) indicate that this loss of trust and confidence in the American healthcare system does not appear to affect satisfaction with one's own physician or dentist, it is likely that relationships with healthcare providers are framed by dissatisfaction with financial uncertainty and risk. Furthermore, these relationships may be affected in ways not yet measured. For example, Kao and colleagues (1998) find that although most patients trust their physicians, fee-for-service indemnity patients have higher levels of trust than patients of physicians who are salaried or receive a capitation fee (as indicated in a telephone interview survey). What needs to be studied further is how the method of payment may influence the process by which providers and patients interact with each other and how this interaction influences the patient–provider dynamic.

PROVIDERS AND FORMULARIES

Managed care has had an impact on how healthcare providers prescribe medications for patients. With the advent of formularies, physicians must limit the brands for which they write to those covered by the drug plan. When the pharmaceutical benefit management (PBM) company initiates a new contract with a pharmaceutical company, the allowed brands of drugs within a given category may change without the physician or patient taking note of the change. When the patient returns to the pharmacy to have the prescription refilled, the pharmacist may change the brand of the drug within class without informing the patient or the physician. Given that all brands within a category are "not created equal," this can cause problems for patients in terms of a drug's reduced ability to achieve the desired effect or its association with side effects not experienced with the previously used agent. This can have profound effects on patient compliance and on patient–provider communication.

Similarly, the presence of formularies necessarily means that physicians are not at liberty to prescribe preferred agents at will. The physician must first ensure that the brand is covered by the plan. Given that a typical physician may have patients from as many as five or more healthcare plans, with as many formularies, this is not a small task. Physicians have commented that the path of least resistance is to "hedge one's bets" by choosing brands most commonly on formularies. This means that sometimes drugs prescribed for patients are chosen to minimize paperwork for the physician rather than based on the careful matching of an agent's benefits to the patient's needs. Patients vary in their ability to understand the role of formularies, and this "nonproximal" but ever-present third-party can become an invisible yet powerful participant in the patient–provider dynamic.

PROVIDERS AND PHARMACEUTICAL COMPANIES

Healthcare providers appear to have a love–hate relationship with pharmaceutical companies. Prescription drugs are largely sold through physicians. Pharmaceutical representatives are paid by drug companies to visit physicians; to inform them of the company's agents, how they work, and how they are efficacious; and to encourage the use of their company's agents over those of the competition's. Although physicians readily state that these "sales calls" need to be treated circumspectly and not taken at face value, a number of physicians appreciate these encounters because they believe that they help the busy physician stay informed with regard to the latest clinical trials and the newest agents. (The reader should be aware that the information drug companies provide to physicians is regulated; claims cannot be made that are not substantiated according to FDA regulations.) An important aspect of this visit is sampling. Representatives leave samples to encourage physicians' use of their brand.

Samples play an important role in physicians' prescribing patterns, and these too have an influence on the patient–provider dynamic and how agents are chosen for a given patient. Many physicians will not start a patient on a new drug unless the patient can be given samples first. The logic is that drugs are expensive, and a physician cannot anticipate how any one patient will react to a particular agent. Thus, rather than have the patient "waste a prescription" on a drug that may be insufficiently effective or cause side effects, the physician is more likely to give the patient samples for 1 or 2 weeks and then judge its appropriateness for this particular patient. If the sample drug appears to be appropriate, a prescription is written; if not, the next brand is sampled. Thus, the absence or presence of samples can have an effect on which agent a physician chooses for first-line therapy.

Direct-to-consumer (DTC) advertising plays a role in the patient–provider dynamic. DTC advertising, also subject to FDA guidelines, provides consumers with information about the availability of prescription drugs that might not otherwise be common knowledge. However, consumers are not always thoughtful in how they interpret DTC advertising and do not always pay attention to details. Some accept the advertisers' claims wholesale and visit their physician demanding the drug by name. Others ask the physician about the advertising but fail to remember the brand name or what was said about the drug. This may create a challenge for the physician who may not be able to respond to patients' requests for information. Historically, most patients were not knowledgeable with regard to prescription drugs, much less able to make informed requests for them. For physicians who are threatened by a proactive patient role, DTC advertising can have a profound effect on the patient–provider dynamic. In these several ways, pharmaceutical companies are now part of the patient–provider dynamic.

HEALTH INSURANCE AND SUBSCRIBERS

Health insurance was originally designed to protect physicians and hospitals from unpaid medical bills during a time when inpatient care accounted for most healthcare costs. As medical care is moving increasingly toward outpatient care and the use of pharmaceuticals in disease prevention and management, the present design of health insurance is meeting fewer and fewer of subscribers' needs. It is now estimated that 50% of all drug costs are borne directly by senior citizens because prescription drugs are not covered by Medicare. The elderly need to purchase private coverage if they desire prescription drug insurance.

When private health insurance was instituted in the United States, there was no awareness that the cost of healthcare would rise as precipitously as it has over the last 20 to 30 years. The reasons for this dramatic rise in cost is severalfold. Modern advances have resulted in the development of more expensive drugs, more expensive equipment, and procedures that are more expensive to perform. There has also been an investment in hospital beds that has proven to be unsound. Even though approval is required before new hospitals are built, substantial numbers of beds go unfilled each year, especially with the increase of outpatient treatment. This represents an investment in capital that is not likely to be recovered. As a nation, people are living longer. The fact that death does not occur as often from "simple" illnesses means that people can live longer with complicated illnesses—illnesses that require more expensive drugs, more complicated procedures, and longer periods of treatment.

Either directly or indirectly, this nation has decided to focus healthcare dollars on the two most expensive periods in life: neonatal care and end-stage disease management. Increasingly, physicians are able to sustain premature babies that are earlier in natal development, at no small cost. Similarly, they are able to sustain life further and further into the terminal stages of illness. It is sometimes unclear at what point the patient has "died." All of these advances have driven up the cost of healthcare as reflected in health insurance premiums and out-of-pocket costs to the consumer.

Unlike the price of other goods and services produced in a capitalist system, the cost of healthcare services has not been affected by market competition and the laws of supply and demand. This is largely because the person receiving the service has not been in a position to negotiate price directly and, under health insurance, does not pay for them directly. Historically, the more services a physician "sold," the more a physician was paid. Managed care was introduced as an effort to put the healthcare provider at some risk for the services provided. However, there is ample evidence that healthcare received in a managed care environment is met with distrust at a level not otherwise found. Although Americans tend to remain confident in their personal physicians, patients worry that their physicians may not recommend care because of the risk of coming under the restrictions of utilization review or because of the risk of loss of incentives for keeping "specialty care costs" at a minimum. For these reasons, among others, Mechanic and Schlesinger (1996) argue that managed care plans themselves, rather than physicians, should be the ones required to disclose financial arrangements as a way to separate the interests of the physicians from those of the health plan organization.

HEALTH INSURANCE AND EMPLOYERS

Given the high percentage of the operating budget that health-care insurance now represents for companies, the increase of just a few percentage points in the amount of monthly premium can make the difference, with regard to profit or loss, especially for small and mid-sized companies. Employers often change health insurance carriers annually. This volatile market is inspiring both insurance carriers and pharmaceutical companies to explore creative financial arrangements to help hold down the cost of health insurance. These arrangements typically include disease management programs and restrictions with regard to which laboratories, radiology services, and hospitals that patients covered by that plan may use. Some plans find it more economically advantageous to fly the patient and a family member to another state for a procedure and pay for room and board than to provide care in a facility that is more geographically convenient for the patient and family. This further affects the patient–provider relationship.

HEALTH INSURANCE AND EMPLOYEES

Most private health insurance is obtained through the place of employment. This means that employees are subject to the contracts that their employers are able to negotiate with health insurance carriers. Employees have virtually no choice of insurance plan or the physician panel associated with it. With each change in carrier, employees are enlisted in new managed care programs. The subsequent plan may not include the patient's present physician, and the patient will be forced to initiate a new relationship: a process that is time-consuming for both the patient and provider and that is fraught with the limitations of each participant's communication skills.

Only a small proportion of employees are offered more than one plan by their employers, and that choice is usually limited to choosing between a traditional (indemnity) or a managed care plan. However, the ability to choose among a number of health insurance plans is not in itself an improvement. For example, federal employees may have as many as five or more plans from which to choose each year. However, these employees are typically overwhelmed by the amount of information they receive from numerous carriers each year and may not even bother to open the envelope containing plan information. Unless they have had a negative experience with their current carrier or hear of a dramatic change in coverage, they appear likely to simply renew the plan they already have. It appears they have no useful system for comparing benefits. Choosing a health insurance plan is a difficult process. Often, subscribers do not appreciate the limits of their insurance until they exceed the benefit. Unfortunately, this typically occurs during an extensive, serious illness.

Managed care plans often seek to standardize care through disease management programs. This means that physicians who treat patients with certain identified diseases and who belong to particular managed care programs must agree to treat according to a predetermined program for patient care. Although these programs are designed to achieve optimal outcomes across a population of patients, physicians and their patients have less autonomy and find there is a "third party" present in the medical relationship.

Increasingly, the confidentiality between patient care and employer access to health information is breaking down. Managed care companies and the employers who subscribe to their benefits have access to patient costs and medical procedures, although those are not typically linked to individual patients. It is not currently clear who sets the rules for privacy with regard to information contained in the medical chart. Certainly, medical, disability, and life insurance companies have access to that information. Patients should know that they can be turned down for coverage if certain diagnoses are listed. For example, patients with a history of depression may not be able to get disability insurance, and patients with a history of having been abused by domestic partners may not be able to get health insurance. The awareness of such risks can restrict the patient's willingness to disclose symptoms and concerns to the provider, a further encroachment on the trust and confidence that is so crucial to the patient–provider relationship.

CONCLUSION

Systems are necessary aspects of social functioning. They exist to ease the course of daily life and to maintain the status quo. One could not drive a car very successfully if, at every corner, one had to determine whether to drive on the right- or left-hand side of the street. If this chapter has focused mainly on the weaknesses in the American healthcare system, it is because the system is in flux and, understandably, resistant to change. Change occurs slowly and is most effective when it is designed to be proactive and take into account all the various forces at play. Change is almost never easy or simple, and the new health-care consumer is demanding difficult, but often reasonable, changes of the system. The system is also demanding difficult, but often reasonable, changes of the patient.

In this age of the "drive through, 90-second hamburger," it is often hard to accept that solutions to difficult problems do not always come in neat packages with straightforward steps for their amelioration. The dynamic between patients and providers is complex, deriving from the multitude of influences and forces previously mentioned: the growing awareness of patients with regard to the cost of medical care and the process of medical decision making, the institution of medical education, the diversity of patients at many levels of social identity, third-party payors and the current system for accessing health insurance, and the role of the pharmaceutical industry in developing new avenues for treatment and in making the public aware of new therapies. Each thread in this "tapestry" has its own history and is mutually influenced by the other "threads." Rather than approaching this dynamic as a "cause-and-effect" phenomenon, I suggest approaching the dynamic as the result of a complex system of institutions and histories that shift and fluctuate with respect to each other. Just as opening the window to cool a room will simply serve to trigger the thermostat to turn on the heater, any change to one aspect of the patient–provider dynamic must be considered in terms of how it is likely to be responded to by all of the other aspects. The patient–provider dynamic is, in turn, influenced by each of these forces acting on the larger system.

This chapter has enumerated a number of forces at play, each holding the other in a dynamic tension, and each responding to the other in an effort to maintain a homeostatic system (Ackoff, 1981). There are steps individuals and single institutions can take to create more positive change on the local level. However, the larger systems that have produced the challenges we now face need to be revisioned at a more macro level. For example, we now have the ability to store, retrieve, and analyze communitywide health data that may suggest steps that communities as a whole can take to improve the health of entire populations. Unfortunately, these data are currently held by private health insurance companies that have competitive reasons for not revealing and not acting on these data.

Just as the public sewage system was historically the single most influential invention that improved public health, data are now available that may suggest other innovations for the wholesale improvement of public health and for wholesale improvement of the patient–provider relationship. The challenge will be to relinquish the culturally held belief that personal health is primarily the responsibility of personal behavior.

REFERENCES

Ackoff R. *Creating the corporate future*. New York: John Wiley & Sons, 1981.

Beckman HB, Frankel RM. The effect of physician behavior on the collection of data. *Ann Intern Med* 1984; 101:692–696.

Beisecker A, Beisecker T. Using metaphors to characterize doctor-patient relationships: paternalism versus consumerism. *Health Communication* 1993; 5(1):41–58.

Blendon RJ, et al. DataWatch: satisfaction with health systems in ten nations. *Health Affairs* 1990; 9(2):185–192.

Brody DS. The patient's role in clinical decision-making. *Ann Intern Med* 1980; 93:718–722.

Calderone KL. The influence of gender on the frequency of pain and sedative medication administered to postoperative patients. *Sex Roles* 1990; 23:11–12, 713–725.

Cohen-Cole SA. *The medical interview: the three function approach*. St. Louis: Mosby, 1991.

DiMatteo RM, et al. Americans' views of health professionals and the health-care system. *Health Values* 1995; 19:23–29.

Engel GL. The need for a new medical model: a challenge for biomedicine. *Science* 1997; 196(4286):129–196.

Frankel RM. Personal communication, 1996.

Friedson E. *Doctoring together: a study of professional social control*. Chicago: The University of Chicago Press, 1975.

Herman R. What doctors don't know about women. In Hicks KM (ed): *Misdiagnosis: woman as a disease*. Allentown, PA: People's Medical Society, 1994:33–45.

Kao AC, et al. The relationship between method of physician payment and patient trust. *JAMA* 1998; 280:19, 1708–1714.

Kauss DR, et al. The long-term effectiveness of interpersonal skills training in medical schools. *J Med Educ* 1980; 55(7):595–601.

Klayman. Unpublished dissertation. Illness as a gendered event: communication behavior reported by women and men diagnosed with chronic conditions. The Graduate School of The Union Institute, 1997.

Kleinman A. *Patients and healers in the context of culture: an exploration of the borderland between anthropology, medicine, and psychiatry*. Berkeley, CA: University of California Press, 1980.

Kleinman A. *The illness narratives: suffering, healing, & the human condition*. New York: Basic Books, 1988.

Kleinman A, Eisenberg L, Good B. Culture, illness and care: clinical lessons from anthropologic and cross-cultural research. *Ann Intern Med* 1978; 88:251–258.

Korsch BM, Gozzi EK, Francis V. Gaps in doctor-patient communication. I: Doctor-patient interaction and patient satisfaction. *Pediatrics* 1968; 42:855–871.

Laurence L, Weinhouse B. *Outrageous practices*. New York: Fawcett Columbine, 1994.

Marvel MK, et al. Soliciting the patient's agenda: have we improved? *JAMA* 1999; 281(3):283–287.

McKegney CP. Medical education: a neglectful and abusive family system. *Fam Med* 1989; 21(6):452–457.

Mechanic D, Schlesinger M. The impact of managed care on patients' trust in medical care and their physicians. *JAMA* 1996; 275(21):1693–1697.

Novack DH, et al. Medical interviewing and interpersonal skills teaching in U.S. medical schools. Progress, problems, and promise. *JAMA* 1993; 269(16):2101–2105.

O'Conner BB. *Healing traditions: alternative medicine and the health professionals*. Philadelphia: University of Pennsylvania Press, 1995.

Oriel KA, et al. Gay and lesbian physicians in training: family practice program directors' attitudes and students' perceptions of bias. *Fam Med* 1996; 28(10):720–725.

Parsons T. *The social system*. Glencoe, IL: Free Press, 1951.

Parsons T, Fox R. Illness, therapy, and the modern urban American family. *J Soc Iss* 1952; 8:31–44.

Rankow L. *Women's health issues: planning for diversity*. Washington, DC: National Lesbian & Gay Health Association, 1995.

Schwenk TL, et al. Where, how, and from whom do family practice residents learn? A multisite analysis. *Fam Med* 1987; 19(4):265–268.

Szaz TS, Hollender MH. A contribution to the philosophy of medicine: the basic models of the doctor-patient relationship. *Arch Intern Med* 1956; 97:585–592.

Wilcox V. Effects of patients' age, gender, and depression on medical students' beliefs, attitudes, intentions and behavior. *J Appl Gerontol* 1995; 14(2):172–192.

Zola IK. Medicine as an institution of social control. *Sociol Rev* 1972; 20:487–504.

8

C H A P T E R

Improving Consumer Health through Disease Management

Marnie LaVigne, Ph.D.

INTRODUCTION

By no means is "disease management" a household phrase among healthcare consumers. Although disease management is not familiar to those outside the medical arena, this recent movement in healthcare capitalizes on consumers as the key to better health outcomes. The high prevalence and growing costs of chronic illness have been a significant catalyst for a consumer-focused shift in healthcare. Improving health outcomes, particularly when chronic illness is involved, requires collaboration between healthcare providers and patients to formulate an appropriate treatment regimen that addresses the full array of contributing factors. In turn, patients must follow the regimen and communicate with their healthcare provider in a manner that allows timely treatment modification to achieve short- and long-term goals. Incorporating this consumer-focus means that "take two aspirin and call me in the morning" no longer applies, at least in the disease management arena.

A growing awareness of the importance of behavioral factors in the development and management of chronic illnesses and the increasing emphasis on quality of life have driven a shift toward new ways of practicing medicine (Feuerstein, Labbe, & Kuczmierczyk, 1986) and measuring outcomes. Consumer-focused healthcare requires taking the patient's perspective. This necessitates understanding an individual's knowledge, capabilities, lifestyle, and motivation. Traditional medical approaches focus mostly on the first factor—knowledge—based on the assumption that better educated patients are healthier patients. However, the more complex the behavior required as part of a medical regimen, the more critical it is to assess the patient's level of motivation, coordinate with the patient's lifestyle, rehearse key behavioral skills, and follow up with the patient to reinforce or redirect treatment recommendations. The consumer-focused approach even extends to measuring the success of treatment through the consumer or patient's eyes. Behavioral science and medicine are collaborating to deliver these consumer-oriented strategies as part of mainstream healthcare. This chapter explores how disease management is being developed, implemented, and evaluated with the consumer in mind.

Disease Management Defined

Disease management was introduced as a new healthcare term in 1993 by the Boston Consulting Group, who described it as a patient care approach that coordinates medical resources across the entire healthcare spectrum (Boston Consulting Group, 1993). Since then, numerous definitions have been offered. In a seminal article on disease management and outcomes research, Epstein and Sherwood (1996) state that this "latest concept in this field, disease management, refers to the use of an explicit systematic population-based approach to identify persons at risk, intervene with specific programs of care, and measure clinical and other outcomes." When reduced to its most common elements, disease management can be understood as the process of improving health outcomes while controlling healthcare costs.

Disease management emerged for a number of reasons. As chronic illness has become the leading cause of morbidity and mortality in the United States, the complexity of conditions such as diabetes, asthma, and congestive heart failure has necessitated a more comprehensive treatment approach. The high cost of healthcare among these patients prompted payors to look from traditional strategies to new approaches. At the same time that cost containment issues were driving disease management, particularly within the managed care arena, there was a call for greater accountability in healthcare. Payors and patients began demanding documentation of value for their healthcare dollar.

Although originally described as oriented toward chronic illness spectrum (Boston Consulting Group, 1993), disease management has expanded to involve many conditions, such as pregnancy, that are not disease entities. A survey published by the National Managed Health Care Congress (NMHCC) in 1996 showed that half of the managed care organizations who responded believed that disease management ideally involves the entire continuum of care, from primary prevention to long-term health maintenance (National Managed Health Care Congress, 1996). *Health management* has been proposed as an alternative phrase, although disease management continues to be the predominant term used.

Given that disease management can be driven by many motivations and operationalized with a variety of components, where does the consumer or patient fit into the picture? The following section reviews those components of disease management programs that are specifically focused on the consumer toward development of cost-effective interventions that help the patient "get" well and stay well.

DISEASE MANAGEMENT PROGRAMS: WHERE THE CONSUMER FITS IN

In many ways, disease management is the healthcare that consumers already believed they were receiving and that practitioners thought they were providing. Aside from expanded data-driven capabilities resulting from technological advances, none of the disease management components listed in Figure 8–1 are

F I G U R E   8–1

Disease Management Spectrum

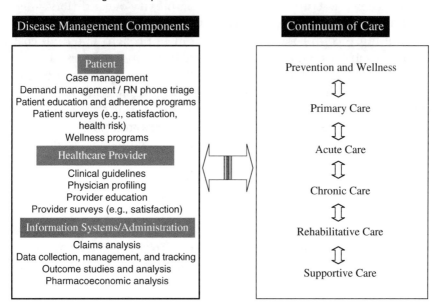

new in healthcare. Rather, it is the coordination of these elements combined with the orientation toward outcomes evaluation on a population level that make disease management a new and distinct approach to healthcare (Epstein & Sherwood, 1996). The disease management components that emphasize the consumer most are those that provide direct patient services or data based on patient self-report. Figure 8–1 lists patient-centered elements versus those targeting healthcare providers or information systems and administration.

The 1996 NMHCC survey previously cited showed that more than 70% of managed care organizations selected the following as core disease management elements: clinical guidelines, clinical outcomes management, provider education, computer data collection and tracking, patient education, outcome studies, benchmarking, and patient satisfaction. The pressure to maintain and intensify the consumer-focused elements is increasing in part because of organizations such as the National Committee for Quality Assurance (NCQA), whose managed care accreditation standards require that disease management programs include (1) a clearly defined and identified population with a chronic condition, (2) the use of data to design an appropriate intervention, (3) a strategy to reach the targeted population, (4) interventions designed to address the continuum of care, (5) a means to involve practitioners, and (6) a strategy to evaluate the effectiveness of the intervention (National Committee for Quality Assurance, 1998).

An example of a comprehensive disease management initiative incorporating patient-centered elements comes from the Lovelace Episodes of Care (EOC) Program, which has modules focused on numerous therapeutic areas, including pediatric asthma (Marosi, Steismeyer, & Faculjak, 1998). The components of this EOC application include development and implementation of practice guidelines; access to care through a pediatric asthma clinic; education of patients, caregivers, and healthcare providers; and outcomes evaluation.

Creating consumer-focused or patient-centered disease management programs involves two dimensions—philosophical issues and practical, or logistical, aspects. This section reviews these two dimensions, beginning with an overview of some leading behavioral theories that, in turn, form the foundation for a better understanding of issues such as compliance and behavior change. These theories emanate from the "biopsychosocial model" of healthcare.

Addressing the Total Patient through the Biopsychosocial Model

In 1977, the biopsychosocial model was introduced as an alternative approach to the biomedical model (Engel, 1977). The traditional medical or biomedical model operates under what is known as a mind–body dualism, where psychological and physical processes are assumed to be mutually exclusive. This reflects a disease focus in which patients are the passive recipients of treatment aimed at eliminating or ameliorating symptoms.

In comparison, the biopsychosocial model is a comprehensive, systems approach to health in which psychological and environmental factors, as well as physical elements, interact to contribute to an individual's health. These nonphysical elements are often broadly termed *psychosocial factors*. The biopsychosocial model focuses on health rather than on disease and, therefore, inherently spans the continuum of care starting with prevention. Patients are seen as proactive agents in promoting positive health outcomes, rather than as passive recipients of treatment as implied by the biomedical model.

To illustrate the biomedical model, consider a patient with asthma who traditionally would receive asthma medication to treat episodes of wheezing and coughing. Following the latest clinical guidelines on pharmacotherapy, a physician ideally would prescribe both long-term control and quick relief medications for a patient with persistent symptoms, but this would be the extent of the healthcare prescription. Similarly, disease management programs based on the biomedical model may easily bypass patient-centered approaches in favor of unidimensional healthcare provider or administrative initiatives such as those listed in Figure 8–1. In this asthma treatment example, a program might be limited to educating physicians about the latest recommendations on asthma medications (healthcare provider component) or conducting a pharmacoeconomic analysis of specific asthma medications (information systems/administration component).

In the biopsychosocial model, the treatment regimen would position the patient as an active partner in developing and maintaining a management plan, including a medication schedule; avoiding or minimizing asthma triggers; self-monitoring asthma symptoms and peak flow meter readings; and building support from family, friends, and community resources. Disease management programs designed from this perspective integrate the patient components with the healthcare provider and information systems/administration elements.

As the biopsychosocial model is gaining ground and stature, clinical guidelines are incorporating comprehensive patient education elements. This is well-illustrated with asthma patients. Recommendations from the First Expert Panel for the

Diagnosis and Management of Asthma, released in 1991, showed an increased focus on preventive pharmacotherapy and proactive patient education elements, such as the patient use of a peak flow meter and a written asthma management plan (National Heart, Lung, and Blood Institute, 1991). The Second Expert Panel's report, released in 1997 (National Asthma Education and Prevention Program, 1997), extends the patient-centric model even further by emphasizing patient and family education immediately upon diagnosis, with thorough instruction on all key self-management information, coupled with a written plan, and follow-up contacts to expand and reinforce the patient education and self-care behaviors.

Patient-Centered Outcomes Evaluation

Outcomes measurement or, simply put, measuring whether the goals of patient care have been achieved on an individual patient and population level, is an inherent part of disease management. While clinical and economic outcomes obtained from medical records and databases have been the standard performance measure in healthcare, the growing consumer focus has expanded the parameters for defining success. Gouveia et al. (1991) describe four types of patient-focused outcomes: clinical endpoints, functional status, well-being, and satisfaction. In this schema, these elements constitute health status from the patient's perspective. Clinical endpoints include symptoms and laboratory values, such as frequency of asthma episodes and spirometry in a person with asthma. Functional status refers to the ability to perform physical, social, and other activities that may be affected by health. This may be measured as an asthmatic patient's ability to attend work or school. Well-being or quality of life is a subjective rating of mood, absence of pain, and overall health, as assessed through a general questionnaire (e.g., Short Form-12 [Ware, Kosinski, & Keller, 1995]), or a disease-specific survey (e.g., Pediatric Asthma Quality of Life Questionnaire [Juniper et al., 1996]). Patient satisfaction refers specifically to perceptions about one's healthcare, including access, convenience, quality, and cost. NCQA has promoted the use of standard satisfaction measures through the specifications in its Health Plan Employer Data and Information Set (HEDIS) (National Committee for Quality Assurance, 1999).

This broad definition of health status includes patient knowledge, patient adherence, patient motivation, and enactment of self-care behaviors. Pharmaceutical companies that are active in the disease management arena have emphasized medication compliance as an outcome target, which has important implications for patients, providers, and payors as well. Compliance with other "behavioral prescriptions," such as appointments for prenatal care, immunizations, and postcardiac event cholesterol testing, is being positioned along with more traditional utilization benchmarks through the HEDIS specifications. The push for greater accountability in healthcare will continue to expand the measurement and use of patient-oriented outcomes.

THE LOGISTICS: IMPLEMENTING CONSUMER-FOCUSED INITIATIVES

As healthcare organizations adopt a patient-focused orientation in daily patient care, they are asking important logistical questions: (1) How do you promote behavior change? (2) How do you reach large patient populations? and (3) What kind of improvement in outcomes should be expected from patient-focused programs? The answers to these questions are still evolving, but the information reviewed in the next section provides significant guidance for developing and implementing successful disease management programs.

How Do You Promote Behavior Change?

As one of the consumer-directed components in disease management, giving patients educational material has been the traditional method for encouraging patients to comply with medical treatment. The premise is that patients who have information about their condition will be motivated to follow treatment regimens ranging from a simple short course of antibiotics to very complex requirements for chronic illnesses such as diabetes. However, providing information does not necessarily translate into behavior change, particularly when significant, long-term lifestyle modification is required. In line with the biopsychosocial model, behavioral and motivational models are being translated from the research environment to real-world clinical settings to enhance the impact of patient education efforts.

Research across a range of chronic conditions, such as asthma (Sullivan et al., 1996), diabetes (Glasgow, 1991), and cardiovascular disease (DeBusk et al., 1994) has shown that programs combining multiple treatment components, versus a single patient intervention, yield the greatest improvement in common behavioral targets, such as medication compliance (Roter et al., 1998). In addition to a foundation of patient education, multimodal programs include ongoing communication between healthcare providers and patients through multiple on-site, phone, and print communications that provide opportunities for redirecting and reinforcing patient behavior. Studies in the chronic illnesses, such as those noted here, have found sustained behavior change as long as a year after patients first enter the intervention program.

The Lovelace EOC Program described previously serves as a good example of a comprehensive multimodal intervention. Rather than depending on generic patient education materials to prompt all the necessary changes, the most comprehensive programs are built around multimodal approaches that draw from various behavioral theories to individually tailor the patient experience.

Some of the leading theories that have migrated from the research laboratories to clinical settings, particularly over the past decade, are presented.

Self-Efficacy and Self-Regulation

Self-efficacy is a concept that has been positioned as the most important prerequisite for behavior change (Bandura, 1977). This concept refers to confidence in one's ability to change a behavior. Research on self-efficacy in the health arena has shown that people who are more confident that they can change a specific health behavior are more likely to adopt the target behavior, such as a new diet, smoking cessation, exercise, and medication adherence (O'Leary, 1985). An important part of building

FIGURE 8-2

Self-Regulation in Health Management

Patient-Focused Measures	Traditional Outcome Measures

Confidence in Managing Disease	Healthcare Utilization
⇕	• Physician Visits
Use of Self-Management Strategies	• Emergency Department Visits • Hospitalizations

self-confidence around health behaviors is for a person to be successful in performing self-care. For example, an asthmatic patient will become more confident about managing this condition if the complex self-care skills can be broken down into smaller steps and rehearsed. A powerful method for enhancing a person's confidence in managing this chronic condition is for a healthcare provider to collaborate with the patient to formulate a written asthma management plan with repeated opportunities to practice each step. The model shown in Figure 8-2 integrates self-efficacy with another behavioral model, the Self-Regulation approach to asthma management (Clark et al., 1994). This integrated model illustrates how greater self-confidence combined with the use of asthma management strategies, such as avoiding asthma triggers, reduces healthcare utilization. This approach has been expanded even further to include social support, in the form of role models and assistance from family, friends, and caregivers, as a way to help individuals make lifestyle changes that affect their health (Glasgow, 1995).

Transtheoretical Stages of Change

One of the most widely evaluated and applied motivational theories is the Transtheoretical Stages of Change model (Prochaska et al., 1994), which classifies an individual's readiness to make a change in diet, exercise, medication adherence, or other health-related behavior. This model is appealing to both health-care providers and consumers because (1) it only requires asking an individual a few brief questions; (2) it can be applied across virtually any health area, including the common concern of medication adherence; (3) it specifies how to intervene with the individual according to his or her "stage of readiness to change"; and (4) it addresses maintenance of long-term behavior change.

In this model, patients' rating of their own readiness to change classifies them in one of five stages, from precontemplation (not interested in changing the target behavior in the next 6 months), contemplation (planning to make changes in the next 1 to 6 months), preparation (ready to make a change in the next month), action (has changed the target behavior for less than 6 months), and maintenance (has sustained changes for 6 months or more). In turn, the intervention strategy is geared to the stage of change. For example, an asthmatic patient who is in the preparation or action stage, beginning to use a peak flow meter, would be given information on how to use the meter and interpret the information as part of an asthma management plan. The same individual who is in the contemplation or pre-contemplation stages would first be encouraged to focus on the benefits of using the meter as part of an overall plan to prevent and treat asthma symptoms, before emphasizing the procedure for proper peak flow meter use. Targeting patient education ma-terials to each of these stages has proven to be more effective than providing one-size-fits-all information in numerous health behaviors, including smoking cessation (Prochaska et al., 1993) and dietary changes (Campbell et al., 1994), both of which are notoriously difficult, but necessary, lifestyle changes for the pre-vention and management of most chronic illnesses.

How Do You Reach Large Patient Populations?

Through the integration of behavioral science and medicine, consumers have a growing number of improved patient educa-tion models to help them make difficult lifestyle changes. However, there is still a question of how these interventions can be delivered to the large patient population that needs to be targeted across the entire continuum of care.

Traditional Patient Education

Traditionally, patient education has occurred through multisession, clinic-based programs between a healthcare provider or other educator and one or more patients. Given the logistics of attending on-site programs, it is not surprising that those who choose to participate are more motivated concerning their health than those who do not participate (LaVigne & Mushlin, 1997). However, it is just as important, if not more so, to reach the very large group of individuals who never receive specialized instruction about managing their health. The next section reviews what can be done to reach those who cannot or will not attend these traditional patient education programs.

Outreach Strategies

Fortunately, outreach methods, including mail and telephone interventions, are gaining acceptance as an alternative to traditional clinic-based approaches to communicate with large patient populations. Research has demonstrated that programs that have been conducted in face-to-face settings can be translated into phone and mail communications. Delivering primary care by phone has been shown to yield superior health status and decreased utilization compared with usual clinic-based care in elderly patients (Wasson et al., 1992).

Automated Strategies

In addition, technology allows these outreach strategies to be automated, so communication can be individually tailored to the patient without requiring a live conversation with a healthcare provider. Figure 8–3 depicts the integration of the positive features of traditional clinical approaches with the efficiencies of public health strategies. Given the limited human resources in today's healthcare settings, automation is an essential way to communicate with large numbers of people, while deploying staff to patients who need more intensive evaluation and care.

Using theories such as the Transtheoretical Stage of Change previously described, mail-based programs tailored via

FIGURE 8-3

Integrated Strategies for Disease Management

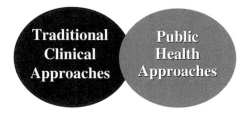

- Individualized care
- Practice guidelines
- Stepped-care
- Provider influence

- Accessibility
- Convenience
- Outreach strategies
- Automation

"demand-publishing" technology yield individualized documents that can be designed to deliver the same type of personalized patient-education messages as a healthcare provider would give in person. Phone contacts can be automated through interactive voice response—ranging from simple reminder messages to more complex, logic-based clinical interview and feedback sessions—to mimic the live interchange that occurs in traditional clinical encounters. Rapidly emerging research has demonstrated that automated phone interventions are both acceptable and effective for reaching and influencing patients across varied therapeutic areas, ranging from immunization reminders to comprehensive disease management initiatives for chronic illnesses (LaVigne & Tapper, 1998). Additional research will serve to identify the most appropriate way to enhance patient care through the combined use of automated and live clinical encounters.

Computer-Based Strategies

Finally, as computer access has grown, health information resources have been widely developed for software and online applications. A Harris poll of more than 1,000 consumers, conducted in January 1999, indicates that as many as 60 million Americans used the Internet in 1998 to obtain health information. One of the few controlled studies of Web-based patient resources showed improvements in quality of life and health service use among users of a breast cancer information and support Web site (Comprehensive Health Enhancement Support System) (Gustafsen et al., 1999). There is a critical need for further research on healthcare applications through the Internet so that the extensive resources being dedicated to this area can be directed to maximize patient outcomes.

A Caveat

The promise of communications technologies for population-based healthcare is tremendous. However, it is important to note that identification of patients is a rate-limiting step in the delivery of any healthcare intervention and, therefore, in the realization of improved outcomes. Even if there is widespread publicity regarding availability of disease management programs, self-referral attracts more highly motivated and severely affected patients. Provider referral creates an unpredictable stream of participants drawn only from patients who are identified as appropriate by healthcare providers. Identification of patients through a database theoretically provides the greatest opportunity to reach the target population. However, disease management programs identifying patients through database extraction have not yielded the anticipated number of patients, in large part because of inaccuracies in patient data (LaVigne & Mushlin, 1997). Analogous to the benefits offered by multimodal patient interventions, a combination of strategies for patient identification and recruitment may provide the greatest access to the target population.

What Kind of Improvement in Outcomes Should Be Expected from Patient-Focused Programs?

The ultimate challenge of any disease management program, particularly one involving significant patient-centered components, is that it must generally meet the burden of providing improved health outcomes and cost savings versus simply being cost-effective or offering a reasonable cost. As previously mentioned, multimodal disease management programs involving intensive clinician–patient communication generally show positive results, but most have not been evaluated for cost impact. Where cost outcomes have been examined, control groups have not typically been included.

For example, a retrospective analysis of a comprehensive diabetes care program, conducted by the Diabetes Treatment Centers of America (DTCA), reported improvements in the proportion of patients receiving care according to recommended clinical practice, as well as a $50 savings per diabetic per month in healthcare costs (Rubin, Dietrich, & Hawk, 1998). Similarly, the Lovelace EOC Program described previously showed improved asthma status, quality of life, and healthcare utilization (Marosi, Steismeyer, & Faculjak, 1998). Without a control group, however, the results of these programs may be suggestive of improved outcomes, but they are inconclusive.

Compared with multimodal disease management programs, controlled research including cost data has been conducted somewhat more extensively with the patient education component. Traditional, clinic-based patient education programs across a broad range of health-related conditions have demonstrated positive results in clinical, psychosocial, and cost outcomes. For example, in asthma management, clinician-led education programs have yielded savings in healthcare expenditures as high as $22.50 for every dollar spent (Bolton et al., 1991; Ghosh et al., 1998). Such figures may be generalized primarily to programs implemented among patients who are motivated to attend on-site sessions and who tend to have a moderate to severe disease.

Much like disease management programs, more recent patient-education programs using communication technology to reach broader populations have fewer examples of controlled evaluations involving cost data. A trial of an automated telephone call-in program for elderly patients versus "usual care" demonstrated improvements in medication adherence and blood pressure at a cost of $0.69 to $3.69 for each 1 mm Hg reduction in diastolic blood pressure (Friedman et al., 1996). However, there was no calculation of the impact on healthcare expenditures. In one of the first randomized controlled trials of an automated program that evaluated the cost impact, colleagues and

I evaluated an interactive asthma management program (CareSense for Asthma) administered to adults with a range of disease severity. The program was administered through interactive voice recognition phone calls and demand-published patient and physician mailings, which delivered communications based on nationally recommended practice guidelines and proven behavioral and motivational models, including those discussed in this chapter (Holt, Mushlin, & Roth, 1999). In addition to improvements in medication adherence, quality of life, motivation, disease status, and healthcare utilization, there was a savings of $7.83 in healthcare costs for each dollar spent on the program.

Empirical research has demonstrated that patient-centered strategies implemented within patient education programs and more comprehensive disease management initiatives enhance clinical and psychosocial outcomes. More recent research also suggests that these approaches can be effectively integrated in large-scale patient education programs delivered through communication technology. Further research is necessary to evaluate the effect of patient-focused strategies in a broader range of patient populations and healthcare settings. It is also critical that this research include evaluation of economic data to expand our understanding of the cost impact.

SUMMARY

Disease management, which has multiple definitions and components, is a recent development in healthcare treatment based on the fundamental elements of improving health outcomes while controlling healthcare costs. The shift toward consumer-centric disease management initiatives has been prompted by several factors, including increased accountability among healthcare organizations for patient-focused outcomes and satisfaction at the population level; increasing healthcare costs; and greater acceptance of the impact of behavioral factors on the management of chronic illness and health.

This chapter has described the consumer-centered aspects of disease management in terms of philosophy and logistics. As healthcare is shifting from the traditional biomedical model to the more recent biopsychosocial approach, there are key differences in the practice of medicine: (1) an emphasis on treatment of disease is counterbalanced with maintenance of overall health and wellness; (2) treatment targets the mind and body not as unrelated entities, but as interactive elements that combine with environmental factors to contribute to one's health; and (3) patients are proactive partners versus passive recipients of care. Just as the approach to treatment reflects a more comprehensive view of the patient and health, disease management outcomes extend beyond traditional clinical and economic measures to patient self-report data across a number of areas, including psychosocial variables and patient satisfaction.

This chapter also reviewed logistical issues surrounding the development and implementation of consumer-focused disease management initiatives. Behavioral science is helping healthcare professionals answer questions about how to change health behaviors. Motivational and behavioral concepts, such as self-efficacy (self-confidence), self-regulation (self-management), and stages of change (readiness to change), present viable models for assessing, educating, and reinforcing patients who are dealing with both short- and long-term treatment regimens. Research supports the impact of these strategies in patient education and disease management.

Another challenge in disease management is how to meet the mandate to affect entire patient populations representing the continuum of care. Clinic-based healthcare can serve only those who are able and willing to access on-site services, which tends to be those who are most motivated and more severely affected by health problems. Fortunately, there are promising research-derived results on the delivery of healthcare through outreach strategies such as phone and mail interventions. Communication technology and computers offer the promise of maximal patient reach and cost-efficiency. Automation through demand publishing, interactive voice recognition, and online services provides a way to integrate the best of individualized patient communication with the efficiencies of public health approaches. In large-scale consumer initiatives, a note of caution is necessary to temper expectations about patient access, given the difficulties of identifying the entire target population.

To design patient-education and disease management programs for a specific application, it is important to consider the research evidence concerning patient-focused strategies. Controlled studies have demonstrated the benefit of multimodal, clinic-based patient intervention programs for enhancing clinical and psychosocial outcomes. However, fewer data are available on the economic impact of these high-intensity programs. It seems intuitive that less intensive strategies, such as those using outreach and automation, would be a cost-efficient way to reach patients across the entire continuum of care. Initial experimental research suggests that computer-based interventions delivered by phone and mail can yield cost savings. Further outcomes evaluation and controlled research of disease management programs will play a vital role in facilitating the implementation of consumer-focused initiatives that provide maximal benefit to patients, healthcare providers, and payors while controlling healthcare costs.

REFERENCES

Bandura A. Self-efficacy: toward a unifying theory of behavioral change. *Psychological Review* 1977; 84:191–215.

Bolton MB, et al. The cost and effectiveness of an education program for adults who have asthma. *J Gen Intern Med* 1991; 6:401–407.

Boston Consulting Group Inc. *The contribution of pharmaceutical companies: what's at stake for America.* Boston: The Boston Consulting Group, 1993: 148.

Campbell MK, et al. Improving dietary behavior: the effectiveness of tailored messages in primary care settings. *Am J Public Health* 1994; 84:783–787.

Clark NM, et al. Patient and family management of asthma: theory-based techniques for the clinician. *J Asthma* 1994; 31:427–435.

DeBusk RF, et al. A case-management system for coronary risk factor modification after acute myocardial infarction. *Ann Intern Med* 1994; 120:721–729.

Engel GL. The need for a new medical model: a challenge for biomedicine. *Science* 1977; 196:129–136.

Epstein RS, Sherwood LM. From outcomes research to disease management: a guide for the perplexed. *Ann Intern Med* 1996; 124:832–837.

Feuerstein M, Labbe EE, Kuczmierczyk AR (eds). Historical perspective. In: *Health psychology: a psychobiological perspective*. New York: Plenum Press, 1986:11–26.

Friedman RH, et al. A telecommunications system for monitoring and counseling patients with hypertension: impact on medication adherence and blood pressure control. *AJH* 1996; 9:285–292.

Ghosh CS, et al. Reductions in hospital use from self-management training for chronic asthmatics. *Soc Sci Med* 1998; 46:1087–1093.

Glasgow RE. Compliance to diabetes regimens: conceptualization, complexity, and determinants. In Cramer JA, Spilker B (eds). *Patient compliance in medical practice and clinical trials*. New York: Raven Press, 1991.

Glasgow RE. A practical model of diabetes management and education. *Diabetes Care* 1995; 18:117–126.

Gouveia WA, et al. Paradigm for the management of patient outcomes. *Am J Hosp Pharm* 1991; 48:1912–1916.

Gustafsen D, et al. Impact of patient-centered, computer-based health information/support system. *Am J Prev Med* 1999; 16(1):1–9.

Holt K, Mushlin A, Roth S. *Improving health, quality and cost outcomes through communication technology: a case study in asthma*. Building Bridges V Research Conference: the health care puzzle using research to bridge the gap between perception and reality. Poster session abstracts: April 11–13, 1999. Jointly presented by the American Association of Health Plans (Washington, DC), the Agency for Health Care Policy and Research (Washington, DC), and the Centers for Disease Control and Prevention (Atlanta, GA).

Juniper EF, et al. Measuring quality of life in children with asthma. *Quality of Life Research* 1996; 5:35–46.

LaVigne M, Mushlin A. Patient identification and recruitment in disease management programs. *New Medicine* 1997; 1:209–217.

LaVigne M, Tapper KA. Interactive voice response in disease management. *Dis Manag Health Outcomes* 1998; 4:1–16.

Marosi A, Steismeyer JK, Faculjak PF. Setting up a multidisciplinary pediatric asthma Episodes of Care™: results from a 1-year study. *Dis Manage* 1998; 1:3–12.

National Asthma Education and Prevention Program. *Expert panel report II: guidelines for the diagnosis and management of asthma*. Bethesda, MD: National Institutes of Health publication, 1997: 97–4051.

National Committee for Quality Assurance. *Surveyor guidelines for the accreditation of managed care organizations.* Washington, DC: National Committee for Quality Assurance, 1998: 72–75.

National Committee for Quality Assurance. *Health plan employer data and information set 1999.* Washington, DC: National Committee for Quality Assurance, 1999.

National Heart, Lung, and Blood Institute. *Expert panel report I: guidelines for the diagnosis and management of asthma.* Bethesda, MD: National Institutes of Health publication, 1991: 91–3642.

National Managed Health Care Congress. *The disease management strategic research study & resource guide.* Waltham, MA: National Managed Health Care Congress, 1996: 7–8.

O'Leary A. Self-efficacy and health. *Behav Res Ther* 1985; 23:437–451.

Prochaska JO, et al. Standardized, individualized, interactive, and personalized self-help programs for smoking cessation. *Health Psychol* 1993; 12:399–405.

Prochaska JO, et al. Stages of change and decisional balance for 12 problem behaviors. *Health Psychol* 1994; 13:39–46.

Roter DL, et al. Effectiveness of interventions to improve patient compliance: a meta-analysis. *Med Care* 1998; 36:1138–1161.

Rubin RJ, Dietrich KA, Hawk AD. Clinical and economic impact of implementing a comprehensive diabetes management program in managed care. *J Clin Endocrinol Metab* 1998; 83:2635–2642.

Sullivan S, et al. National asthma education and prevention program working group report on the cost effectiveness of asthma care. *Am J Respir Crit Care Med* 1996; 154:S84-S95.

Ware JE, Kosinski M, Keller SD (eds). *SF-12: how to score the sf-12 physical and mental health summary scales,* 2nd ed. Boston: The Health Institute, New England Medical Center, 1995.

Wasson J, et al. Telephone care as a substitute for routine clinic follow-up. *JAMA* 1992; 267:1788–1793.

9

CHAPTER

The Drug Benefit: Design and Management

Tim R. Covington, M.S., Pharm.D.

INTRODUCTION

American society is in a period of unprecedented and rapidly accelerating change regarding how healthcare is financed and delivered. Turf wars are raging, pricing and cost sensitivity is acute, and competitiveness is intense. In this dynamic healthcare marketplace, many major forces are fostering constructive change: issues of value to payors, confidentiality of patient information, information management, consumer preferences, accreditation, credentialing, provider profiling, performance measurement, access to healthcare, and application of technology in the public interest.

Change in the healthcare delivery and financing system is being driven primarily by the process known as managed care. Managed care is often maligned, perhaps because selected insurers and other forms of managed care organizations (MCOs) have made some highly visible tactical errors driven by an overemphasis on cost reduction.

Managed care is thought by some to be a recent innovation. In reality, healthcare has been "managed" forever. In the past, healthcare providers (e.g., physicians, pharmacists, nurses) were the primary managers of healthcare; however, they imposed little accountability upon themselves. Medical and pharmaceutical accountability, in a fee-for-service environment, did not increase substantially until the mid-1970s. Healthcare accountability and fiscal and clinical management systems began to evolve rapidly in the late 1980s and early 1990s, as healthcare costs skyrocketed and annual expenditure growth rates were 10% or higher. Payors developed "sticker shock" and empowered fiscal managers to control cost escalation. Cost of care escalation slowed in the early and mid-1990s; quality of care received short shrift in some cases, but physician–patient care preferences were delivered and paid for 97% of the time.

The process of managed care is a complex system of interrelated procedures that seek to manage the delivery of high-quality healthcare in a cost-effective manner. Managed care now takes a more balanced view of the primary elements of healthcare—access, cost, and quality.

This balanced approach will be assured as ultimate payors (e.g., employers, Medicare, Medicaid) and individual consumers become more prudent purchasers of healthcare goods and services. Successful providers will be consumer-driven, customer (patient)-oriented, and payor-friendly. More balanced partnerships will replace traditional relationships in the patient–provider–payor triad. Value-based, cost-efficient, patient-focused, outcome-oriented healthcare is becoming the true, dominant differentiating denominator of success in the contemporary system of healthcare delivery and financing.

THE ROLE OF MODERN DRUG THERAPY IN MANAGING DISEASE

Informed and responsible consumerism in managing illness with drug therapy is needed. Healthcare providers and patients are often too casual about their drug therapy. Drug selection, use, and monitoring are often neglected. Drug therapy is often undervalued by patients, providers, and payors. Insurers and other models of managed care often view the drug benefit in its own distinct silo as a "cost center" and do not recognize how crucial it is in overall medical management.

Of the approximately $1.1 trillion annual healthcare expenditure, drug therapy consumes only 9% to 12% of the total. What is compelling, however, is the fact that 85% to 90% of patients with acute or chronic illness get well or have their chronic disease managed and its progression slowed with drug therapy. Most patients do not have their diseases managed solely by surgery, radiation therapy, acupuncture, chiropractic therapy, or herbal therapy. Prescription and nonprescription drug therapy is central to the management of most diseases. The return-on-investment (ROI) from drug therapy relative to healing, symptom management, quality of life, and reduction in consumption of other healthcare resources is vast.

Prudent payors of the nation's healthcare bills should be educated and encouraged to view the drug benefit and drug therapy in its proper context. The drug benefit and drug therapy management issues are pervasive and cross virtually all organizational, programmatic, and healthcare boundaries. Although the drug benefit and drug therapy require active management by payors, healthcare providers, and patients, they should not be viewed as components of healthcare to be manipulated and micromanaged in isolation.

Drug benefit management has tended to focus on overutilization and cost (Cassak, 1995; Covington, 1996; Gurnee, 1995). The simplistic and logically flawed approach to escalating drug expenditures by some fiscal managers has simply been to decrease utilization. Underutilization, as well as overutilization, of drug therapy is associated with great risk. The key is to intellectually empower and financially incentivize healthcare providers and patients to not underutilize or overutilize drug therapy, but rather to appropriately utilize drug therapy.

In-depth analysis of clinical and economic drug benefit management issues generally leads to the conclusion that proper investments in appropriate drug therapy and drug benefit management processes will ensure effective drug use and optimal health outcomes at a reasonable cost. Dividends from proper investments in the drug benefit and active cognitive involvement in drug benefit management processes by physicians, pharmacists, and patients are often seen in the medical component of healthcare. These drug therapy management dividends manifest themselves in a variety of ways, including the following:

- Fewer prescriptions issued
- Fewer trivial or follow-up office visits
- Decreased utilization of diagnostic/laboratory testing
- Fewer after-hours visits to emergency departments and ambulatory care centers
- Fewer hospitalizations
- Shorter hospitalizations
- Fewer nursing home admissions
- Improved occupational productivity
- Improved health status and quality of life
- Lower drug-associated morbidity and mortality rates

SYSTEM FAILURES IN DRUG BENEFIT MANAGEMENT

In stating that a properly managed drug benefit is perhaps the "best buy" in American healthcare, one must express appropriate caveats. The key phrase in the previous statement is "properly managed." How are the collective *we* (e.g., physicians, pharmacists, patients) doing in optimizing drug therapy in the disease management process? The answer is that *we* are not doing nearly as well as *we* should and could. *We* are not doing as well as *we* should and could in the drug selection, use, and monitoring process because prescribers, dispensers, and consumers of medication are not doing enough to ensure safe, appropriate, effective, and economical drug use.

A little-appreciated fact is that our nation spends approximately $2 managing the complications of drug therapy for every $1 we spend on drugs (Johnson & Bootman, 1995). Thus, we are spending approximately $200 billion annually managing problems associated with drug use. Many of the complications associated with drug overutilization, underutilization, misuse, and/or abuse are preventable if physicians, pharmacists, and patients would make fewer erroneous assumptions regarding what the other is doing, become more knowledgeable about the pharmacotherapy of prescription and nonprescription drugs, and communicate and partner more effectively with one another.

The following are but a few examples that illustrate the compelling need for higher levels of pharmaceutical care (Covington, 1996; Johnson & Bootman, 1995):

- Approximately 30% to 50% of the 2.8 to 3.0 billion prescriptions dispensed annually are taken incorrectly by the patient. These compliance errors manifest themselves as underutilization, which predisposes to therapeutic failure, or overutilization, which increases the probability of drug-induced toxicity.
- Approximately 7% to 10% of all new prescriptions are never presented to the pharmacist to be filled. This represents the ultimate noncompliance error.
- The annual direct cost of therapeutic noncompliance and subsequent therapeutic failure or drug-induced morbidity or mortality is estimated to be $70 billion to $90 billion per year. The indirect cost (e.g., lost productivity, lost wages) of therapeutic noncompliance is estimated to be at least $60 billion per year.
- The economic consequences of managing the complications of inappropriate or mismanaged drug therapy exceeds the annual cost of all diabetes care (more than $60 billion) and approaches the cost of managing all cardiovascular disease (approximately $150 to $190 billion annually).
- As many as 28% of all hospital admissions (more than 8.0 million per year), at a cost in excess of $50 billion annually, are attributed to drug-related morbidity.
- Approximately 10% to 20% of nursing home admissions (at an annual average cost per person, per year of $41,000 to $45,000) can be linked to failure to reliably manage medication use at home.
- Approximately 120 million physician office visits per year (more than 17% of all physician office visits), at an

annual cost of more than $10 billion, result from drug-induced problems.

- The strict compliance rate to prescribed antihypertensive drug therapy in patients diagnosed 3 years or more is only 32%. The damage associated with poor antihypertensive compliance (e.g., strokes, heart attacks, decreased kidney function, vision change) is vast.

- Of the 44% of Americans age 45 or older, 29% stop taking medication before it "runs out." This is a problem in managing any acute condition and is a particular problem in treating an infectious disease.

- Of antibiotic use in hospitals, 24% to 66% is either unnecessary or otherwise inappropriate as judged by expert panels of infectious disease physicians.

- Well over 25 million workdays are lost annually because of medical complications associated with noncompliance to prescribed drug therapy.

- Failure to take drugs properly results in 125,000 to 140,000 deaths annually in the United States. This mortality rate is approximately three times (300%) greater than the annual death rate from both breast cancer and prostate cancer. Breast cancer and prostate cancer awareness and treatment are national health priorities. Drug-induced deaths are not.

The strategic position of drug therapy in managing disease creates a moral, ethical, and professional imperative to develop new and improved methods and models for delivering health-care. New methods and models should emphasize patient-focused provision of drug therapy that involves not only effective drug distribution but also the provision of informational, intellectual, educational services designed to achieve positive health outcomes and improved quality of life.

Properly delivered pharmaceutical care is highly dependent on the physician, pharmacist, and patient working together as a team to accomplish the following (Hawkins, 1997; *Pharmaceutical Care*, 1997):

- Achieve safe, effective, appropriate, and economical drug use.
- Produce optimal therapeutic outcomes by achieving precision in drug therapy management.
- Deliver highly cognitive, problem-based, outcome-oriented drug therapy services by maximizing the benefit of drug therapy while operating to prevent, identify, and resolve drug-related problems and therapeutic misadventures.

COMMODITY COST-DRIVEN (FIRST-GENERATION) DRUG BENEFIT MANAGEMENT PROCESSES AND SYSTEMS

Management of the drug benefit in the contemporary healthcare system has evolved through two generations of sophistication. Most first-generation drug benefit management systems focus on reducing commodity costs and drug utilization rates. Efforts are directed toward purchasing drugs at the lowest possible cost, paying the pharmacist the lowest acceptable dispensing fee, fostering prudent generic drug utilization, encouraging compliance to the formulary or preferred drug list, limiting days supply or dosage units per defined period, and using the least expensive drug distribution system.

Components of commodity-based cost avoidance and cost minimization processes are easier to implement and administer than second-generation drug benefit management systems; thus, they are generally thoroughly developed before moving to the more sophisticated, clinically based, second-generation management systems. First-generation commodity-based cost reduction measures will, however, reach a point of diminishing returns if they are overly aggressive and insensitive to proper disease management and clinical outcomes. The "hassle factor" for healthcare providers and patients should not be overly restrictive because provider and patient relations may suffer. Insensitivity to reasonable provider and patient access to key drugs can cause medical and hospital costs to soar.

Mature insurers and the various models of MCOs (e.g., HMOs, PPOs) are approaching or have achieved the maximum commodity (drug) cost reductions that can be realized from first-generation drug benefit management processes. Selected examples of these processes are included in the following sections.

Prudent Purchasing and Contracting Strategies to Achieve Lowest Ingredient (Drug) Cost

Because most insurers/MCOs use a formulary or preferred group of drugs, they can determine (within limits) what drugs are prescribed by physicians. When this is done, the MCO can help increase the market share of a particular drug. This gives the pharmaceutical manufacturer of the formulary or preferred drug a competitive advantage. Under these circumstances, the pharmaceutical manufacturers of brand name drugs with high-profit margins are generally willing to contract to pay a rebate on the price of the drug to the plan (insurer/MCO). These rebates are usually based on performance, meaning the rebate percentage goes up as the market share or utilization rate of a particular drug within a plan goes up. Low utilization might produce a rebate of 2% to 3% on a drug. The percentage rebate may grow in percentage increments, or tiers, as utilization or market share within a drug class increases. For example, in the antidepressant category, if a contracted drug (e.g., Zoloft) had a 5% utilization rate in the plan, the rebate might be 2% to 4%. If utilization grew to 10%, the rebate might increase to 5%. A 20% utilization rate might warrant a 7% to 10% rebate. Higher utilization thresholds and rebates could also be negotiated.

Negotiating Discounts and Lowest Possible Dispensing Fees with the Pharmacy Provider Network

All insurers/MCOs use a network of pharmacy providers that meet certain credentialing criteria. Plans contract with independent and chain pharmacies to provide prescriptions at a predetermined rate of reimbursement. That rate of reimbursement is typically the average wholesale price (AWP) of the drug less a percentage of the AWP (discount), plus a dispensing fee. A typical reimbursement rate to a pharmacy is AWP less 10% to 14% plus a dispensing fee of $2.00 to $2.75. This allows a very small margin of profit per prescription for pharmacies and is becoming a serious issue between the profession of pharmacy and insurers/MCOs.

Applying Maximum Allowable Cost Pricing on Multisource (Generic) Drugs

Maximum allowable cost (MAC) is the maximum level of reimbursement a plan will pay for a particular generic drug. For example, if a particular generic drug was available from 12 different sources and the prices ranged from $9.00 to $14.00 per 100 dosage units, the plan might set the MAC at $12.00 per 100 dosage units ($0.12 per dosage unit). Any submitted charge above the MAC limit (plus dispensing fee) would be denied. Plans are careful not to set MAC prices too low because they want generic drug use to be as high as possible. In 1997, the average cost of a prescription filled with a generic drug was $16.04; the average cost of a prescription filled with a brand name product was $47.00. The $31.00 price difference between the average generic versus brand name prescription produces a powerful incentive to use high-quality generic drugs when appropriate.

Management of Formularies or Preferred Drug Lists

Management of formularies and preferred drug lists serves to (1) maximize generic drug utilization and (2) ensure a high degree of formulary/preferred drug list compliance to maximize performance-based rebates on brand name drugs (*AMCP Position Statement,* 1997; American Society of Hospital Pharmacists, 1992; Bailey & Ferro, 1998; Baskin, 1998; Carroll, 1999; Curtiss, 1996; *Formulary Management,* 1998; Jackson, 1997; Shornick, 1998; *Survey Reveals . . . ,* 1997; Ulmishek, 1998). Formularies and preferred drug lists are often maligned by prescribers and brand name pharmaceutical manufacturers, but they are a fundamental and essential drug benefit management tool. A formulary or preferred drug list is an ever-changing, limited list of drugs selected by an expert panel of healthcare practitioners, predominantly physicians and pharmacists, serving as members of an organizationally sanctioned Pharmacy and Therapeutics Committee, or its equivalent. This committee is carefully selected by the MCO and also recommends policy and procedures that protect the economic viability of providers and the MCO, create value for the payor, and serve the best health interest of patients.

Some drugs are much better than others. Without a formulary or preferred drug list, a plan would be obligated to pay for any of more than 6,000 prescription drugs available. A Pharmacy and Therapeutics Committee that deliberates objectively and places clinical considerations of drug safety and efficacy above cost considerations will serve patients well. All other things being equal (e.g., safety, efficacy), however, it makes no sense to pay a premium for the highest priced brand name drugs when lower-cost alternatives are available as either generic drugs or lower-cost brand name drugs. The formulary system fosters quality drug use at a reasonable cost with a minimum of external influence.

Providing Coverage of Selected Nonprescription (Over-the-Counter) Drugs as a Part of the Drug Benefit

More and more plans are paying for certain nonprescription drugs when the prescription drugs in the same pharmacological class offer little or no therapeutic advantage over the nonprescription version for certain uses. Many nonprescription drugs are powerful and effective therapeutic agents that were, until recently, available only with a prescription. The fact that a drug has moved from prescription to nonprescription status does not, in any way, devalue a drug or suggest it is any less effective. It simply means the drug has been proven safe enough to be made available to the general public without going to a physician for a prescription. Physicians can and do prescribe nonprescription drugs when appropriate.

Nonprescription drugs are highly effective in the management of scores of medical conditions. Some examples are headache, allergic rhinitis, nasal congestion, heartburn/dyspepsia, gastritis, indigestion, cough, fever, sprains, strains, myalgia, arthralgia, diabetes mellitus, vaginal candidiasis, acne, head lice, athlete's foot, superficial wounds, motion sickness, canker sores, cold sores, premenstrual syndrome (PMS), dysmenor-rhea, smoking cessation, nausea, and nutritional deficiencies. Nonprescription drugs, at an average cost of $7.00 to $10.00 per package unit, represent a very-low-cost alternative to pre-scription drugs, and particularly brand name prescription drugs.

Implementing Prior Authorization Procedures for Nonformulary or Nonpreferred Drugs

Just because a drug is not on a formulary or preferred drug list does not mean it cannot be a covered benefit paid for by the plan. A formulary system or prior authorization program is not designed to usurp the physician's prescribing prerogatives or de-prive patients of necessary drug therapy. The prior authoriza-tion process is simply a method of ensuring that certain nonfor-mulary or nonpreferred drug use is medically justified (Smalley et al., 1996). It is a form of prescriber accountability. A pre-scriber has to assure a plan that the patient and the medical sit-uation meet predetermined clinical criteria of the prior autho-rization program. If those criteria are met, the plan will generally pay for the requested nonformulary/nonpreferred drug less predetermined co-payments and deductibles.

Limiting Days' Supply of Prescribed Medication

Many medical conditions are acute and self-limited. For an MCO to pay for a 30-day supply of a prescription medication to manage a medical condition whose symptoms will last for only hours to a few days is wasteful, inefficient, and clinically and economically irresponsible. Examples of clinical situa-tions in which the days' supply per prescription may be lim-ited include injury associated pain (e.g., sprains, strains), nausea and vomiting associated with viral gastroenteritis, symptoms associated with viral upper respiratory infections, situational anxiety or insomnia, episodic heartburn, cough, fever, and superficial infections.

Establishing Maximum Units Per 30-Day Period for Selected Drugs

Seldom do individuals require dosages of prescription medication that exceed the upper limit of the daily dosage range published in the package labeling (package insert) and approved by the FDA. Through electronic edits at the point-of-sale (the pharmacy), an MCO has an opportunity to alert pharmacists that the maximum number of dosage units prescribed per 30-day period has been exceeded. A "hard edit" would require an intervention by the pharmacist or the MCO to explore with the prescriber the clinical circumstances as to why the prescription request for preestablished maximum units was exceeded. These circumstances are evaluated against predetermined clinical criteria. If medical justification is appropriate, the drug is dispensed in a quantity above the maximum. If medical justification is not adequate, the prescription is dispensed at the level of the predetermined maximum.

Increasing Coinsurance through Variable Co-Payments and Deductibles

Co-payment and deductible strategies are designed to shift a reasonable degree of cost awareness and responsibility to the patient. Drug benefit deductibles range from $50 to hundreds of dollars per year. Employers are beginning to realize that with escalating healthcare costs, low deductibles and co-payments do not generally provide an adequate financial risk or disincentive to patients to prevent them from overusing healthcare goods and services. For example, a $10 patient co-payment on a $120 prescription rarely causes a flinch on the part of the patient. If patients do not appreciate drug cost issues, they will seldom ask for or allow use of lower cost, but therapeutically equivalent, generic alternatives. Recent drug benefit design innovation is focused more on the co-payment structure than on the deductible structure. The three-tiered co-payment structure is evolving as an industry standard. This co-payment structure requires the lowest co-payment (e.g., $5 to $10) for multisource (generic) prescriptions, an intermediate co-payment (e.g., $15 to $25) for prescriptions filled with formulary or preferred brand name drugs, and a high co-payment (e.g., $35 to $50) for prescriptions filled with nonformulary or nonpreferred brand name drugs. If the cost of the prescription is less than the co-payment, the patient assumes full responsibility for the cost of the prescription.

As drug costs and utilization escalate, and nonprescription (OTC) drugs are being added as a covered benefit, a five-tiered co-payment structure may evolve. A likely scenario is projected below.

Drug Group	Projected Patient Co-Payment Range
Covered nonprescription (OTC) drug generated by a physician prescription	$0 per prescription
Multisource (generic) prescription	$5 to $10 per prescription
Formulary or preferred prescription filled with a brand name drug	$15 to $25 per prescription
Nonformulary or nonpreferred prescription filled with a brand name drug	$35 to $50 per prescription
Ultra high cost (e.g., $150 to $1000 per prescription or per month of therapy) in formulary, nonformulary, preferred or nonpreferred status	30% to 70% of total prescription cost

There is a limit to what healthcare benefits employers and other payors can afford. Shared financial responsibility with the patient will assist in preserving broad-based healthcare benefits and the crucial drug benefit.

Engaging in Retrospective Drug Utilization Review Activity to Detect Misutilization of Drug Therapy

A review of aggregate, prescriber-specific and patient-specific drug utilization patterns is very helpful in detecting drug overutilization, underutilization, and otherwise inappropriate use (Covington, 1993; *Drug use evaluation,* 1999; Klink, 1998;

McGuffy, 1998). Drug utilization norms are established and can be woven into the claims adjudication process. Edits, which address issues such as early refills, late refills, duplicated prescriptions, and drug interactions, can be addressed by the pharmacist before the prescription is dispensed. This quality assurance process fosters appropriate prescribing and drug therapy monitoring.

Providing Alternative Channels of Drug Distribution at Lower Cost

Mail-order drug distribution via pharmacy benefit management (PBM) companies, traditional MCOs, or Internet pharmacies is a cost-effective drug distribution channel for providing chronic maintenance medications to ambulatory patients. Automation, purchasing power, and other economies of scale increase the cost-competitiveness of mail-order pharmacies. MCOs may offer a variety of co-payment incentives to patients to encourage use of mail-order drug distribution when appropriate. For example, patients may be required to pay only one or two co-payments for a 3-month (90-day) supply or one co-payment for a 2-month (60-day) supply. Mail-order pharmacy continues to grow at the expense of traditional community pharmacy-based drug distribution.

Providing Financial Incentives to Medical and Pharmacy Providers to Assist in Drug Benefit Management Strategies

The managed care industry has not been overly creative in engaging physicians and pharmacists in a true partnership with patients and the MCO to optimize the safe, appropriate, effective, and economical use of drug therapy (Allawi, 1997; Covington, 1998; Dillabough, 1997; Findlay, 1996; Kalies, 1995). Most strategies have been more punitive (e.g., physician profiling, physician capitation, physician withholds, low compensation of pharmacist providers) than collaborative. Pharmacists assist MCOs in meeting drug benefit management goals (e.g., optimal generic drug utilization, formulary compliance, drug utilization review [DUR] edits) by interpreting, enforcing, and communicating MCO policy and procedures to both physicians and patients. These services are provided by pharmacists in an environment of declining reimbursement involving greater percentage discounts off the average wholesale price of prescription drugs and lower dispensing fees.

Physicians and pharmacists can and should be financially incentivized by MCOs with reasonable professional fees, rebate sharing, and/or a percentage of the savings that inure to the MCO from particular actions (e.g., conversion from brand to generic prescription drug, conversion from nonformulary to formulary drug, detection of duplicated prescriptions from multiple prescribers, conversion from prescription to nonprescription [OTC] drug). The lack of proper financial incentives for healthcare providers deters the provision of optimal pharmaceutical care.

Miscellaneous Commodity-Based Cost-Avoidance and Cost-Minimization Strategies

Three other cost-containment strategies focus on drug utilization. These are fraught with a great deal of risk relative to clinical outcomes and include the following:

- Capping payment of prescriptions per patient per month at a defined number of prescriptions
- Limiting prescriptions per beneficiary per year
- Capping the drug benefit at a certain dollar amount per patient per year

In highly visible situations in which these strategies have been applied, they have failed. In most cases, when drug coverage is inappropriately restricted, medical costs (e.g., office visits, emergency room visits, hospitalizations, length of hospitalizations) have increased greatly. Medical and pharmaceutical needs within a given month or year cannot be predicted. Excessive constraint on the drug benefit is generally a false economy.

HEALTH OUTCOMES–DRIVEN (SECOND-GENERATION) DRUG BENEFIT MANAGEMENT PROCESSES AND SYSTEMS

Once first-generation, commodity-based cost-avoidance and cost-minimization processes have been implemented and refined, MCOs generally direct attention and resources to clinically focused, intellectually based, health outcomes–oriented drug benefit management processes. Many health economists believe that far greater financial and clinical dividends can be achieved through cognitive interventions and the clinically driven achievement of optimal health outcomes than from focusing on commodity (drug)-based cost and utilization reductions, although both strategies are appropriate and deserve time and resources.

Selected examples of health outcomes–driven drug benefit management processes and systems are included in the following sections.

Disease-Specific Outcomes Management Activity

There are many components to a comprehensive disease management program, and successful delivery involves not only the physician but also other healthcare providers (e.g., pharmacists, nurses) and the patient (*Disease state management,* 1997; Greengold, 1998; MacKinnon, 1998). Drug therapy is central to most disease management programs.

Most contemporary disease management initiatives focus on high-cost chronic diseases with measurable endpoints so that the value of therapeutic interventions can be more easily assessed. Disease management initiatives usually include, but are not limited to, the following medical conditions:

- Asthma
- Diabetes mellitus
- Congestive heart failure
- Depression
- Hyperlipidemia
- Hypertension
- Migraine

A thorough presentation of disease-specific outcomes management methodologies is beyond the scope of this chapter.

Prudent Use of Practice Guidelines, Critical Pathways, or Treatment Algorithms

Use of these "best practices" tools is highly complementary of disease-specific outcomes management initiatives (Berg, Atkins, & Tierney, 1997; Hlatky, 1995; Shaneyfelt, Mayo-Smith, & Rothwangl, 1999). Scores of sanctioned practice guidelines and treatment protocols are available. The universal and complete application of such guidelines is arguable, however.

Physicians, pharmacists, case managers, and other providers of healthcare goods and services often view the algorithmic approach to disease management, which uses branching logic, to be "cookbook" medicine. Some believe that overreliance on treatment algorithms and protocols precludes adequate consideration of "shades of gray" and the near-infinite confounding factors associated with co-morbidities, polypharmacy, and biological variability of the species.

Although valuable in many instances, organizationally sanctioned practice guidelines and their "cousins" (e.g., critical pathways, treatment algorithms) cannot substitute for human logic, unique patient factors, and clinical judgment. Furthermore, the clinician must always be mindful of the currency of the guidelines. Although valuable tools, overdependence on such guides is generally discouraged.

Appropriate Use of Provider Profiling Methodology

Provider profiling is often referred to as "report carding." Reliable provider profiling requires good computer technology and information systems. The most sophisticated provider profiling systems integrate pharmacy claims data with medical claims data and evaluate the impact and value of certain medical and pharmaceutical interventions. Most MCOs, however, currently possess information systems of intermediate sophistication and capability. Therefore, most of today's provider profiling focuses on drug utilization by physician prescribers.

Individual physician prescribing patterns are evaluated and compared with peer prescribing patterns and drug utilization norms of the MCO. Items often evaluated using the pharmacy claims database are average per member per month (PMPM) drug charges, generic drug utilization rate, and formulary compliance rate. Medical claims data can profile a physician relative to such things as frequency of patient office visits, cost per patient for diagnostic laboratory testing, patient emergency room visits, patient hospitalizations, and length of patient hospitalizations. An interface of medical claims data with pharmacy claims data can evaluate the efficacy, or lack thereof, of certain drug therapies relative to clinical outcomes.

Patient populations must be stratified by disease types, degree of acuity, expense of therapies, co-morbidities, and other clinical factors to correct for adverse selection (i.e., a disproportionately high number of "sicker" patients). After all population-based adjustments are made, physicians who are considered outliers relative to drug utilization will likely be targeted by the MCO for education and other interventions designed to change prescribing behavior to more appropriate drug therapies.

Provision of Provider Education

Provider education is also referred to as academic detailing. As with provider profiling, provider education focuses on the prescribing practices of individual physicians who fall sufficiently outside of established prescribing norms (Frazier et al., 1991; Henahan, 1991; Shulkin, 1994; Stern, 1996). Provider education relative to drug therapy tends to be highly educational and nonpunitive. Provider educators from the MCO create a communication stream on relevant matters of pharmacotherapy with prescribers. The focus is often on drug therapy options and "best practices." Issues such as generic drug utilization, compliance with the formulary or preferred drug list, appropriate use of practice guidelines or their equivalent, and compliance with health management and case management strategies and priorities of the MCO are often presented for consideration. Communication may occur via fax, e-mail, telephone or face-to-face communication. Prescribing behavior changes are usually positive from both a clinical-outcomes and cost-of-care perspective.

Use of Prospective Drug Utilization Review Processes and Systems

DUR is a criteria-based ongoing, planned, organizationally authorized, systematic process for monitoring and evaluating the prophylactic, therapeutic, and empiric use of drugs to ensure that they are prescribed and used safely, appropriately, effectively, and economically (Covington, 1993; *Drug use evaluation,* 1999; Klink, 1998; McGuffy, 1998). The goal of DUR is to optimize clinical outcomes with drug therapy. Prospective drug utilization is a very valuable quality-of-care process. Prospective DUR should occur before the patient consumes the first dose of prescribed medication.

Prospective DUR requires application of information technology that allows certain criteria and edits to be visualized in the pharmacy where the prescription is presented. The focus of prospective DUR is detection of drug overutilization and/or underutilization (e.g., dosage, quantity dispensed, frequency of dose, interval between prescriptions, duration of therapy) and/or inappropriate drug therapy (i.e., appropriate indications are met, contraindications to drug use, patient risk factors, age criteria, gender considerations, concurrent drug use that may lead to drug–drug interactions). Prospective DUR is not generally used to the full extent technologically possible. This is primarily because MCOs have not demonstrated the willingness to compensate pharmacists who are positioned to enforce drug use criteria and take the labor-intensive action necessary to contact prescribers, explore clinical circumstances, and remediate prescribing deficiencies. Pharmacists provide some DUR services to MCOs *gratis.* These usually involve early and late refills, duplicated prescriptions, and drug–drug interactions; DUR services provided by pharmacists that go beyond these would generally require additional compensation.

Provision of Disease-Specific Case Management Services

Optimal use of drug therapy is a core element of a successful case management program. MCO-based case management is generally directed toward a defined population of high-cost, high-risk patients (e.g., transplant recipients, cancer patients, dialysis patients, AIDS patients, elderly patients with advanced stages of multiple diseases) (*Disease state management,* 1997; Greengold, 1998; MacKinnon, 1998). Supplemental patient management designed to ensure optimal health outcomes is generally viewed as cost-effective.

Provision of Patient Education on Prescribed Drug Therapy in the Pharmacy

Patient education and counseling by a pharmacist regarding prescribed drug therapy is obligatory for Medicaid patients under the provisions of OBRA-90, and the offer to counsel all patients about their prescription drugs is generally a provision of individual state pharmacy practice regulations. This represents another "unfunded mandate" for the pharmacist, but the argument that patient education and counseling by the pharmacist is a core professional responsibility is compelling. In fact, since 1990, the pharmacy profession has responded favorably to patient education and counseling expectations, both through verbal and print communication. The pharmaceutical care movement, which focuses on nondistributive, cognitive professional functions in pharmacy, is contributing substantially to improved patient care without imposing significant cost-of-care increases on the healthcare system.

Miscellaneous Health Outcomes–Driven Drug Benefit Management Services

In the section of this chapter addressing system failures in drug benefit management, it is obvious that *patient nonadherence / noncompliance* to prescribed drug therapy is an extremely significant clinical and economic public health dilemma (Bates, 1998; Berg et al., 1993; Jackson, 1997; Meade, 1996; Murphy & Coster, 1997; Rogers & Ruffin, 1998). Patient comments such as "I stop taking the prescription when I start feeling better," "I cannot afford the medication," or "I take it only when I need it" are often associated with minor, moderate, severe, and even fatal health consequences.

A host of factors contribute to therapeutic noncompliance by patients, but two of the most important are (1) patients do not adequately understand their disease and (2) if they do not adequately understand their disease, they tend to not understand the importance of their drug therapy. Achievement of higher levels of patient adherence to prescribed drug therapy should become a national health priority. Aggressive health policy at the state and national levels is needed to address non-compliance/nonadherence issues. The keys to success are (1) enhanced recognition of this problem by healthcare providers, payors, and patients and (2) educational initiatives focused on patients that assist them in better understanding their diseases and the importance of their drug therapy. This job belongs to all healthcare providers, payors, insurers, MCOs, and public health enterprises. MCOs are strategically positioned to coordinate drug therapy compliance initiatives.

Another key drug benefit management service involves monitoring for *drug-induced adverse effects*. The system failures section of this chapter reveals clearly that consequences associated with drug therapies can produce profound morbidity, requiring physician office visits or hospitalizations. Because the positive side of drugs is so heavily marketed by the pharmaceutical industry with four-color print ads in medical, pharmacy, and lay publications, and direct-to-consumer ads in print and electronic formats, the "dark side" of drugs often goes underappreciated.

All drugs should be viewed as "two-edged swords" with the potential to not only do great good but also inflict substantial harm under certain biological or behavioral circumstances. If healthcare professionals would review the pharmaceutical package insert periodically, their index of suspicion regarding the adverse effects of drugs would be enhanced. This needs to occur. Aside from the brief indications section of drug package labeling, most of the text addresses negative or precautionary elements (e.g., contraindications; warnings; risk factors; adverse effects; drug interactions; special considerations in administration and dosing the drug in light of factors such as age, pregnancy status, lactation, renal function, liver function, co-existing or previous pathologic condition).

The adverse drug reaction dilemma, like the noncompliance/nonadherence dilemma, cannot be adequately addressed in isolation by one group. Adverse drug reaction monitoring and management is a collective responsibility of healthcare providers, payors, and patients. MCOs, serving as coordinators of care, can be leaders in fostering policy development, educational initiatives, and behavioral changes in healthcare providers that will minimize the risk and consequences of drug-induced adverse effects.

THE DRUG BENEFIT: ADMINISTRATIVE AND PAYMENT PROCESSES

Healthcare providers, payors, and others must be knowledgeable about the intricacies of drug benefit design, administrative procedures, and payment processes. Contracts with MCOs must be balanced appropriately between quality of care and cost of care. Premiums charged by insurers/MCOs and payments made to providers for services rendered must be fair and equitable. Negotiations between providers and payors are critically important. Both macroissues and microissues must be thoroughly addressed by both parties.

Selected administrative and payment processes related to the drug benefit have been addressed piecemeal throughout this chapter. A brief summary of their various components follows.

Administrative Services

Administration of the drug benefit is complex, largely because so many healthcare transactions are involved in its delivery. Administrative services address (1) developing the pharmacy provider network and (2) contracting with and coordinating the activity of the pharmacy provider network. Elements of these services are included below (Covington, 1996; *The Essential Guide . . . ,* 1994):

Provider Network Development

- Establish pharmacy and pharmacist eligibility criteria.
- Recruit the pharmacy provider network.

- Contract with the pharmacy provider network.
- Advise enrollees of the availability of the pharmacy provider network.

Note: The size and type of the pharmacy provider network will depend on the nature of the insurer/MCO and patient preferences.

Provider Network Contracting and Coordination

A network of qualified pharmacy providers should be sufficient to provide convenient access for insured patients. Drug benefit management elements to be contracted and coordinated may include the following:

- Definitions of contract terminology
- Confidentiality provisions
- Criteria for enrollee eligibility
- Claims submission and adjudication procedures
- Provisions for auditing pharmacy records
- Scope of the drug benefit
- Limitations of the drug benefit
- Exclusions from the drug benefit
- Pharmacist education provisions
- Patient education provisions
- Provider education provisions
- Co-payment/co-insurance provisions
  - Enrollee deductibles
  - Enrollee co-payments
  - Out-of-network service and payment provisions
  - Enrollee drug benefit limits
- Pharmacy reimbursement provisions
  - Assignment provisions
  - Basis for ingredient cost (e.g., average wholesale price [AWP], wholesale acquisition cost [WAC], estimated allowable cost [EAC], maximum allowable cost [MAC])
  - Discount off ingredient cost
  - Dispensing fee
  - Differential fees for cognitive services

- Capitation provisions (if any)
- Timeliness of payment to pharmacy
- Pharmacy performance incentives
  - Formulary compliance
  - Generic utilization rate
  - Per member per month cost reduction
  - Prior authorization intervention
  - Maximum units and days' supply intervention
  - Drug utilization review activity
  - Compliance services
  - Adverse drug reaction monitoring
  - Disease management services
  - Patient-specific case management services

Once a contract is executed between the MCO and the provider network, pharmacy services may be rendered to eligible patients. Some of the services just listed may be subcontracted or outsourced by the MCO to an administrative services organization (ASO) or its equivalent. Self-insured employers may choose to provide and manage administrative elements of the drug benefit themselves.

Payment Processes

Pharmacy reimbursement provisions are addressed in the contracting process (see previous discussion) (Findlay, 1996; Kalies, 1995; *The Essential Guide . . . ,* 1994). The pharmacy provider universe, as a whole, has not been highly sophisticated or aggressive in negotiating payment for pharmaceutical goods and services. This has produced significant erosion in what MCOs pay for a prescription. Pharmacy profit margins have slipped substantially. Cost shifting by pharmacy from a third-party payor to uninsured private-pay patients is no longer feasible as the private-paying population is shrinking and the uninsured are often indigent and unable to pay.

Capitation is receiving considerable attention as a payment vehicle in several parts of the United States. This financial risk-sharing arrangement between patient and provider, which provides a fixed payment for a defined set of services, usually paid monthly and in advance on a per capita or per beneficiary basis, adds new meaning to the term *risk*. Healthcare providers should thoroughly understand that fee-for-service and capitation are at the two extreme ends of the provider payment spectrum. In a fee-for-service payment environment, the temptation for the provider is to overutilize patient care goods and services to maximize revenue and profit. Fixed-dollar capitation can produce the temptation to underutilize patient care goods and services to maximize revenue and profit.

In the current environment, the drug benefit is not typically capitated as a stand-alone service. When the medical benefit is capitated, it usually includes the drug benefit. This arrangement fosters collaboration between the physician and pharmacy provider networks because drug therapy is one of the most significant components of effective disease management and optimal health outcomes. Interventions focused on quality of care and optimal health outcomes are crucial to financial success in capitated arrangements.

Capitation of the drug benefit in isolation to the pharmacy provider network is extremely high risk for the following reasons:

- Pharmacists have limited control over the demand, use, and cost of services they provide because the physician typically generates the prescription.
- Financial risk is greatly increased by adverse selection.
- The MCO may not have developed processes, systems, and services that are appropriately focused on improving health outcomes or controlling drug utilization at reasonable levels.
- Pharmacists may reduce time-consuming patient interventions if capitation is linked to drug cost reduction only.
- Pharmacists will have difficulty managing patient care and financial risk if patients change pharmacies on a whim.
- The MCO or pharmacy provider network may not have set aside adequate reserves or purchased adequate reinsurance to cover possible financial losses.

- If appropriate risk corridors are not negotiated and
  established between the MCO and the pharmacy
  provider network in order to limit losses to a fixed
  percentage of actual losses (e.g., 5%, 10%, 15%), the
  pharmacy provider network could be held liable for the
  full loss experienced under a capitated contract.

Contracting always favors the side that has clearly defined
goals and objectives, sophistication regarding how all moving
parts of healthcare delivery and financing articulate with one
another, operational and financial maturity, and advanced negotiating skills. Providers, on the road to becoming prudent contracting entities, have signed many contracts with MCOs that
are unfavorable to providers. Parity in contracting knowledge
and skill between MCOs and providers is emerging but continues to require vigilance and high understanding of all facets
of healthcare delivery and financing. In the information age, one
"wins" by being smarter.

CONCLUSION

Healthcare will grow increasingly complex over time. Issues of
technology application—access to care; quality of care; information management; confidentiality of health information; limits
on healthcare coverage by employers, government, and other ultimate payors; role reconstruction of healthcare providers; coordination of care; and affordability of healthcare—will dominate
thinking. Pressures will increase to further "manage" or coordinate healthcare.

True management of healthcare requires responsible behavior and accountability for that behavior by all those involved
in the delivery and receipt of healthcare. The three most vital
"players" in a contemporary and efficient system of healthcare delivery and financing are value-based ultimate purchasers/payors
of healthcare goods and services, providers of healthcare goods
and services (e.g., physicians, hospitals, pharmacists), and patients themselves.

These groups, their primary interests, and the public interest are poorly coordinated today. Nowhere is coordination of

care and shared accountability more critical than with the drug benefit. Prescription and nonprescription drugs are often overutilized, misused, and/or abused. These powerful chemicals can do great good when properly prescribed and used; they can also produce substantial harm when improperly prescribed and/or misused by the patient. Furthermore, drug therapy is expensive and often unnecessarily so. As emphasized earlier, the cost of managing the complications associated with inappropriately prescribed or utilized drug therapy is approaching $200 billion per year.

Despite a host of drug therapy dilemmas and therapeutic misadventures, the drug benefit holds the greatest promise of all the high-cost components of healthcare to be effectively managed. Many tools for efficiently and effectively managing the drug benefit are presented in this chapter, and others are available. These processes and systems need to be more fully understood and implemented. Employers and HCFA (Medicare, Medicaid), as ultimate payors of approximately 80% of the nation's healthcare bill, should consider or require the effective utilization of many of the processes and systems presented in this chapter when contracting with their HMO, PPO, Blue Cross/Blue Shield plan, network of physicians, or whatever entity is contracted to manage/deliver/coordinate healthcare.

Finally, patients need to more fully appreciate their role in managing illness. They are often in the final position to determine whether a therapy, particularly drug therapy, will produce the optimal positive health outcome. If drugs are overutilized or underutilized, the health consequences can be extremely negative. Patient responsibility in the tripartite arrangement involving ultimate payor, healthcare providers, and the patient produces a phenomenally powerful synergy that has not yet been achieved on a large scale or consistent basis.

Change characterizes healthcare over the previous decade. Healthcare delivery and financing periodically morphs into new forms. This change reflects, more fully than ever, that the drug benefit is a primary component of healthcare, is not to be delivered casually, and requires active management. This chapter attempts to place the drug benefit in its proper context and describe and define key elements of the drug benefit management process.

REFERENCES

Allawi SJ. Five irresistible forces. *Healthcare Forum Journal* 1997; 40(1):48–51.

AMCP Position Statement. Formularies. Alexandria, VA: Academy of Managed Care Pharmacy. 1997.

American Society of Hospital Pharmacists. ASHP guidelines on formulary system management. *Am J Hosp Pharm* 1992; 49:648–652.

Bailey M, Ferro K. Innovative drugs formulary management through computer-assisted protocols. *J Managed Care Pharm* 1998; 4:246–252.

Baskin L. Pharmacoeconomics and the formulary decision-making process. *Formulary* 1998; 33:459–466.

Bates DW. Drugs and adverse drug reactions—how worried should we be? *JAMA* 1998; 279:1216–1217.

Berg AO, Atkins D, Tierney W. Clinical practice guidelines in practice and education. *J Gen Intern Med* 1997; 12(Suppl 2):525–533.

Berg JS, et al. Medication compliance: a healthcare problem. *Ann Pharmacother* 1993; 27(suppl):2–19.

Carroll NV. Formularies and therapeutic interchange: the health care setting makes a difference. *Am J Health Syst Pharm* 1999; 56:467–472.

Cassak D. Pharmacy benefit management's second generation. In vivo. *Bus Med Rep* 1995; 13:48–57.

Covington TR. Drug use evaluation for managed care. *Pharm Ther* 1993; 18:225–226, 236–242.

Covington TR. Healthcare megatrends for strategic thinkers. *DrugLink* 1998; 4:31.

Covington TR. The pharmacy benefit: trends and issues in healthcare delivery and financing. The Mylan Institute of Pharmacy. *Continuing Education Series* 1996; 2:1–15.

Curtiss FR. Drug formularies provide a path to best care. *Am J Health Syst Pharm* 1996; 53:2201–2203.

Dillabough EM. Managed care and pharmacy practice: are they compatible. *AACP District III annual meeting.* 1997.

Disease state management. Academy of Managed Care Pharmacy. Concepts in managed care. Second in a series. 1997.

Drug use evaluation. Academy of Managed Care Pharmacy. Concepts in managed care pharmacy. Fifth in a series. 1999.

Findlay S. Can capitation save the world? *Bus Health* 1996; 14:44–55.

Formulary management. Academy of Managed Care Pharmacy. Concepts in managed care pharmacy. Third in a series. 1998.

Frazier LM, et al. Can physician education lower the cost of prescription drugs? A prospective, controlled trial. *Ann Intern Med* 1991; 115:116–121.

Greengold NL. *Disease state management: Strategies for continuous improvement.* Annenberg Center for Health Sciences at Eisenhower and Glaxo Wellcome Inc. Monograph. 1998.

Gurnee M. The evolution of pharmacy benefit management. *Managed Care Pharmacy Practice* 1995; 38–45.

Hawkins PR. The pharmacist as a health education coordinator. *Am J Health Syst Pharm* 1997; 54:1497–1499.

Henahan S. Kaiser educates M.D.s and reduces pharmacy costs. *Drug Top* 1991; 135:56.

Hlatky MA. Patient preferences and clinical guidelines. *JAMA* 1995; 273:1219–1220.

Jackson RA. Practice guidelines, physician groups and drug formularies. *J Managed Care Pharm* 1997; 3:489–492.

Johnson JA, Bootman JL. Drug-related morbidity and mortality: Cost-of-illness model. *Arch Intern Med* 1995; 155:1949–1956.

Kalies RF. Reimbursement in the managed care era: Placing a value on pharmaceutical care. Applied Communications Inc. and Roche Laboratories. *Continuing Education Series.* 1995.

Klink B. Utah Medicaid DUR program proves effective cost-saver. *Drug Top* 1998; 142:54.

MacKinnon NJ. A systems approach to the evaluation of a disease state management program. *Formulary* 1998; 33:769–770, 775–778, 787–788.

McGuffy EC. Computerized DUR alerts: Boon or bane to pharmaceutical care? *J Am Pharm Assn* 1998; 38:122, 124.

Meade V. Expanding pharmacy's role to reduce drug-related problems. *Q Lett* 1996; 8:1–11.

Murphy J, Coster G. Issues in patient compliance. *Drugs* 1997; 54:797–800.

Pharmaceutical Care. Academy of Managed Care Pharmacy. Concepts in managed care pharmacy. First in a series. 1997.

Rogers PT, Ruffin DM. Medication non adherence—part I: the health and humanistic consequences. *Managed Care Interface* 1998; 11:58–60.

Shaneyfelt TM, Mayo-Smith MF, Rothwangl J. Are guidelines following guidelines? The methodological quality of clinical practice guidelines in the peer-reviewed medical literature. *JAMA* 1999; 281:1900–1905.

Shornick JK. Using a drug-benefit help desk to manage the formulary benefit plan: experiences at an HMO. *Formulary* 1998; 33:471–474.

Shulkin DJ. Enhancing the role of physicians in the cost-effective use of pharmaceuticals. *Hosp Formul* 1994; 29:262–273.

Smalley WE, et al. Effect of a prior authorization requirement on the use of nonsteroidal antiinflammatory drugs by Medicaid patients. *J Managed Care Pharm* 1996; 2:158–164.

Stern CS. Academic detailing: what's in a name? *J Managed Care Pharm* 1996; 2:88–90.

Survey reveals continued HMO shift toward closed and partially closed formularies. *Formulary* 1997; 32:781–782.

The essential guide to pharmacy benefits—a view from the experts. Managed Care Communications Inc. and Glaxo Health Management. 1994.

Ulmishek M. Cost-effectiveness drives the decision when MCOs draw up formulary lists. *Managed Healthcare* 1998; 8:29–32.

10

CHAPTER

The Role of Self-Care and Nonprescription Drug Therapy in Managing Illness: The Rx-to-OTC Switch Movement

Mary Pat Manfredi, MPH

Tim R. Covington, M.S., Pharm.D.

INTRODUCTION

"I spend $13 million a year on [Prilosec®] and I don't even know who is selling it. Now imagine that. Is there any other business where you would have a $13 million expenditure and have no idea about the company?"

Woodrow A. Myers, Jr., M.D., MBA
Director of Healthcare Management
Ford Motor Company

The healthcare system is rapidly evolving, in large part to address the transformation and progression of contemporary consumer needs and expectations. Employers and managed care organizations (MCOs), in particular, are finding themselves at the crux of this "consumerism" movement. Direct-to-consumer (DTC) advertising and other market forces have produced a tidal wave of consumer interest in and demand for prescription drugs—a demand that is draining drug budgets of many MCOs and self-insured employers. Many employers, such as Ford Motor Company, are facing double-digit annual increases in prescription drug costs. As drugs such as Prilosec and Claritin are topping the lists of most advertised and, consequently, most prescribed drugs, MCOs and employers are facing tough choices. Such drugs "can be taken for decades to smooth the rough edges of life more than to eradicate disease," one observer noted (Hensley, 1999), making them detrimentally costly. Payors are being compelled to alter their health benefit design, reduce coverage, or further restrict formularies. There is a solution, at least in part, to this cost dilemma for employers and MCOs: the availability of safe, effective, clinically comparable, and low-cost alternatives to high-cost prescription drugs. Such alternatives are the "Rx-to-OTC switches"—those prescription drugs that have switched from prescription-only to nonprescription status—and they are the focus of this chapter.

For MCOs in particular, over-the-counter (OTC) drugs can provide enormous benefits, including cost savings, increases in member satisfaction, and competitiveness with other plans in a fierce healthcare marketplace. When you compare a $0.30/dose cost for Pepcid AC, for example, with $3.59/dose for Prilosec to treat episodic, uncomplicated heartburn, cost savings opportunities are tremendous. Increasingly, MCOs are taking note of switch products and are incorporating them into the drug benefit design (see Heartburn Case Example). Providing consumers the self-medication option of using nonprescription drugs is a positive, cost-effective move consistent with the powerful consumerism movement.

The Manual of Policy and Procedures (MaPP) of the FDA defines an Rx-to-OTC switch as "the OTC marketing of a drug that was once a prescription product for the same indication, and at the same strength, dose, duration of use, dosage form, population, and route of administration" (Smith, 1998). Key switches that sparked this movement include the Rx-to-OTC switch of topical hydrocortisone (0.5%) in 1979 and ibuprofen in 1984. Critically important, the switch of many drugs that were formerly available only with a prescription has fostered consumer empowerment and broadly based healthcare decision making. Now, 60% of all medications sold are nonprescription (Food and Drug Administration, 1999). The Consumer Healthcare Products Association (CHPA), formerly the Nonprescription Drug Manufacturers Association (NDMA), estimates that more than 600 current nonprescription drug products use ingredients or dosages that were available only by prescription 20 years ago. More Rx-to-OTC switches are expected.

Switched OTC drugs have impacted the pharmaceutical market significantly. The annual retail market value of switch drugs is estimated to reach $4.6 billion by the year 2001 (Business Communications Company, Inc., 1998). The Rx-to-OTC switch movement provides the consumer with greater access to drug therapy, allows patient involvement in critical decision making, and fosters patient responsibility and accountability. Furthermore, in its evolution, the impact of the Rx-to-OTC switch movement has extended beyond the individual consumer to MCOs, physicians, pharmacists, employers, and others.

Following an examination of the historical prologue to the Rx-to-OTC switch movement, this chapter examines the benefits of the switch movement for various groups, particularly MCOs, and conveys the urgency with which these groups must adapt their thinking, tactics, and strategies to accommodate consumerism. This chapter also explores several implications of the switch movement for the patient–provider relationship, and the opportunities for pharmacist intervention and collaboration with other healthcare professionals. A case example of heartburn is presented from the "switch" perspective. Finally, this chapter reviews the projected future of the Rx-to-OTC switch movement.

SELF-MEDICATION: A HISTORICAL PERSPECTIVE

Healthcare Professionals: Initial Concern, Gradual Acceptance

Self-care is one of the most basic and timeless health practices in our society, and publications addressing the topic date back centuries. Self-medication has been the topic of many research studies and "expert musings" in historical literature. By the 1960s, a diversity of opinion regarding consumer ability to use nonprescription medications properly, and the related or unrelated effects on physician authority, was manifest in the professional literature. This literature is now in sharp contrast with the strides that have been made in consumer self-care empowerment. Some healthcare self-interest groups labeled self-medication as "an increasing public health problem" (Friend, 1964); others delineated boundaries between "folk" medicine and "professional" medicine (Self-Medication Practices, 1967). Some historical professional literature openly discouraged self-medication, fearing severe disruption of the traditional physician-dominated healthcare model. Patient input and ability to participate in the medical healthcare process was understated, if not ignored.

In 1972, the FDA initiated a review of nonprescription drugs that, for the first time, spotlighted and validated the critical presence of OTC drugs in the consumer marketplace. The FDA's OTC Drug Review, or monograph process, stated specifically that "OTC drug monographs should be created for the various therapeutic classes of drugs and that each monograph would establish the conditions under which a category of OTC drugs is generally recognized as safe and effective and not misbranded" (Gilbertson, 1978). The OTC Review created more scientific interest in documenting the safety and efficacy of nonprescription drugs and self-medication, and it gave precedence to switching drugs from prescription to OTC status, a change that would allow patients more control over their own care. The reclassification of drugs, from prescription to OTC, weighed such factors as, "Is the condition self-diagnosable?" "Is the condition self-treatable?" "What is the product's toxicity?" and "Can the labeling be read and understood by the ordinary individual?" (Covington et al., 1996). Experts have pointed to the receptive economic, political, and cultural climate surrounding the OTC Review that fostered the progression of the prescription to nonprescription switch movement (Rosenau, 1994).

One result of the OTC Review was the successful switch of topical hydrocortisone from prescription to OTC status. Since then, many successful "switches" have been made, dating from

FIGURE 10–1

Selected examples of switched drugs and year of switch.

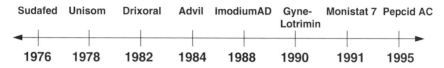

the 1970s to the present (Figure 10–1). Today, switches are initiated primarily by the pharmaceutical manufacturers, and accordingly, the Rx-to-OTC switch movement has become a significant trend within the pharmaceutical industry. The switch process entails many strategic considerations for the pharmaceutical company, including the clinical trial process, consumer research and use studies, adherence to FDA criteria, physician acceptance of the switch, market dynamics, competition, and product marketing. It is particularly essential for the company to be *first to market* with the Rx-to-OTC switch product. In addition to many successful Rx-to-OTC switches, there have also been several switch petitions that were *not* ultimately successful, such as for OTC status for acyclovir, metaproterenol, and cholestyramine.

A New Role for Consumers

By the 1990s, healthcare consumers had made significant strides from the passive roles once expected of them to more informed and assertive roles in the management of their healthcare. A running theme of a symposium of the Proprietary Association (now CHPA) in 1980 was "give the consumer credit"—referring to their self-care aptitude and assertiveness in the healthcare arena (Welsh, 1980). The evolution of consumerism in healthcare and the Rx-to-OTC switch movement has afforded consumers increasing opportunities to demonstrate prowess in assisting in the management of their own healthcare. Consumers have demonstrated their ability in evaluating and interpreting healthcare information directed toward them via mass media print and electronic advertising for both nonprescription and prescription drugs.

Changing Sources of Information

Consumers have become educated and informed about self-care and nonprescription drugs through a variety of sources, particularly evolving mass media vehicles. In the past, radio and print were the primary media by which people could obtain information about health-related products and self-care, aside from healthcare professionals. Eventually television expanded the pool of information resources. With the Internet, we are now witnessing a surge of readily retrievable information accessible to most anyone in the United States. With the proliferation of health-related Web sites, now numbering nearly 50,000, the Internet has unfolded as a major source of reliable information, education, and management processes about a variety of medical conditions and their treatment.

Self-care guidelines and nonprescription drug therapy are among Internet-provided topics; as such, healthcare consumers have greater access to health-related information and support in their self-care practices, use of nonprescription medications, and quest for better management of their medical conditions. The proliferation of online health resources providing information on virtually every disease state has helped advance consumer knowledge. Pharmaceutical companies that manufacture nonprescription drugs have Web sites, and on these sites, consumers can find product-specific information. Furthermore, as with Johnson & Johnson • Merck's "Physicians' Corner" Web site, healthcare providers can get information about a number of products. Medical information has become increasingly more consumer-friendly, assisting healthcare consumers in drug selection and use. Publications devoted solely to Rx-to-OTC switches, such as SWITCH Newsletter, reflect an increased focus on the Rx-to-OTC switch movement.

OTCs Today

Today, approximately 100,000 nonprescription drug products are on the market that, by science-based FDA standards, are not only safe and effective but also appropriate for treating many medical conditions once only treatable by prescription medication (Consumer Healthcare Products Association, 1998). In fact, the American Pharmaceutical Association (APhA) estimates that nearly 60% of the more than 2 billion health problems treated annually are treated with nonprescription drugs as primary therapy or major adjunctive therapy (American Pharmaceutical Association, 1998). The OTC market has progressed from a $3 billion market in 1972 to well over $30 billion today (Johnson et al., 1976; Consumer Healthcare Products Association, 1998). Consumers have numerous nonprescription drug therapy options to self-treat a variety of conditions, including cough, cold, and allergy; fever; heartburn; gastrointestinal distress; diarrhea; candidal vaginitis; functional aches and pains; sprains and strains; a variety of dermatoses; and smoking cessation. With so many OTC options available and so much health-related information at their fingertips, today's consumers expect to participate in their own treatment. Armed with this knowledge, MCOs can design plans to maximize benefits for both the consumer and themselves.

IMPLICATIONS OF THE RX-TO-OTC SWITCH MOVEMENT FOR MANAGED CARE

The Rx-to-OTC switch movement affects MCOs in several important ways. Coupled with the self-care trend, Rx-to-OTC switch products provide the MCO with opportunities for cost savings, increased member satisfaction and loyalty, reduced demand for high-cost services, and benefit design enhancements.

Cost Savings

Prescription medication costs can account for 15% or more of total medical costs for some health plans (Meyer, 1998). A number of health plans and self-insured employers have experienced annual pharmacy cost increases of 15% to 25% (Frazier, 1997; McCarthy, 1998). Some plans have responded to this problem by assigning tiered co-payment levels for "preferred" or "nonpreferred" prescription drugs. The percentage of dollars allocated to prescription drugs is staggering, and rising. One plan spokesman recently predicted that proton pump inhibitors (PPIs), antiallergens, and antidepressants will consume 25% of their drug budget by the year 2000 (Hensley, 1999). Thus, they are scrambling to do something about it. To add to the dilemma, the list of new, and very expensive, drugs, such as the COX-2 inhibitors for treatment of osteoarthritis and rheumatoid arthritis, cost up to 20 times more than the traditional therapy of ibuprofen, naproxen, ketoprofen, or aspirin (Hensley, 1999). Nonprescription drugs and specifically switch drugs can provide a cost-effective, value-added "solution" to some of these drug cost "crises" affecting health plans and, ultimately, payors (e.g., corporate America, Medicaid).

Increased Member Satisfaction and Loyalty

Modern consumers are demanding health-related information, and it is available from a variety of sources. Surveys have revealed that 86% of individuals with mental and physical health problems attempted to obtain information about their health problem, and 79% of adults are interested or somewhat interested in general health information (Deering, 1996). A study by the accounting firm KPMG and Northwestern University in Chicago found consumer information-seeking about medications or prescriptions ranked second behind consumer information-seeking regarding benefits provided by healthcare plans (KPMG & Northwestern University, 1998).

MCOs must better understand the global health needs of their member population; they must also respond to their members and keep them satisfied. Patient satisfaction is the area that MCOs measured the second most frequently in 1997 (InterStudy, 1997). It has been shown that when an MCO implements a program to educate members on self-care and on the array of products and resources available to them, member satisfaction with their plan increases (Johnson & Johnson, 1996). Accordingly, health plans, in this modern age of information technology, should better connect with their enrollees by offering them healthcare tools and knowledge through diverse media that foster effective self-care and health maintenance.

For plans such as Aetna U.S. Healthcare, provider compensation is tied in part to patient satisfaction. For these network physicians, the level of patient satisfaction can often determine part of their payment. In 1998, the company distributed more than 3 million patient satisfaction surveys and, based on results, gave its capitated physicians bonuses "of up to 3%" (Larkin, 1999). Patients' voices can make a difference, demonstrated here by their tangible economic impact on healthcare providers.

MCOs that recognize the growing consumerism trend can achieve or increase member satisfaction and loyalty. In the fiercely competitive healthcare market, healthcare plans strive to attract new clients/enrollees and to retain current enrollees. More than half of U.S. HMOs lost money in 1998 (Weiss Ratings Inc., 1999). Plan annual disenrollment rates range up to 40% in highly competitive markets (Reese, 1997). The HSM Group Ltd. estimates the financial impact of voluntary disenrollment as ranging from nearly $7 million for a 143,000-member plan to more than $55 million for a 995,000-member plan (HSM Group Ltd., 1999). MCOs seek to retain members to reap long-term cost savings achieved from their various disease prevention/management programs. If membership turnover is high, this can cloud their clinical and economic outcomes. Teaming with the provider and employer to address how to better effect prudent nonprescription drug use can give an MCO some leverage in retaining members. Consequently, employers may be more willing to renew their contracts.

Benefit Design Enhancements

Managed care plans should be encouraged to devise unique and creative ways to address consumerism and cost-effective healthcare by promoting appropriate use of nonprescription drugs. A recent pharmacy benefit report found that pharmacy benefit managers (PBMs) and MCOs increasingly recommend OTC products as part of step-care protocols and member education materials (Novartis Pharmacy Benefit Report, 1998). Many health plans and PBMs have provided coupons and free samples of OTC medication to members, a result of working with pharmaceutical manufacturers. PBMs with prescription drug cost caps have also encouraged members to use OTC products to avoid hitting their coverage cap (Muirhead, 1995).

Prudent OTC drug use can be a critical component of the disease management and demand management programs of MCOs. The *Disease Management Strategic Research Study & Resource Guide* reveals that almost 95% of surveyed organizations predicted greater utilization and influence of disease management programs within their organization during the next 3 years (Rauber, 1999). In addition, MCO and employer investment in disease prevention–focused programs is predicted to increase, narrowing the gap between such programs and those focused on treatment. This increased preventive focus can be assisted by the strategic deployment of certain nonprescription drugs. Furthermore, Rx-to-OTC switches of the future should increasingly address chronic conditions such as osteoporosis and hypercholesterolemia. Lorig and colleagues at Stanford University have worked extensively with patient self-management programs for chronic diseases such as arthritis. Four-year results for the arthritis program showed a 40% reduction in outpatient visits for arthritis and a 20% reduction in pain (Lorig et al., 1993). As part of an MCO *demand* management program, such as a nurse telephone triage service, OTC drugs can be recommended to callers with appropriate symptoms.

The Rx-to-OTC switch movement and the concomitant influx of safe and effective drugs into the OTC market have implications for MCO reimbursement strategy. Opportunities for reimbursement reside within creative benefit design, perhaps through innovative technology or incentive programs (e.g., swipe card, coupons). Providing reimbursement for switch drugs such as OTC famotidine (Pepcid AC) for heartburn has shown promising financial benefit for the MCO (Nash, 1999). In addition to cost containment, MCOs can demonstrate their commitment to member self-care, thereby gaining a market advantage over other plans.

Independent Health, a plan with more than 430,000 members and based in Buffalo, New York, instituted a Pepcid AC conversion program in March of 1998. In just the first quarter of implementation, which involved automatically switching prescriptions written for Pepcid to Pepcid AC, the plan realized a total decrease in per member per month (PMPM) H_2-blocker costs of 73%. Over the course of the year, the plan sustained a 72% decrease in PMPM H_2-blocker costs. Furthermore, adjusting for membership fluctuations, the program did not inflate prescription use (and costs) for other H_2-blockers or PPIs. Strategic elements of the program's success have included consistent communication from plan administration to network physicians; a sales force pull-through collaboration on the part of Johnson & Johnson • Merck communicating the switch opportunity to physicians; and, based on initial success, the consideration of an expanded program focusing on decreasing overuse of high-cost PPIs.

Pepcid AC is covered by 22 state Medicaid programs, an initiative that has been highly successful, particularly in Alabama and Connecticut. Medicaid-derived sales of Pepcid AC provide relief from high prescription drug costs in the acid/secretory therapeutic category. Success from the Medicaid initiative can be applied to commercial healthcare plans with a little innovation and commitment to reducing high prescription drug costs.

Case Example: Heartburn

THE SUCCESS AND BENEFITS OF THE SWITCH OF FAMOTIDINE (PEPCID) TO OVER-THE-COUNTER STATUS (PEPCID AC)

BACKGROUND

Ninety-five million Americans per year experience heartburn at varying frequencies. It is estimated that 15 million Americans have heartburn symptoms every day (American College of Gastroenterology, 1998). U.S. heartburn sufferers spend more than $3.7 billion annually on heartburn medications (Utley, 1996). Famotidine (Pepcid AC), an H_2-receptor antagonist (H_2RA) was switched to OTC status in 1995. Clinical studies have demonstrated both the efficacy and safety of low-dose OTC famotidine in managing uncomplicated heartburn (Decktor et al., 1998; Feldman, 1998; Kunz et al., 1996; Simon et al., 1995).

COST SAVINGS

A study by Kunz et al. demonstrated an estimated $6 million savings over 5 years in a 26,000-member MCO. Savings were calculated by assigning appropriate patients to *nonprescription* famotidine for treatment of mild heartburn/nonulcer dyspepsia. The savings accrued from a decrease in physician office visits, prescriptions, and laboratory tests (Kunz et al., 1996).

Estimated healthcare costs:	*$1.2 billion*
▪ Office visits	$480 million
▪ Prescriptions	$720 million

continued

Case Example: Heartburn *(continued)*

36% of Rx H$_2$RAs are written for heartburn
Relative cost—retail:

- OTC Pepcid AC 10 mg: $.30/dose
- Rx Zantac 150 mg: $1.48/dose
- Rx Prilosec 20 mg: $3.59/dose

(Sources: IRI, Nov 1997; Red Book Update, Nov 1997; IMS America, Sept 1997)

TREATMENT AND PREVENTION

In a recent telephone survey of 2,000 men and women who experienced heartburn, nonprescription medications comprised the leading method of treatment *and* prevention of heartburn. More than 76% of respondents take a nonprescription medication to treat heartburn; nearly half take nonprescription medications to prevent heartburn as well (Oliveria et al., 1999)

In a report delineating successes from failures of switch drugs, Tom Lom lists Pepcid AC as a winner, beating out other OTC H$_2$RAs because of several key criteria, among them, its effectiveness toward heartburn prevention (Lom, 1997). Also key to the success of Pepcid AC has been its brand identity, specifically toward prevention, which had a year head-start on other switch drugs in the same therapeutic category.

PLAN COVERAGE

Pepcid AC provider education programs in state Medicaid programs were initiated in 1997 and have proven to be an overwhelming success. Pepcid AC is now a covered drug benefit of 22 state Medicaid plans. Medicaid-derived sales of Pepcid AC grew from $125,000 in 1997 to nearly $1 million in 1999. Also covering the product is Independent Health, a 430,000 + member managed care plan in Buffalo, New York, which instituted a Pepcid AC conversion program in March of 1998. Other plans covering Pepcid AC include WellCare (Florida) and Univera (New York). The PBMs, RxAmerica, Pequot, and ProCare also have contracts.

THE PROBLEM WITH PPIS

In addition to being both safe and effective, OTC H$_2$RAs provide a low-cost alternative to costly prescription H$_2$RAs and PPIs for managing episodic, uncomplicated heartburn. Compared with 10-mg famotidine, at $0.30/dose, the brand name, patent-protected Rx H$_2$RA is nearly 6 times (600%) greater in price, and the PPI is nearly 13 times (1300%) greater in price at $116 to $178 for a month's supply (Lagnado, 1998). Prilosec and Prevacid are expensive and, for mild-to-moderate heartburn (grade 0 to grade 1 gastroesophageal reflux disease), can be substituted with a cost-effective option such as Pepcid AC or other OTC H$_2$RAs. Steele states that patients without documented esophagitis or another significant complication (i.e., asthma) should be managed aggressively with stage I therapy avoiding *long-term* prescription H$_2$RA or PPI therapy (Steele, 1996).

RX-TO-OTC SWITCHES: CONSUMER BENEFITS

Opportunities for Active Consumer Role in Healthcare

The switch of many medications from prescription to OTC status has afforded consumers an opportunity to take a more active role in their healthcare. According to a 1997 survey commissioned by *PREVENTION* and the APhA, self-treatment was most common for headache (80%), upset stomach (76%), and coughs/colds (73%); as more products are now available OTC, there is increased potential and resources to self-treat (Navigating the Medication Marketplace: How Consumers Choose, 1997). Not only are consumers performing the act of self-medication to a greater extent, they are entirely capable of doing so, and studies have demonstrated this fact. The CHPA published a compilation of thirteen national consumer studies, confirming that consumers are demonstrating responsible behavior in using OTC drugs, including reading labels and using the medications for the appropriate indications (Consumer Healthcare Products Association, 1996). To illustrate this fact, women have proven their abilities in self-diagnosing vaginal candidiasis, thus allowing manufacturers of vaginal antifungal products to receive FDA approval to switch them to OTC status. A recent paper by Lipsky and Waters of Northwestern University drives home this point, stating, "despite physicians' concern, there has been little objective evidence of serious harm resulting from this [vaginal antifungal] switch, and overall, it appears that the OTC availability of antifungal preparations may be beneficial" (Lipsky & Waters, 1999). Through their extensive research on the Rx-to-OTC switch movement, the researchers emphasize the need for enhanced education for consumers as well as healthcare professionals (Northwestern University, 1999).

Improving Health and Lifestyle

Rx-to-OTC switches provide consumers an opportunity for better health and quality of life. For example, smoking is a significant public health problem in this country, evidenced by 45+ million nicotine-dependent Americans. This addiction can be addressed, at least partially, through nonprescription nicotine replacement therapy via products such as the Nicotrol transdermal nicotine patch. Such a product, in combination with behavioral modification techniques, provides a convenient and inexpensive pharmacologic strategy for smoking cessation and confronts this large-scale public health menace in an innovative way. The Nicotrol transdermal nicotine patch, switched to OTC in July 1996, was shown to be used successfully by consumers in clinical studies. McNeil Consumer Healthcare, the manufacturer, demonstrated smoker labeling comprehension, including warnings and directions for its proper use. In addition, more than 80% of consumers used the behavioral modification materials, including handbooks, an audiotape, and toll-free help-line (FDA, 1996). Cigarettes can be purchased in virtually any retail outlet, yet individuals were not given the same wide retail access to treatment before the switch of nicotine replacement therapy to OTC status.

For mild-to-moderate heartburn, OTC famotidine (Pepcid AC) and other OTC H_2RAs, in addition to diet and lifestyle changes, have helped millions of heartburn sufferers treat symptoms effectively as well as prevent episodes of heartburn. For symptom management of coughs and colds, individuals can select one of many formulations available in numerous retail outlets. Consumers can access many OTC drugs capable of providing rapid and effective symptom relief, allowing routine activity.

Convenience and Choice for the Consumer—Saving Time and Money

In this day and age, convenience, choice, and immediacy are core values of American consumers. It is common to hear consumer complaints about the wait in physicians' offices and the "hassle factor" associated with managed care. Internet companies are seizing on convenience-minded consumers, as evidenced by the rapid growth of e-commerce and the ability to purchase products and services with the use of a personal computer. Rx-to-OTC switch products have afforded consumers this desired convenience and choice. A competent individual, recognizing his or her symptoms, can reach into the medicine cabinet or visit the nearest pharmacy or grocery store to select a safe and effective nonprescription product to treat certain medical conditions. The consumer can achieve immediate relief, depending on the OTC switch product and medical condition being treated, and generally continue with daily activity. Although many conditions and/or symptoms require a medical evaluation, many can be managed safely and appropriately by the proactive healthcare consumer who prudently selects and uses nonprescription drugs.

Another attribute of the Rx-to-OTC switch movement is the realization of cost savings for the consumer. When physician office visits, waiting times, laboratory work, and unnecessary prescriptions are eliminated, the consumer and the insurance premium payor (e.g., employer) ultimately save money. OTC drugs are relatively inexpensive and have been proven to work as effectively as prescription drugs for many conditions. In the early 1980s, it was estimated that, after being available for 2 years as a switch product, 0.5% topical hydrocortisone had saved consumers and payors $400 million (Murphy, 1985) through the avoidance of unnecessary physician office visits and associated costs. Availability of OTC medications reportedly saves the nation more than $20 billion per year that otherwise would have been spent for prescription drugs and doctor visits and that would have accrued from lost time away from work (Kline & Company, 1997).

Forging Partnerships with Healthcare Professionals

Historically, self-care has been regarded with trepidation concerning its potential to undermine and/or usurp the authority of the physician. Increasing numbers of Rx-to-OTC switches have entered the market, inevitably changing this dynamic. Attitudes of acceptance have emerged toward some of these once-controversial switches (e.g., ibuprofen, cimetidine), and opportunities to self-medicate have increased. Such opportunities do not, of course, represent a declining need for the physician; however, they can provide heightened opportunities for partnerships between patients, physicians, and pharmacists in particular.

Specifically, the physician's role is evolving more toward an educator/facilitator for patients. Conceptual frameworks surrounding this role have been explored, focusing on "clinical health promotion" (Caraher, 1998). Health education is vitally important, and physicians have a major role in helping patients decipher correct from misleading information, especially concerning Internet-based medical information (Bader & Braude, 1998). Not all such information is factual, as shown by a study involving the University of Michigan Health System, which found that more than 40% of Web sites reviewed for information about Ewing's sarcoma contained questionable, nonvalidated medical information (Biermann et al., 1999; Study finds much . . . , 1999). The self-treating patients' healthcare decision making can be bolstered and supported by the physician's and pharmacist's role in health education.

HEALTHCARE PROVIDERS AND THE EFFECTS OF THE SWITCH MOVEMENT ON RELATIONS WITH PATIENTS

The Rx-to-OTC switch process impacts healthcare providers and the patient–provider relationship in several positive ways. As the slogan of one retail store chain, the Syms Corporation, declares, "An educated consumer is our best customer"—this applies equally to the relationship between the modern, informed, and proactive healthcare consumer and the enlightened healthcare provider, particularly the physician and pharmacist. Patients are increasingly self-medicating with nonprescription drugs, searching for medical information, and using alternative and complementary therapies. The availability of Rx-to-OTC switch drugs for consumers enhances these trends and offers healthcare providers numerous opportunities to communicate and interact effectively with this new type of patient. Moreover, when self-medicating patients do not need the services of a physician, the physician has more time for addressing health needs of more severe cases. In a capitated reimbursement climate, providers benefit from having patients who can appropriately self-manage less severe, self-limited medical conditions.

The Importance of Communication

The availability of increasing numbers of nonprescription drugs and line extensions validates the need for physicians and pharmacists to be well-informed about self-care relevant to their patients' self-medication activities. Goals of medication management include selecting the proper drug and dosage for the appropriate indication, minimizing side effects, improving compliance, reducing complications, and avoiding drug–drug interactions and complications (Todd & Nash, 1996). It is equally important for healthcare providers to be aware of the nonprescription products that patients may consume so that they can note them in the patient's medical and medication history. Specifically, effective physician and pharmacist communication skills remain essential to effective patient care, including safe patient self-medication and other self-care practices (Braddock et al., 1997; Layne & Seibert, 1998; Quill & Brody, 1996). Incorporating effective communication skills can elicit, for example, a more detailed patient history and patient drug profile that is inclusive of all medications and relevant dietary/lifestyle behaviors. As providers are aware, not all patients inform them of their use of "other medications," including OTC drugs (Hensrud, Engle, & Scheitel, 1999). Providers must continue to probe with appropriate questions to extract such information. For example, patients may be wearing a nicotine patch for smoking cessation or may be regularly taking herbals/supplements and OTC drugs and not consider these as medications. Compliance with any and all treatment plans is important to overall health outcomes, and effective patient–provider communication is a key element of any behavior/lifestyle modification attempts by the healthcare provider.

It is no surprise that physicians can have a very strong influence on patient drug utilization patterns. In one survey, 74% of consumers ranked doctor's recommendation as the most influential factor in deciding whether to purchase an OTC drug (Navigating the Medication Marketplace: How Consumers Choose, 1997). The proliferation of resources designed to empower patients engaging in self-care behavior emphasizes the need for "two-way" communication.

Pharmacy Risk Sharing Implications

Physicians are increasingly practicing under "pharmacy risk arrangements," particularly in California, where it is estimated that up to two-thirds of all (capitated) physician organizations participate in some form of pharmacy risk (Grandinetti, 1999). One medical practice had to return more than $1 million to health plans for prescription drug costs in excess of their "drug budgets" (Grandinetti, 1999). With such financial ramifications for providers, reasonably and competitively priced nonprescription drug use makes a tremendous amount of sense. Providers have an array of excellent OTC drugs from which to select and recommend to patients. In addition, physician and pharmacy providers can provide samples or coupons to patients, along with "self-care" plans, instead of a costly prescription. Providers can and should demonstrate a commitment to appropriate self-care, rational OTC drug use, and the patient's ability to manage his or her health concern to a higher degree.

Partnering Opportunities

The Rx-to-OTC switch movement enhances the opportunities for provider partnering, both with patients and with other health professionals, in the care of the patient. Advances in communication technology, such as the Internet and e-mail, have fostered development of more viable provider–patient partnerships. A recent survey by Healtheon found that of 10,000 doctors surveyed, more than one-third have used e-mail to communicate with patients (Mangan, 1999). In the time-constrained physician office, such tools, combined with more astute, self-medicating patients, can enhance the patient–provider relationship.

Pharmacists, nurse practitioners, physician assistants, and allied health professionals are playing increased roles in patient care. Many believe that they improve quality of care, as discussed in *Physicians Financial News* (Delmar, 1999). Such extensions of the physician can allow more time for patients, during which issues such as self-medication can be addressed more thoroughly. In addition, pharmacists, nurse practitioners, and physician assistants can facilitate communication between the medical provider and patient on such topics.

THE PHARMACIST'S EXPANDING ROLE

A Proprietary Association (now CHPA) symposium in 1980 was titled "Self-Medication: The New Era." A theme of this event was that the key to good care lies in making the best use of resources. The pharmacist is one such resource. One expert is quoted as saying, "[healthcare] information itself will become a commodity—and pharmacists valuable traders" (Welsh, 1980). Pharmacists have also been referred to as "self-care consultants" (Newton et al., 1996).

Historically, a great deal of literature has focused on the pharmacy profession, urging pharmacists to assert themselves professionally (Knapp & Beardsley, 1979; Schoen, 1996). The nonprescription drug area was, and remains, a specific opportunity to advance the pharmacist's role in the management of patient therapy. In 1974, APhA sponsored a program called "Over-the-Counter Intelligence: Your Pharmacist Has It" (Griffenhagen, 1974). The program's goals included educating consumers about nonprescription drugs as well as publicizing the unique expertise, professional role, and availability of the pharmacist in assisting patients in the safe, appropriate, effective, and economical selection and use of nonprescription drugs. In 1984, APhA's position on the Rx-to-OTC switch process recommended that newly switched drugs be dispensed by pharmacists only for a "transition period" (Penna, 1985). Although the Rx-to-OTC switch drug "transitional" category was never labeled a third class of drugs and is still debated, pharmacists have developed expanded roles and responsibilities as effects of the switch movement evolve.

This trend continues today, as pharmacists nationwide are being sought out by consumers as learned intermediaries for advice about the nonprescription drugs lining the nonprescription drug aisles of the pharmacy. A recent *PREVENTION*/APhA survey revealed that 70% of consumers depend on the pharmacist for information about OTC products (Navigating the Medication Marketplace: How Consumers Choose, 1997). As numerous drugs have moved from prescription to OTC status, the pharmacist's role has been augmented to accommodate consumers' inquiries about these products and their appropriate use.

To broadcast and enhance the role of the pharmacist, many community pharmacy chains are developing programs in which the pharmacist takes a central role in patient management. CVS, for example, sponsors a "Pharmacy Outreach Program" making pharmacists available for presentations and education of members of community and business groups (Gross, 1999). Many chains (e.g., Eckerd) sponsor disease management programs in which the pharmacist plays a central role, particularly for conditions such as hypertension, asthma, and hypercholesterolemia. "Project IMPACT: Hyperlipidemia," supported by Merck & Co., Inc., and administered by the APhA Foundation, is "designed to demonstrate that pharmacists who act as disease state managers for patients with dyslipidemias can improve persistence and compliance with therapy" (American Pharmaceutical Association, 1998).

Much of this activity illustrates a broader movement within the pharmacy profession, known as "pharmaceutical care," and is defined as an approach to patient care that motivates pharmacists to constantly seek and obtain the skills and resources necessary to ensure patients receive the maximum benefit from their medications (National Wholesale Druggists' Association, 1999). The APhA and others have documented the "human and financial cost of drug therapy misadventures, the need for improved pharmaceutical care services, and the documented clinical and economic impact of pharmacists who have taken on the job of providing pharmaceutical care" (American Pharmaceutical Association, 1999). Therapeutic areas highlighted by the APhA include management of asthma, diabetes, drug therapy compliance, dyslipidemia, hypertension, and pain, and the value of such activities has been presented in the literature (Fincham, 1998).

Pharmacists are increasingly being involved in what is known as "collaborative practice arrangements" with physicians. These arrangements are defined as, "a voluntary, written agreement between a pharmacist and a prescriber that permits expanded authority for the pharmacist, such as the ability to initiate or modify drug therapy and order laboratory tests." Such collaboration is intended to optimize patient care outcomes, and may use protocols, practice guidelines, critical pathways, care plans, and formulary systems (American Society of Consultant Pharmacists, 1997). These arrangements focus on cognitive services that foster optimal outcomes from both prescription and OTC therapies.

Pharmacists certainly have an extraordinary opportunity to advance their profession while serving the public interest by capitalizing on the Rx-to-OTC switch movement, and as such, to build their professional service repertoire in patient management.

EMPLOYERS: SWITCHES CAN BENEFIT

A recent survey found that employer costs for health benefits for both active and retired employees topped the $4,000 per-employee per-year mark, at $4,164 per employee, for the first time during 1998 (Mercer/Foster Higgins, 1999). The same survey found that employers plan to adopt programs that will better manage their drug costs (Tanouye, 1998). Employers, faced with annual premium increases of up to or in excess of 15%, are confronted with difficult choices: absorb the costs, change to better-managed health plans, or cost-shift to employees. More than one-third of large employers (with 500+ employees) altered their prescription drug benefit for plan years 1998 or 1999. These large employers generally increased employee cost-sharing (18%) or made formulary modifications (9%). Regarding the overall healthcare cost burden for employers, the Washington Business Group on Health (WBGH) member survey of 35 companies (2.1 million employees) projected that overall healthcare costs would increase 8.1% for employees and 9.6% for retirees in the year 2000 (Large employers to absorb . . ., 1999).

The Rx-to-OTC switch movement benefits employers. A wide range of effective nonprescription products offers employees cost-effective choices for addressing many health-related problems and necessary treatment. When employees must see a doctor and take time off from work, the employer realizes a loss in work time and productivity. Furthermore, the Rx-to-OTC switch movement provides employers the opportunity to enhance their existing wellness or health promotion programs by offering employees guidance on selecting appropriate OTC drugs. A 1997 study by Hewitt Associates LLC found that almost 90% of surveyed employers had a health promotion program in place, as well as an increasing focus on patient-specific programs, such as health risk appraisals, individualized wellness programs, and use of financial incentives/disincentives (Zablocki, 1997). Work site health and wellness programs, inclusive of nonprescription drugs, are truly synergistic with the self-care movement and could be a value-added benefit in the eyes of potential employees.

RX-TO-OTC SWITCHES: THE FUTURE

> "Managed care will increasingly promote the use of OTC medications as part of health-maintenance programs and as effective, cost-limiting alternatives to prescription drugs."
>
> *D. Vaczek (Vaczek, 1996)*

The environment of nonprescription drug therapy, a realm primarily for management of symptomatic, self-limited conditions, now has the *potential* (pending FDA approvals) to extend self-medication with nonprescription drugs to asymptomatic, chronic conditions, such as hypercholesterolemia. Nonprescription drug therapy for mild asthma, osteoporosis, migraine, hypertension, incontinence, and other medical conditions may proceed down a similar path.

As the Baby Boomer generation ages and life expectancy increases, more conditions will be treatable by OTC switch products. Older Americans comprise 13% of the population, yet purchase almost 30% of nonprescription drugs (Cameron, 1997). Many OTC and OTC switch drugs on the market treat the symptoms of conditions afflicting the elderly, such as muscle and joint pain and insomnia.

Experts proclaim that the "easy" switches are over; now it is time to approach the more complex switches, addressing more chronic health conditions (Breu, 1999). This should only increase the attention to consumer self-care through self-medication with such drugs. In addition, self-diagnosis will be augmented through the development and introduction of new home diagnostic products. At a recent Drug Information Association conference, titled "OTCness: Changing the Paradigm," Randy Juhl, Ph.D. of the School of Pharmacy at the University of Pittsburgh predicted the future this way, "As social and economic trends move [force] consumers to become more self-reliant, in sickness and in wellness, they will demand OTC science-based products and information. . . . To meet this need, the industry, the medical and scientific communities and the FDA will need to pick up the pace" (Juhl, 1998).

Managed care organizations can commit to the worth of switch products by making them a *covered* benefit for members. Several plans do this already, and more will in the future. Tom Ferguson, M.D., an expert on self-care, came up with "seven laws of self-care" (Ferguson, 1997). The sixth law is, "the principal goal of a healthcare system should be to help people take care of themselves." The Rx-to-OTC switch movement makes a powerful contribution toward consumer self-care and empowerment, and healthcare professionals and inter-industry professionals can learn and benefit from this movement.

REFERENCES

American College of Gastroenterology. 1998. From www.acg.gi.org.

American Pharmaceutical Association. 1999. From www.aphanet.org.

American Pharmaceutical Association. In Consumer Healthcare Products Association *OTC Facts and Figures* 1998. From http://www.ndmainfo.org/facts/factsFrame.html.

American Society of Consultant Pharmacists. 1997. From www.ascp.com.

Bader SA, Braude RM. "Patient informatics": creating new partnerships in medical decision making. *Acad Med* 1998; 73:408–411.

Biermann JS, et al. Evaluation of cancer information on the Internet. *Cancer* 1999; 86(3):381–390.

Braddock CH, et al. How doctors and patients discuss routine clinical decisions: informed decision making in the outpatient setting. *J Gen Intern Med* 1997; 12:339–345.

Breu J. Drug firms hope for end in slump in Rx-to-OTC product switches. *Drug Topics* July 19, 1999; 143(4):47.

Cameron KA. Over-the-counter and into the home. United Seniors Health Cooperative, Summer 1997, Special Report 48.

Caraher M. Patient education and health promotion: clinical health promotion—the conceptual link. *Pat Educ Couns* 1998; 33(1):49–58.

Consumer Healthcare Products Association. American consumers support self-medication and practice it responsibly: a compilation of thirteen national consumer studies. 1996.

Consumer Healthcare Products Association. *OTC Facts and Figures.* 1998. From http://www.ndmainfo.org/facts/factsFrame.html.

Covington TR, et al. (eds). *Handbook of nonprescription drugs*, 11th ed. Washington, DC: American Pharmaceutical Association, 1996.

Decktor D, et al. *Can single-dose omeprazole prevent heartburn: a comparison of omeprazole 10mg and 20mg and famotidine 10mg on meal-induced heartburn symptoms?* Boston: Program of the American College of Gastroenterology 63rd Annual Scientific Meeting, October 12–14, 1998.

Deering MJ. Consumer health information demand and deliver: implications for libraries. *Bulletin of the Medical Library Association* 1996; 84(2):209–216.

Delmar D. Physician extenders boost efficiency. *Physicians Financial News* 1999; 17(9):S8.

Feldman M. Comparison of the effects of over-the-counter famotidine and calcium carbonate antacid on postprandial gastric acid: a randomized controlled trial. *JAMA* 1998; 275(18):1428–1431.

Ferguson T. The seven laws of self-care. 1997. From HealthWorld Online: http://www.healthy.net/hwlibraryjournals/self%2Dcarearchives/7lwssc.htm.

Fincham JE. Pharmaceutical care studies: a review and update. *Drug Benefit Trends* 1998; 10(6):41–45.

Food and Drug Administration. 1999.

Food and Drug Administration. From Web site: "9–0 vote for OTC Nicotrol," 1996. http://www.verity.fda.gov.

Food and Drug Administration. Manual of policy and procedures. In Smith MC (ed): Rx-to-OTC switches: reflections and projections. *Drug Topics* July 20, 1998; 42:70–79.

Frazier G. Strategies to tackle the recent surge in pharmacy costs. *Drug Benefit Trends* 1997; 9(11):31–49.

Friend DG. Self-medication: an increasing public health problem. *Clin Pharmacol Ther* 1964; 5:533–536.

Gilbertson WE. The OTC Drug Review—FDA's viewpoint. *Agents & Actions* 1978; 8(4):422–424.

Grandinetti DA. Drug costs could come out of your pocket. *Medical Economics* April 12, 1999; 76(7):178–190.

Griffenhagen GB. Editorial—over-the-counter intelligence—do you have it? *JAPhA* 1974; 14(3):115.

Gross J. Pharmacist care management program enters region. *Physician's News Digest: Delaware Valley Edition* June 1999; XII(8):1, 4, 19.

Hensley S. Prescription costs become harder to swallow. *Modern Healthcare* August 23, 1999; 29(34):30–34.

Hensrud DD, Engle DD, Scheitel SM. Underreporting the use of dietary supplements and nonprescription medications among patients undergoing a periodic health examination. *Mayo Clinic Proceedings* 1999; 74(5):443–447.

HSM Group Ltd. In: 1999 Bayer Retention Report: relationships in harmony: striking new chords in member loyalty. Advertising supplement to *Managed Healthcare*. July 1999, p. 27.

Johnson & Johnson. Independent Johnson & Johnson survey of 725 members of an HMO. 1996.

Johnson RE, et al. Reported use of nonprescription drugs in health maintenance. *Am J Hosp Pharm* 1976; 33: 1249–1254.

Juhl, R. Impact of the changing healthcare paradigm on Rx to OTC switch. Presentation by Randy Juhl, PhD at the Drug Information Association "OTCness" conference, Washington, DC, September 16–17, 1998.

Kline & Company. 1997. From Consumer Healthcare Products Association Web site: "OTC Facts & Figures" http://www.ndmainfo.org/facts/factsFrame.html.

Knapp DA, Beardsley RS. Put yourself into the OTC picture—professionally. *American Pharmacy* 1979; NS19(10):37–39.

KPMG, Northwestern University Institute for Health Services Research and Policy Studies. *Consumerism in healthcare: new voices* 1998.

Kunz K, et al. Economic implications of self-treatment of heartburn/nonulcer dyspepsia with nonprescription famotidine in a managed care setting. *J Manag Care Pharm* 1996; 2:263–271.

Lagnado L. Drug costs can leave elderly a grim choice: pills or other needs. *The Wall Street Journal* November 17, 1998; A1, A15.

Large employers to absorb big health cost hikes. August 1999; 13(9). *Employee Benefit News.* From www.benefitnews.com.

Larkin H. Satisfaction pays: happier patients can bring fatter wallets. *AMNews* August 9, 1999; 42:35.

Layne BA, Seibert DJ. Center expands drug education focus. *Pennsylvania MEDICINE* February 1998; 101:12.

Lipsky MS, Waters T. The "prescription-to-OTC switch" movement: its effects on antifungal vaginitis preparations. *Arch Fam Med* 1999; 8:297–300.

Lom T. Caveat switcher! *Medical Marketing & Media* March 1997; 32(3).

Lorig KR, et al. Evidence suggesting that health education for self-management in patients with chronic arthritis has sustained health benefits while reducing healthcare costs. *Arthritis and Rheumatism* 1993; 36:439–446.

Mangan D. Save time and please patients with e-mail. *Medical Economics* July 12, 1999; 76:155–165.

McCarthy R. Rx ads hit consumer bull's-eye. *Drug Benefit Trends* 1998; 10(1):23.

Mercer/Foster Higgins National Survey of Employer-sponsored Health Plans, 1999.

Meyer H. The pills that ate your profits. *Hospitals & Health Networks* February 5, 1998; 72(3):19–22.

Muirhead G. Coverage for OTCs? *Drug Topics* August 21, 1995; 139(16):38.

Murphy DH. Taking the chance out of the Rx-to-OTC switch. Comment refers to presentation by Peter Temin at Rx-to-OTC symposium, 1982, sponsored by the Proprietary Association. *American Pharmacy* 1985; NS25(1):41–45.

Myers WA. Ford's $13 mil. annual Prilosec spend partly due to DTC ads, executive says. *First!* May 9, 1999.

Nash DB. The case for covering Rx-to-OTC switch products: the H2-receptor antagonist example. *Formulary* 1999; 34:452–454.

National Wholesale Druggists' Association. From www.nwda.org/pharm/what.htm.

Newton G, et al. Rx-to-OTC switches: from prescription to self-care. *J Am Pharm Assoc* 1996; NS36(8):489–495.

Northwestern University Institute for Health Services Research and Policy Studies. *Findings* Summer 1999; 1(1):2.

Novartis Pharmacy Benefit Report: Trends and Forecasts. East Hanover, NJ: 1998.

Oliveria SA, et al. Heartburn risk factors, knowledge, and prevention strategies: a population-based survey of individuals with heartburn. *Arch Intern Med* 1999; 159:1592–1598.

Penna R. A transitional category: how APhA's policy would work. *American Pharmacy* 1985; NS25(1):46–50.

PREVENTION, American Pharmaceutical Association. Joint Survey, *Navigating the medication marketplace: how consumers choose.* 1997.

Quill TE, Brody H. Physician recommendations and patient autonomy: finding a balance between physician power and patient choice. *Ann Intern Med* 1996; 125:763–769.

Rauber C. Disease management can be good for what ails patients and insurers. *Modern Healthcare* March 29, 1999; 29(13):48–54.

Reese S. Disenrollment: what it costs, how to stop it. *Business & Health* Special Report, "Treatment Compliance," 1997; 40–44.

Rosenau PV. Rx-to-OTC switch movement. *Medical Care and Review* 1994; 51:429–466.

Schoen MD. Lipid management: an opportunity for pharmacy service. *J APhA* 1996; NS36(10):609–619.

Self-medication practices. *California Medicine* 1967; 107(5):452–454.

Simon TJ, et al. Acid suppression by famotidine 20 mg twice daily or 40 mg twice daily in preventing relapse of endoscopic recurrence of erosive esophagitis. *Clin Ther* 1995; 17(6):1147–1156.

Smith MC. Rx-to-OTC switches: reflections and projections. *Drug Topics* July 20, 1998; 142:70–79.

Steele GH. Cost-effective management of dyspepsia and gastroesophageal reflux disease. *Gastroenterology* 1996; 23(3):561–576.

Study finds much of the consumer health advice on the Internet is wrong. *Modern Healthcare* August 9, 1999; 29(32):78.

Tanouye E. U.S. has developed an expensive habit: now, how to pay for it? *The Wall Street Journal* November 16, 1998; A1, A10.

The InterStudy Competitive Edge HMO Industry Report. Version 7.2. Minneapolis: InterStudy Publications, 1997.

Todd W, Nash DB. *Disease management: a system approach to improving patient outcomes.* Chicago: AHA Press, 1996.

Utley DS. *Stop the heartburn.* Woodside, CA: Lagado Publishing, 1996.

Vaczek D. The second arena: pharmacy faces surge of Rx-to-OTC switches. *Pharmacy Times* March 1996; 62:31–32, 35.

Weiss Ratings Inc. (data). *Employee Benefit News*, August 1999; 13(9). From www.benefitnews.com.

Welsh JS. Stepping up to positive health—consumers and professionals take the lead. *American Pharmacy* 1980; NS20(6):16–18.

Zablocki E. Employers: offering help along the way. *Business & Health* Special Report, "Treatment Compliance," December 1997; 19–23.

C H A P T E R

Empowering Consumers to Make Informed Choices

David Lansky, Ph.D.

Christina Bethell, Ph.D., MBA, MPH

INTRODUCTION

Observers of the American health system are concerned that quality of care is inconsistent and somewhat poor. Research reports often highlight patterns of inadequate care, but virtually no one—doctors, managers, or patients—is able to determine who provides the best care for any particular problem, and virtually no organizations—hospitals, health plans, or medical groups—receive any financial reward for providing high-quality care.

The Foundation for Accountability (FACCT) was formed in 1995 to introduce new mechanisms to measure and reward quality care. FACCT was created by purchasers and consumers who sought better information about the quality of the care they were buying or receiving and who believed that widely available quality information would mitigate marketplace trends that rewarded low prices but seemed to ignore the quality of care provided. They sought to create a market in which excellence would be rewarded, and healthcare organizations would have an incentive to improve.

FACCT's mission is to ensure that Americans have clear, accurate information about quality they can use to make better healthcare decisions. To accomplish this goal, FACCT has defined numerous consumer-focused quality measures, implemented them in market regions across the United States, and developed tools for helping people interpret and use the information. These three activities are tightly related: quality measures are no good unless the data are widely and reliably collected, and the data are not useful unless decision makers—purchasers and consumers—care about it and can understand what it means. This chapter examines one approach to sharing information about healthcare quality with the American public and argues that a common, rigorous approach can rapidly achieve desirable changes in the healthcare marketplace.

RATIONALE

Since 1965, the United States has experienced repeated efforts at healthcare reform, typically engineered around attempts to extend insurance coverage or constrain expenditures. The nation has enjoyed some success in these efforts, most notably the creation of Medicare and Medicaid, the recent Children's Health Insurance Program, and the introduction of prospective payment and managed care financing arrangements. In 1993 and 1994, President Clinton attempted to extend these successes with comprehensive reform, which he characterized as an effort to ensure "health security" for all Americans (Health Security Act of 1993).

Many of these national reform initiatives included design features that were intended to ensure that Americans received high-quality care. Yet these elements of the reform package were typically of secondary importance and have not proven effective (Brook, Kamberg, & McGlynn, 1996; Milgate, 1994). In March 1998, the President's Advisory Commission on Consumer Protection and Quality found the following:

Several types of quality problems in health care have been documented through peer-reviewed research. They include the following:

Avoidable errors: Many Americans are injured during the course of their treatment and some die prematurely as a result. For example, a study of injuries to patients treated in hospitals in New York State found that 3.7% experienced adverse events, of which 13.6% led to death and 2.6% permanent disability. A national study found that from 1983 to 1993, deaths due to medication errors rose more than twofold with 7,391 deaths attributed to medication errors in 1993 alone.

Underutilization of services: Millions of people do not receive necessary care and suffer needless complications that add to healthcare costs and reduce productivity. For example, an estimated 18,000 people die each year because they did not receive beta blockers following a heart attack.

Overuse of services: Millions of Americans receive healthcare services that are unnecessary, increase costs and often endanger their health. For example, an analysis of hysterectomies performed by a sample of health plans in 1990 found that nearly one in five was inappropriate.

Variation in services: There is a continuing pattern of wide variation in healthcare practice including regional variations and small-area variations. This is a clear indicator that the practice of healthcare has not caught up with the science of healthcare to ensure evidence-based practice in the United States (President's Commission, 1998).

More recently, the Institute of Medicine Roundtable on Managed Care reported the following:

Serious and widespread quality problems exist throughout American medicine. These problems, which may be classified as underuse, overuse, or misuse, occur in small and large communities alike, in all parts of the country, and with approximately equal frequency in managed care and fee-for-service systems of care. Very large numbers of Americans are harmed as a direct result. Quality of care is the problem, not managed care. Current efforts to improve will not succeed unless we undertake a major, systematic effort to overhaul how we deliver healthcare services, educate and train clinicians, and assess and improve quality (Chassin & Galvin, 1998).

Remarkably, these comments only repeat and amplify observations that were initially made around World War II. Millenson recently summarized the failure of the health professions and institutions to correct persistent, serious quality deficiencies (Millenson, 1997).

NEED FOR PARADIGM SHIFT

Today, we again are grappling with difficult decisions in organizing care and arranging for its financing, and we remain reluctant to address the quality deficiencies of the healthcare system. Healthcare administrators and purchasers are attempting to fine-tune managed care and make modest adjustments in financing arrangements, but they do so without serious attention to the remarkable social, cultural, and technological forces that are reshaping American life. One reason for this disconnect between health services and other aspects of economic and social life is the persistent exclusion of American consumers from the evaluation and design of healthcare.

In addition, medical technology and biomedical information have grown at an exponential rate. Today, there are 4,000 or more peer-reviewed scholarly publications, and any illusion that an individual physician can be master of all relevant clinical information has been retired (Hunt & Newman, 1997; Rennie, 1998). Similarly, the growing complexity of medicine mandates that effective care requires partnerships among diverse and substantial teams, which in turn require coordination and management.

Finally, these trends are compounded by growing consumer activism and impatience. The interest of state and federal legislators in managed care regulation and the "patient bill of rights" testify to the influence of an anxious public. Public concerns about the quality of care at the end of life (Lo, 1995; Lynn et al., 1997; The SUPPORT Principal Investigators, 1995), about patient safety and medical error (Ross, 1999), and about access to emergent treatments all reflect the urgency of engaging the American consumer in a more candid dialogue about the quality of healthcare services.

Healthcare leaders have responded to some of these trends with piecemeal experiments. The quality improvement movement has imported industrial management and analytic techniques, and it has some important psychological and local impact. However, the broad patterns of healthcare delivery and outcome appear to be unaffected (Blumenthal & Kilo, 1998; Shortell, Bennett, & Byck, 1998). Hospitals and managed care plans have been subject to elaborate and expensive accreditation programs that examine structural and procedural conditions, but even advocates of these programs have noted their modest impact on ensuring and improving quality. The federal government and the AMA have made a serious effort to document best practices and encourage conformity to practice guidelines; both initiatives have been shelved.

PARAMETERS OF CHANGE

What mechanisms can now be considered for reengineering U.S. healthcare to put it on the road to higher-quality care and service? How can the decades-long pattern of variable and inadequate performance be corrected? It is worth noting that all attempts, until now, have relied on the insights and goodwill of healthcare and policy leaders. The approach has been limited to a "top-down" strategy of quality improvement and healthcare reform. Despite well-intentioned efforts, no leading healthcare organizations have demonstrated their ability to help patients achieve outcomes of recognized importance to the public. Perhaps it is time that these questions are put to the public to humbly ask for instruction on how best to meet their needs.

Ethically, sociologically, and clinically, the U.S. healthcare system cannot improve until consumers are able to become full partners in its management and operation. The healthcare system can provide quality care only when it learns to listen to the needs of the people it serves and is prepared to reorganize its resources in response to those needs.

To achieve this objective, the healthcare system must work with its public to establish a quality lexicon. We will need a common language to discuss our expectations of those who provide healthcare services, and a common metric will be needed that tells us if those expectations are being met. Most important, this vocabulary and set of metrics must be defined by those served. The healthcare system will not be altered if professionals persist in conversing only with those who share their training, values, and expertise.

By establishing a common vocabulary and measurement language, we can begin to support individuals' ability to seek the healthcare arrangements that they judge best. Patients, consumers, and families can be permitted to select where to seek their care based on relevant, understandable information about quality performance. In the face of clear and relevant information about public expectations, providers and plans will seek to excel on those dimensions used by consumers and purchasers to make selections.

This approach to building a consumer-centered, market-based healthcare system assumes that we can solve several daunting problems:

- Learn what the public cares about.
- Develop reliable, valid measures of the desired quality and service constructs.
- Gather relevant data across all relevant service entities.
- Compile and represent the data in a way that is understood and used by a critical mass of Americans.
- Communicate quality and service performance in a realistic personal choice context that addresses concerns about costs, benefits, and plan rules.
- Communicate personal decision-making information in a context that addresses broader societal healthcare challenges and shapes a successful national health policy.

A FRAMEWORK FOR COMMUNICATING WITH THE PUBLIC ABOUT QUALITY HEALTHCARE

What Does the Public Want?

In 1996, HCFA engaged FACCT to develop an organizing framework for the representation of quality performance information (Bethell, Lansky, & Read, 1997). To develop this Consumer Information Framework, FACCT first researched all available consumer communication templates. These were analyzed and condensed into four conceptually distinct approaches, organized as follows:

1. Health states model (e.g., getting better, living with illness, staying healthy)
2. Type of measure model (e.g., process, outcome)
3. System competencies (e.g., prevention, acute care)
4. Satisfaction concepts only

These models were tested with more than 400 consumers drawn from a variety of settings across the United States, including Medicare and Medicaid beneficiaries, commercially insured consumers with both managed care and non–managed care experience, and people both with and without chronic disease. These investigations identified five quality constructs of widespread public interest (Box 11–1, p. 272). These five quality domains are inclusive; that is, they accommodate all of the important quality concerns as indicated by respondents.

Each of these five domains can be deconstructed into component concepts, each of which may be represented by quantitative measures. The "Living with Illness" domain, for example, is made up of four subcategories that address important competencies of chronic disease care:

- *Appropriate care:* conformity to practice guidelines and commonly accepted standards of care
- *Education and teamwork:* effectiveness of patient and caregiver teaching
- *Help for daily living:* helping patients minimize adverse symptoms and maximize daily functioning
- *Experience of care:* patient ratings of access, communication, and service quality

Each of these subcategories is in turn comprised of individual performance measures. "Appropriate care," for instance, could include whether severe asthmatic patients possess and know how to use a peak flow meter or inhaler, or whether diabetic patients have had regular assessments of their feet or hemoglobin A_{1c} level.

B O X 11–1

THE BASICS

Delivering the basics of good care—doctor care, rules for getting care, information and service, satisfaction

STAYING HEALTHY

Helping people avoid illness and stay healthy through preventive care, reduction of health risks, early detection of illness, education

GETTING BETTER

Helping people recover when they are sick or injured through appropriate treatment and follow-up

LIVING WITH ILLNESS

Helping people with ongoing, chronic conditions (e.g., diabetes, asthma) take care of themselves, control symptoms, avoid complications, and maintain daily activities

CHANGING NEEDS

Caring for people and their families when needs change dramatically because of disability or terminal illness—with comprehensive services, caregiver support, hospice care

This hierarchical structure has several advantageous features:

- Users with particular interests may populate the structure with measures of special relevance to them, while retaining the conceptual and methodological integrity of the model.
- Users with interest in greater detail may use layered technologies—such as Internet Web sites—to probe performance issues of personal concern.

- Users with differential abilities to gather data may implement selected branches of the hierarchy and phase in additional content areas over time.

Tailoring: How Can We Develop Measures?

The Consumer Information Framework can be effective only if the information content it conveys is meaningful, relevant, and sound. A nine-stage process is recommended for qualifying measures for inclusion in the Framework. Critical qualification tasks include the following:

1. Assess relevance of topic to consumers and purchasers.
2. Compile expert opinion on quality measurement in topic area.
3. Solicit consumer and patient judgments on dimensions of quality for topic area.
4. Synthesize expert and consumer quality criteria.
5. Develop technical measurement definitions, including case identification, measure specifications, and methods recommendations.
6. Review measurement proposal with experts and consumers.
7. Conduct field trials in different types of settings.
8. Revise measurement proposal as necessary.
9. Publish technical specifications for data collection and communication of quality measures.

Two elements of this process are most important. First, the question "what is quality care?" must have a working definition that reflects the values, preferences, and experiences of patients, families, and the community at large. Typically, patients will include a strong desire for quality measures to reflect expert judgment regarding best practices and contemporary standards of care. They will also emphasize an involvement of patient and family in decisions, the quality of communications between providers and patients, and the commitment of the providers to help patients manage their own care. In addition, patients often highlight the effectiveness of care in achieving desired outcomes, such as symptom relief, functioning, and clinical benefit to a greater degree than do experts.

As one AIDS patient stated:

> Overall health status is what's really important because that's a function of the anti-(retro)viral treatment. It's a function of having mental health services. It's a function of preventing opportunistic infections. All those come together to indicate to me that everything is being done but without mental health coverage or care, I would get depressed. I'm on antidepressants. Without that kind of situation, I think that would make my physical health worse and I know it does. So, it's all interrelated (FACCT focus group, 1998).

Second, emphasis is placed on the importance of testing data collection methods and reporting strategies before publication of measurement specifications, and the need to conduct such trials in multiple settings. As the healthcare system continues to change, quality measures must be available to permit comparisons across settings of care and types of financing systems, both to help consumers understand systematic consequences of alternative structures and to help policy makers evaluate alternative strategies. If the content of quality measures is based on patients' experiences and their values, they will remain relevant as the financial and delivery system arrangements evolve.

Where's the Data?

Some authorities argue that systematic quality assessment and public disclosure must await improvements in clinical information systems (Eddy, 1998). This argument reflects two fallacies. First, it presumes that relevant quality information is principally available in the record-keeping systems of providers and health plans and that such information is more relevant or reliable than alternatives. The authors are unaware of any evidence to support this view. On the contrary, clinical record keeping in paper charts is notoriously incomplete and inaccurate, often reflecting economic incentives, variations in clinical interpretation, and competing administrative requirements (Palmer & Nesson, 1982; Romano & Mark, 1994; Solberg et al., 1990). The clinical record typically fails to document quality in the domains of concern to patients, such as functioning, symptom level, independence, counseling, or communication. The medical record often fails to record public health interventions of substantial concern to purchasers, such as immunizations, cholesterol checks, or mammograms that may be provided by various community service agencies (IPRO, 1998). Second, the clinical record may report activities of healthcare professionals without noting if they ever reached the patient or had the intended consequences. Medications may be prescribed and not taken; specific counseling provided but not understood (Ickovics & Meisler, 1997; Morse et al., 1991; Sackett, & Haynes, 1976). Whether the impact of professional interventions should be considered as a performance measure (policy versus technical) is an issue unto itself. However, relying solely on the clinical record for capturing information on effectiveness would be a deterrent to any quality strategy.

Instead, we recommend that performance data be gathered from multiple sources that respond to different needs: transaction data that describe key services rendered, medical chart data that reflect objective biological measures, and patient reports that reflect symptoms, functioning, and the patient's experiences of care.

Across studies, patients report that they value each of these types of information. In a series of studies, FACCT asked patients to rate the relative importance of alternative types of quality performance information. In each study, patients were shown proposed quality measures of specific, relevant aspects of care. For persons with diabetes, for example, proposed measures included frequent testing for the hemoglobin A_{1c} and lipid levels, the attainment of desirable levels of hemoglobin A_{1c}, and adequacy of access to specialists and necessary medical materials, such as test strips. Patients provided ratings of their relative importance as follows:

- Whether or not recommended care processes are followed: 1.00 (index)

- Whether or not the desired patient outcomes are achieved: 0.81
- Whether or not patients report satisfaction with care: 0.60

This approach suggests that the evolution of measurement approaches should happen simultaneously, not in sequence. We should develop and implement measures of processes, outcomes, and experience of care in parallel in an effort to minimize bias. If society focuses exclusively on one or another domain, it will present a distorted picture of healthcare performance to the public and possibly influence markets in undesirable ways.

Communicating Quality Performance to the Public

The Consumer Information Framework involves the aggregation of discrete performance data into summary scores that are relevant and understandable to the general public. The process of organizing individual measures into consumer "information" involves these major steps:

- Organizing individual measures into reporting categories and subcategories
- Transforming each item into a standardized value that permits comparison and summation
- Aggregating multiple items into summary scores
- Reporting summary scores to the public in one or more media

Each of these activities involves both policy and methodological decisions, each of which may affect the ranking of healthcare organizations and, ultimately, their economic success. These are summarized briefly here to suggest both that public healthcare performance information can be produced in a systematic and logical fashion and that legitimate policy debates may be necessary.

Organizing Measures into Categories

There are many ways to define the conceptual categories to be used for presenting information to the public: (1) based on characteristics of the organizations being profiled, (2) based on the nature of the reported data, (3) based on expert theories about healthcare quality, or (4) based on consumer healthcare experiences or values. The categories in the Consumer Information Framework provide a uniform vocabulary that is accessible and interpretable to most consumers. It is a template that accommodates most currently available performance measures as well as those in development. Over time and for various audiences, users can add or drop measures and retain a stable approach to communicating with the public.

The top-level categories of the Framework provide potential standards for public information, but they are not adequate for any but the most superficial reporting systems. Many consumers prefer more detailed performance information than those available at the highest level of aggregation. FACCT has developed a second-level set of (sub)categories that map three or four subcategories associated to each top-level category. A robust design feature of the framework is the flexibility it affords each data collection/reporting project. Individual reporting projects may have reasons to develop alternative subcategories that better meet the needs of specific audiences. For example, a target population with established diseases may wish the "Living with Illness" category to accommodate subcategories such as overall ratings of "diabetes care," "asthma care," and so on.

Once a set of policy-defined reporting categories has been established, the available performance measures must be assigned to each category. The assignment is nontrivial. For example, is the HEDIS measure of *whether beta blocker medications are prescribed following myocardial infarction* properly regarded as an intervention for a chronic disease—thus belonging to "Living with Illness"—or an expected element of acute care best grouped with "Getting Better"? Is *counseling asthma patients about important lifestyle changes* a dimension of "Staying Healthy" or "Living with Illness"?

When measures are matched to reporting categories, psychometric analyses (e.g., measures of reliability and factor analysis) must then be conducted for the proposed groupings. Users need to be confident that the summary categories they report send an accurate signal to consumers about the information they actually contain.

Transform Raw Performance Data into Standardized Scores

The goal at this stage is to transform individual quality measures to a common metric and common scale before aggregation. This often includes two steps:

1. *Standardization of individual scores to a common metric:* This is especially necessary when combining rate- versus score-based measures.

2. *Translation of each standardized score to a common scale so that it is appropriate for entry into the summarization and weighting process:* Translation is also important so that the score for each plan is easily understood.

Translating standardized scores to an understandable scale—such as a 0 to 100 scale—will usually involve the determination of which value should represent a "0" performance score (bottom end of the scale) and which value should represent a "100" score (top end of the scale). One option is to assign the *best score* (100) to the best performing organization in a region, and assign the *worst score* to the worst performing organization. Such relative anchor scores can be misleading, particularly if the absolute differences in performance are small. A second option is to assign the *highest value* to a computed "best possible" score (e.g., if every respondent answered "excellent" to every question asked, that organization would achieve 100). Consumers generally prefer the second approach because it provides absolute performance information, but it can be difficult to establish a "best possible" score for some clinical measures (e.g., cholesterol level).

Selection of the comparison benchmarks and the anchor values for transforming the data can have a substantial impact on the consumer's perception of healthcare system performance. As health plans, providers, and consumer advocates understand these decisions, they often become significant policy debates.

Figure 11–1 illustrates the different apparent performance of seven health plans in caring for asthmatic patients, based on the use of relative or absolute anchor values.

Aggregate Individual Scores into Summary Scores

Each performance measure has presumably been assigned to an appropriate category and the data has been standardized and is

FIGURE 11-1

Apparent performance of seven healthcare plans in caring for asthmatic patients. **A,** Relative comparison; **B,** absolute comparison.

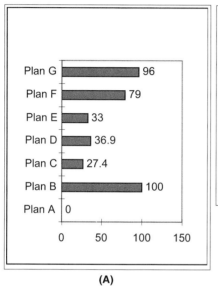

(A)

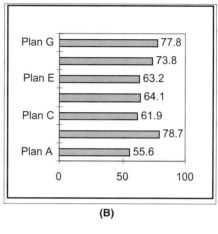

(B)

now scored on a 0 to 100 scale. In general, it is assumed that measures will be combined using a simple additive model of the form:

$$\text{Score} = (\text{wt}_1 \times \text{measure}_1) + (\text{wt}_2 \times \text{measure}_2) + \ldots$$

Determining the appropriate weights is a sensitive and powerful policy decision, because the ultimate ranking of organizational performance will be affected by the relative importance of each component measure.

At least three types of criteria could affect the assignment of weights:

1. Consumer (user) utilities
2. Expert valuation
3. Statistical properties of the measure

Some experts express concern that consumers will give preference to measures of customer service rather than to measures that reflect conformity to best clinical practices or achievement of desired outcomes. In FACCT's early investigations, we found high agreement between experts and consumers (approximately 85%), with the latter giving modestly higher weight to functional outcomes and elements of communication and relationship with providers. In the case of patients diagnosed with HIV and AIDS, for example, there was strong agreement on the importance of measures of viral load testing and the availability of antiretroviral therapies, but patients argued that poor relationships with providers compromised their willingness to comply with any clinician recommendations and thus deserved primacy in the weighting scheme.

A policy commitment to assess and incorporate consumer utilities in the weighting scheme raises additional questions. Should a quality report, targeted for a particular insurance class or cultural group, use weights generated specifically by that group? Should personal decision aid technology (e.g., interactive Internet sites or computer kiosks) permit each person to assign his or her own weights?

Expert weighting could be applied and based on a variety of criteria. Clinicians tend to advocate weights proportional to expected physiological impact—so maintenance of a diabetic patient's low blood glucose is rated more important than patients' rating of physician communication skills. Social scientists may assign weights based on expected public health impacts or relative cost-benefit, so mammograms for women aged 50 to 64 are weighted higher than well-child visits for grade school-age children.

In addition, weights may be determined by *attributes of the measures* themselves. For instance, the reporting system may choose to systematically weight clinical outcomes higher than overall satisfaction. If the reporting agency wishes to reward organizations that achieve consistency in their performance—as well as high average performance—measures may be weighted inversely by the variance in the distribution of the measure. For example, two health plans may each achieve an average satisfaction rating of 75%, but one does so by having higher numbers of members offering ratings of "very good," whereas the other has a wider range of members across the entire range from "excellent" to "poor" and thus a higher standard deviation associated with the same mean. These variances could be used to give additional weight to the more consistent performer.

The selection of these weights does have a meaningful impact on public rankings. In one comparison of using equal weights (.33, .33, .33) versus unequal weights (.2, .5, .3) when aggregating three measures into an asthma score for seven health plans, the choice of weighting schemes altered relative ranks either one or two places for all but the first- and second-ranked plans.

Symbolism and Reporting of Summary Scores

Given a set of performance scores, users still face numerous design decisions affecting the communication of the data to the public. Key issues include the following:

- Should data be presented as numbers, as symbols, or as words? People vary widely in their comfort and understanding of each of these formats. If data are represented numerically, publishers must be careful to avoid misrepresentation of small differences as statistically meaningful or different. Consumers often indicate an interest in being told which performance levels indicate good or poor performance. If data are represented with symbols, publishers must recognize that they are losing data. Auto workers, for example, have complained that a reporting system using one, two, or three stars (where one or three represent statistically significant differences from the mean) hides absolute performance and inevitably clusters too many health plans into an uninterpretable "two-star" category.
- Should publishers indicate confidence intervals or sampling errors? Attempts to represent measurement uncertainty seem important to researchers and the health plans that are being compared, but confuse most consumers. When applied to aggregate scores, these adjustments require additional, complex decisions regarding the treatment of unequal sample sizes, treatment of within-plan variation, and the calculation of composite standard errors. These convoluted analyses

can create perverse incentives for health plans, encouraging smaller sample sizes and even lower performance. By adding uncertainty to the consumer's ability to interpret the data, these adjustments also have the unfortunate consequence of lessening the consumer's confidence in the entire reporting enterprise (Hibbard, Slovic, & Jewett, 1997).

- Should publishers tell a story when presenting data? Communications theorists agree that data without context is not helpful (Rodgers, 1999). Yet providing an interpretive context inevitably reflects the publisher's own agenda. Important policy questions need to be addressed to guide the presentation of data. Should the "story" indicate that quality performance is generally lower than desired or that it varies inexplicably? Should it provide the consumer with tools and ideas for self-advocacy when navigating the health system? At a minimum, quality categories and the words used to describe them must be carefully tailored to accurately reflect the information content being presented. We can easily mislead people into thinking information is included in scores when it is not and vice versa.

HOW CAN QUALITY INFORMATION BE INTEGRATED WITH OTHER IMPORTANT FACTORS?

Most consumers evaluate numerous aspects of a product or service when making a decision. Price, features, and quality are all important. For health plan or provider decisions, additional constraints may come into play—such as the number of choices made available by their employer or public sponsor, specific geographic and access considerations, or the importance of maintaining current relationships. Quality information must be arrayed in a specific choice context.

In general, four categories of information should be presented to consumers when making these marketplace decisions, and consumers should be aided in evaluating the trade-offs among these four considerations. In addition to quality information, consumers should understand the following:

- *Costs:* What will each of the available options cost the consumer, including co-pays, deductibles, and premium contributions? Optimally, this information can be estimated for the individual subscriber, based on previous utilization experience.
- *Benefits:* What coverage is available from each of the available options?
- *Rules:* What barriers to care exist that may affect the subscriber? Particular concern has been voiced about continuity with current doctors, access to preferred medications, and opportunities to see specialists without primary care referral.

Numerous initiatives are under way to develop decision models and decision support systems to assist consumers in evaluating their own needs and selecting health plans and provider relationships. Some efforts involve computer-assisted decision aids; others involve in-person "choice counseling" either one-on-one or through a "town hall" format.

HOW CAN CONSUMER DECISION MAKING SHAPE SUCCESSFUL NATIONAL POLICY?

This chapter argues that consumers can be given substantial, relevant, and valid information upon which to make important healthcare decisions. We identify a concise framework for organizing performance information and discuss both the methods for constructing meaningful performance scores and the context within which such data should be communicated.

There is a risk that consumers are not interested in quality information, have not valued such information as has been made available, or may overvalue service performance at the expense of clinical performance. These are serious concerns and heighten researchers' obligations to evaluate the impact of consumer information strategies, both to improve the various technologies described here and to avoid unnecessary or irresponsible policy initiatives.

Yet the mere tabulation and presentation of individual performance data is unlikely—*prima facie*—to stimulate new

marketplace behaviors. Consumers have not previously been informed about the workings of healthcare or the legitimacy of
their expectations for high-quality care. They have not been encouraged to inquire about performance or to make meaningful
decisions about their care.

FACCT continuously conducts interviews, focus groups, and
quantitative surveys of American consumers. We are constantly
reminded of the pressing and anxious desire of consumers for
guidance on navigating the healthcare system and for ensuring
that they can get high-quality care. Over time, we have seen that
a simple framework, reflecting careful technical work, can help
people gain a common understanding of how healthcare works
and how they can look for the best care for themselves.
Numerous organizations have embraced the Consumer
Information Framework—ranging from the State of Michigan to
the "big three" auto companies to *Newsweek* magazine. Despite
slow progress in improving the availability of quality data, there
seems to be great interest in using a common vocabulary and
technical toolkit for educating the public about quality.

However, the inadequacy of quality data presents a profound challenge. Communications messages without meaningful content is just "spin." Government agencies and purchasers will need to explore new ways of acquiring quality
information that matters to people. Certainly, the Internet will
provide an opportunity for broad distribution of quality data
and, perhaps, for inexpensive collection of patient evaluations of
their care. But the likelihood that quality data will be slow in
coming suggests that quality leaders will need to start focusing
their efforts on educating patients to advocate for themselves, to
give them tools to recognize and demand high-quality care in
their own lives, and thereby send a message to providers, insurers, employers, and governments that their accountability
remains to the public and for the public's well-being.

The present market environment poses serious barriers to
effective consumer choice and to the prospect of rewarding excellence in healthcare. A strategy of systematic disclosure of
healthcare system performance, coupled with coordinated and
thoughtful public education, has the potential to accelerate necessary changes in the healthcare system.

REFERENCES

Bethell C, Lansky D, Read D. *Reporting quality information to consumers. A report to the Health Care Financing Administration.* Portland, OR: Foundation for Accountability, December 1997.

Blumenthal D, Kilo CM. A report card on continuous quality improvement. *Milbank Quarterly* 1998; 76(4):625–648.

Brook RH, Kamberg CJ, McGlynn EA. Health system reform and quality. *JAMA* 1996; 276(6):476–480.

Chassin MR, Galvin RW. The urgent need to improve healthcare quality: Institute of Medicine National Roundtable on healthcare quality. *JAMA* 1998; 280:1000–1005.

Eddy DM. Performance measurement: problems and solutions. *Health Affairs* 1998; 17(4):7–25.

FAACT focus group. San Francisco, CA, August 15, 1998.

Health Care Security Act of 1993. A bill to ensure individual and family security through healthcare coverage for all Americans in a manner that contains the rate of growth in healthcare costs and promotes responsible health insurance practices, to promote choice in healthcare, and to ensure and protect the healthcare of all Americans.

Hibbard JH, Slovic P, Jewett JJ. Informing consumer decisions in healthcare: implications from decision-making research. *Milbank Quarterly* 1997; 75(3):395–414.

Hunt RE, Newman RG. Medical knowledge overload: a disturbing trend for physicians. *Health Care Management Review* 1997; 22(1):70–75.

Ickovics JR, Meisler AW. Adherence in AIDS clinical trials: a framework for clinical research and clinical care. *J Clin Epidemiol* 1997; 50:385–391.

IPRO. Audit Report: 1997 Medicare HEDIS® 3.0/1998 Data. http://www.hcfa.gov/quality/3i2.htm

Lo, B. Improving care near the end of life: why is it so hard? *JAMA* 1995; 274(20):1634–1636 (editorial).

Lynn J, et al. Perceptions by family members of the dying experience of older and seriously ill patients. *Ann Intern Med* 1997; 126(97):97–106.

Milgate K. Health reform and accountability for quality. *QRC Advis* 1994; 10(7):8.

Millenson ML. *Demanding medical excellence: doctors and accountability in the information age.* Chicago: The University of Chicago Press, 1997.

Morse EV, et al. Determinants of subject compliance within an experimental anti-HIV drug protocol. *Soc Sci Med* 1991; 32:1161–1167.

Palmer RH, Nesson HR. A review of methods for ambulatory medical care evaluations. *Medical Care* 1982; 20(8):758–781.

President's Advisory Commission on Consumer Protection & Quality in the Health Care Industry. Quality First: Better Health Care for All Americans. Final Report, March 13, 1998. http://www.hcqualitycommission.gov

Rennie D. The present state of medical journals. *Lancet* 1998; SII:18–22.

Rodgers AB. *Making quality count: a national conference on consumer health information. Conference summary.* February 1999. HCFA contract 500-97-P511.

Romano PS, Mark DH. Bias in the coding of hospital discharge data and its implications for quality assessment. *Medical Care* 1994; 32(1):81–90.

Ross PE. Nine mistakes doctors make. *Forbes* 1999; 9:116–118.

Sackett DL, Haynes RB (eds). *Compliance with therapeutic regimens.* Baltimore: Johns Hopkins University Press, 1976.

Shortell SM, Bennett CL, Byck GR. Assessing the impact of continuous quality improvement on clinical practice: what it will take to accelerate progress. *Milbank Quarterly* 1998; 76(4):593–624.

Solberg LI, et al. The Minnesota project: a focused approach to ambulatory quality assessment. *Inquiry* 1990; 27:359–367.

The SUPPORT Principal Investigators. A controlled trial to improve care for seriously ill hospitalized patients: the study to understand prognoses and preferences for outcomes and risks of treatment (SUPPORT). *JAMA* 1995; 274(20):1591–1598.

12

C H A P T E R

The Ascendancy of the Employer as Consumer Advocate in Healthcare

Suzanne Mercure

INTRODUCTION

Employers have historically played an important role as providers of healthcare and medical coverage for employees, their dependents, and retirees. Over time, this role has evolved from being fairly exclusively focused on occupational health and safety, to that of healthcare information source and wellness advocate, in line with employees' expanding awareness of and demand for healthcare choices. This historical context will provide a background for better understanding the current purchaser role, including how employers influence healthcare market change and promote the advance of consumer information. In the process, the potential synergies between employers and providers will be identified.

HISTORICAL PERSPECTIVE: BACK TO THE FUTURE

In some respects, the employer's role is going back to the future. That is, many of the same issues that employers focused on in the last half century are being addressed again today. The techniques and approaches may have changed, yet many of the basic problems—getting employees to work, achieving high levels of productivity, controlling costs, and improving quality—have remained the same. A review of the development of health coverage from the employer perspective will provide the historical "stepping stones" taken by the employer, as a purchaser of healthcare. Significant events or turning points therein are highlighted in the following narrative timeline (Figure 12–1).

1860–1900

In this early role, employers hired company doctors whose roles were limited to dealing with industrial accidents and injuries. Paul Starr, in his book *The Social Transformation of American Medicine* (Starr, 1982), describes the role of the employer in employee health starting at the time of the Civil War.

1900–1950

In the beginning of the twentieth century, states began to enact Workman's Compensation laws, spurred by worker protection needs because of high rates of industrial injury and by physicians' dislike for business control over doctor selection. As a result, employers expanded their occupational focus—treatment of employees from accident and injuries—to preventive medicine. The goals of preventive medicine were to improve industrial hygiene and avoid worker injuries before they occurred.

Employers in the first half of the twentieth century were focused on ways to enhance productivity (Starr, 1982). The predominant school of thought centered on analysis of the production processes and motivational behavior. In time and efficiency studies, productivity was measured in terms of physical motion. The turn of the century novel, *Cheaper by the Dozen*, written by Frank Gilbreth and Ernestine Carey and made into a popular movie, depicts in a humorous manner the work of these industrial hygiene and medical engineering experts.

Another force in the early 1900s that helped shape employers' roles was a growing interest and trust in medical knowledge. Before the commonly held belief that medical treatment could be effective, employers' main objective was to select healthy workers. Starr contends that this change in attitude

Historical Progression of Employer Role Concerning Consumers' Healthcare

Time Period	Employer Role in Healthcare	Employer Interaction with Consumer (Employee, Retiree, Dependent)
1860–1900	Company physician for accidents especially in hazardous industries.	Support for injuries while on the job.
1900–1950	On-site medical facilities for occupational health and safety. Companies begin to focus on accident and injury prevention.	Workers' compensation programs for accident and injury treatment; on-site industrial physician.
1950–1970	Health insurance becomes common employee benefit.	Insurance coverage for accidents and illness on and off the job. Coverage extended to dependents of the employee. Health plan coverage information provided.
1980–1990	Cost containment programs, including utilization review, second surgical opinion, health promotion, and wellness. Introduction of flexible benefits programs. Growth of business groups on health.	Insurance coverage for preventive services through HMOs, corporate education on health promotion, and work site programs for prevention and wellness. Information on rationale for controls provided.
1990–2000	Accountability for quality and cost with measures used for performance monitoring and health plan selection. Emphasis on accountability and value.	Information on plan choice includes quality measures. Nurse help lines introduced. More information on maintenance of health status. Increased consumer "self-service" tools including Internet.

about the "usefulness of medical knowledge" caused employers to demonstrate a higher degree of interest in the use of on-site medical facilities. Employers in more hazardous industries, such as railroads, mining, and lumbering, were motivated to minimize financial and legal liability. For example, according to the

Interstate Commerce Commission, in the railroad industry in the year ending June 30, 1900, 1 of every 28 employees sustained an injury and 1 of every 399 employees died while working. Rural locations with few accessible medical professionals led some employers to pay the salary for a physician to live and provide health services in that area. A few employers used the provision of medical programs as one of the mechanisms to promote loyalty.

Employer-sponsored medical clinics focused on employee health for the job. These clinics paved the way for the formation of industrial medical programs, providing a controlled environment for access and services. The preventive medical aspects included work site treatment for on-the-job injuries, physical examinations for job applicants, and workplace hygiene programs. Services were not extended to family members, nor was health insurance provided.

The labor movement began the fight for health insurance benefits in the 1930s and 1940s. In 1929, the Los Angeles Department of Water and Power employers established an arrangement with two physicians to provide healthcare services for 2,000 members. In 1933, Sidney Garfield and his associates set up a similar arrangement for 5,000 aqueduct building workers. In 1938, Garfield extended health services in another program for workers for Henry J. Kaiser at the Grand Coulee Dam. Similar programs were established by others in Washington, Oregon, and Texas.

At the same time these early prepaid medical programs were being established, hospitals and physicians organized as Blue Cross and Blue Shield, respectively. Blue Cross service plans were well established in the 1940s due to special enabling acts by states that allowed the creation of tax-exempt corporate structure. Starr presents the history of the development of these two organizations, including the politics that impacted the formation of "The Blues."

1950–1970

After World War II, the rise of labor unions and the tax deductibility of healthcare coverage for employers greatly influenced the development of health insurance as an employee benefit. As the unions negotiated for larger contributions by employers, employers had more incentive to address the issue of healthcare cost.

The health insurance coverage of this period was designed for catastrophic illness and accident. Prevention and chronic condition management were not addressed. Early programs had additional coverage riders that could be purchased for polio, cancer, and other "dread diseases." The expansion of the healthcare delivery system, with the introduction of Medicare and Medicaid programs in the 1960s, led employers to begin to look at the capacity of the healthcare system and the need for additional facilities. For example, some employers began to get involved in the regional certificate of need review programs to understand the issues and processes used in making informed decisions to increase services or capacity.

The HMO Act of 1973 was introduced as an attempt to control spiraling healthcare costs and initiate a national health plan. The Act, which required employers with more than 25 employees to offer a federally qualified HMO as a health coverage option, was met with resistance by employers, mainly because of the government's mandate approach to the issue. Employers found ways to avoid or delay compliance or to make the option unattractive to their employees. Only 10 million Americans were enrolled in HMOs in 1980.

1980s

By the 1980s, employers began to experience significant cost escalation in their healthcare programs. Initial reactions were to address the financing arrangement for health insurance. Employers also began to introduce programs to contain costs in their fee-for-service benefit plans. These programs required reviews (e.g., "second opinion," case management review) before surgery or use of other services. Consumers and providers viewed these programs as being driven by cost and as barriers to effective, timely care. Denials of payment for services were regarded with somewhat less vehemence by consumers than were the review programs because the medical benefits design related to coverage for defined services and categories of providers. The third-party payment was distanced from the actual provision of care that exists today, with financing and services intermingled. This payment system insulated consumers from the costs of services. The distinction of insurers paying only for services began to erode as insurers started entering the realm of medical decision making with the introduction of managed care.

A few employers began to provide information to their employees to support the rationale for these review programs. The introduction of Jack Wennberg's variation in provider practice data in 1973 had alerted employers (in addition to the healthcare professions) to the vagaries of health services consumption, highlighting how little was known about the complex issues within healthcare (Wennberg & Gittelsohn, 1975). A decade later, employers were using the small-area variation analysis-type information developed by Wennberg, and similar tools, as ways to educate their employees about employers' imperative to control costs, with attendant changes in health plan options and premium contributions. Reduction in variation is a tenet for quality improvement. The variation data were influential as a basis for the later work of employers in quality. Employers endeavored to highlight consumer choice in the process, providing avenues to help employees make informed choices. An example of innovative approaches by an employer in mobilizing resources to educate employees was Boston-based Wang Laboratories. Wang developed its list of procedures for obtaining a second opinion based on the small-area variation data developed in Massachusetts by the Health Planning Council for Greater Boston with the Massachusetts Health Data Consortium.

Polaroid and the former New England Telephone, also Boston-area employers, participated in the Health Planning Council for Greater Boston. The planning councils reviewed certificates of need for facility and service expansion and helped educate purchasers and consumers with data about new procedures and equipment as well as the variation in practice, such as surgical procedure rates. Potential over and underutilization of healthcare services were reviewed by service area. Employers learned from this involvement and began to frame their questions about quality and cost based on this knowledge.

Some employers introduced health promotion and wellness programs for their employees, including general health education, on-site screening and health fairs, exercise programs and facilities, health assessments, and self-help materials. This movement was aligned with a growing philosophy of prevention as a way to keep employees healthy and out of the hospital, concomitant with shifting the locus of care from inpatient to outpatient settings. This approach to prevention differed from that of the early 1900s, when the focus was restricted to injury and hygiene only. The success of these programs was often assessed by the corresponding reduction in absenteeism resulting from the programs. Some employers were able to focus targeted care management programs based on the results of screening to help employees who were most at risk.

By this time, many large employers had moved to self-funded financing for medical benefits. This funding arrangement allowed the company to maintain any reserve for unpaid and incurred claims and to avoid premium tax required in most states for insured programs. In addition, self-insuring allowed the employer to limit utilization. Other ways that employers sought to gain control of their costs, in addition to self-insuring, included developing catastrophic case management programs to avoid potentially costly and complex situations.

During the 1980s, consumer choice was extended to an array of benefit options as many employers introduced flexible benefit programs. These programs are designed to provide tax advantages for employees and to allow employers to define dollar amounts that will be provided by the company for the employee to "spend" on benefits—usually health, disability, and life insurance. These programs also provide a mechanism to educate employees about the cost of their health benefits program.

Employees with spouses who had coverage elsewhere were encouraged with cash incentives to opt out of the program by a minority of employers. This effort was designed to eliminate the duplication of benefits and the need to coordinate with another insurer. In addition, this approach put some degree of price sensitivity back on the employee because 100% coverage was not being encouraged.

As more companies moved to employee contributions through flexible benefit programs, managed care plans became the favored choice for employees because of fewer out-of-pocket expenses, broader coverage for preventive services, and lower contribution requirements. With more employees in managed care programs, employers experienced a reduction and stabilization of cost that was shown in benefit surveys. In addition, for employers with retiree health obligations, the liability that was now required to be reported under Financial Accounting Standards Board rules decreased significantly. The reduction in liability resulted from the comparatively lower cost escalation that was expected with managed care versus traditional fee-for-service indemnity plans.

During this time, employers began to come together to wield their collective leverage in health plan purchasing. Business groups on health began to proliferate at both the local and national level. Today, their popularity as an avenue for collective strength and bargaining is undiminished from a decade ago. Given the sheer numbers of covered lives a large employer (e.g., Fortune 500 or 100) is responsible for, their clout is indeed considerable and health plans have been obliged to negotiate accordingly. Pacific Business Group on Health, which includes such employers as Chevron, Bank of America, and GTE, was one of the earliest groups. Although leveraging purchasing power is the implicit aim of these groups, their respective goals—ranging from employee education to data collection and analysis (to learn more about health outcomes of their employees and to improve healthcare quality)—are as varied as the employers who fill their ranks. More than 100 such organizations exist today.

Over time, with an increasing awareness of what drives their costs, employers have honed their activities to reflect the real drivers, for example, by focusing on claims that represent the highest percentage of costs. Increasingly, quality, rather than cost, has become the predominant concern of employers, who, in tandem with the healthcare system today, adhere to the premise that quality care is, or can be, cost-effective care.

In 1989, the Health Plan Employer Data and Information Set (HEDIS), which was developed to measure HMO quality performance, was launched. A first-of-its-kind initiative, the pioneering group consisted of GTE, Xerox, Digital Equipment, and Bull Information on the purchaser side, and an association of staff and group model nonprofit HMOs, which composed the HMO Group. HEDIS originated because employers had no way to measure HMO performance or to compare the effectiveness of HMO plan participation with indemnity plan participation for their employees. A decade later, the National Committee for Quality Assurance (NCQA), a nonprofit "watchdog" organization, manages the development, change, and implementation of HEDIS. Today, HEDIS remains the "gold standard" not only for quality measurement but also for health plan quality accreditation, accrediting more than three-quarters of American health plans. Through HEDIS, NCQA has helped employers become engaged in the development of quality "report cards." These report cards are used for employer decision making as purchasers and are extended to consumers (i.e., results are shared with employers' employees). The communication to consumers is multipurpose. Employers want to begin to educate employees about healthcare quality and to provide information so that consumers can make an informed choice of health plan. General Motors and GTE are two companies who, in part, base their corporate contribution for health plans on the result of their health plan quality assessment from these report cards.

The 1990s and Beyond: Purchasers in an Age of Consumerism

At the end of the twentieth century, four areas demonstrate the purchaser focus on consumers: (1) accountability, (2) information and education, (3) evidence-based healthcare, and (4) value.

Accountability

Accountability generally connotes shared responsibility. In healthcare, this means that the goals of the health plan, provider, employer, and community are aligned in the direction of consumer-based systems of care, with the consumer at the center. Although great progress has been made in health plan accountability, employers as purchasers of healthcare have been disappointed with the results. Costs continue to escalate, many quality issues have yet to be addressed, providers have not really changed their practices, and many avoidable errors still occur. The transition to managed care promised to control costs within a framework of quality. The premise was that care would be managed with a systemic approach based on the needs of the patient and the population. Yet, purchasers encountered another reality. Some employers would say that what occurred was managed cost and not managed care. The accountability that employers desired has not yet occurred in widespread fashion at the provider or health system level.

Information and Education

Employers are seeking and using more information for corporate decision making about health benefit plan management and negotiation as well as for employee education. The employee education includes individual healthcare choices as well as health plan and provider selection. Another component of education is lifestyle management for optimal health. Preventing disease and maintaining health are critical elements for the employer to control cost and have a productive workforce. The role of information and education further extends to the marketplace—how employers work with health plans and providers for quality improvement.

Evidence-Based Healthcare

To improve value, thereby affecting both cost and quality, employers are promoting evidence-based healthcare. This work means closer alliance with providers and consumers. Consumers must be educated and informed about, and providers must use, evidence-based healthcare. This means broad-based implementation of the findings from research indicating which medical procedures and services are effective and appropriate. The overuse of antibiotics is one example of not using the evidence and of patient demand from lack of knowledge.

Value

"Value" equates to cost-effective healthcare. The value equation considers such variables as indirect costs (e.g., lost work time), functional status, and the direct cost for healthcare premiums or claims, coupled with quality of care and service. Assessing value entails measuring cost and quality and begins to build the case for differentiation of health plans and providers based on outcomes.

HOW ARE EMPLOYERS MEASURING VALUE, AND WHAT ARE THEY DOING TO PROMOTE IT FOR THEIR EMPLOYEES?

Shopping for Accredited, Consumer-Centered Health Plans

The demand for increased accountability has produced strong accreditation and measurement systems. Many employers require health plan accreditation by NCQA, as previously mentioned. NCQA accreditation and HEDIS form the basis for many employers in health plan selection and performance management. Quality Compass '99, the NCQA report of HEDIS measures, found that health plans that consistently report HEDIS demonstrate the best results and that consumer satisfaction is higher in plans with better clinical performance.

The Joint Commission on Accreditation of Healthcare Organizations (JCAHO) has taken on the important issues of working to improve quality and eliminate errors that occur in hospital settings.

The American Medical Accreditation Program (AMAP) is working with NCQA and JCAHO on the coordination of measures so that providers and plans will not be inundated with myriad quality measurement requirements. Providers must be involved in the development of measures to improve systemic clinical quality and service. At the root of developing reliable, valid instruments is the dearth of good information systems. Employers are supporting the definition of uniform data reporting and requirements and are looking for the healthcare industry to make the necessary investments.

Although the quality focus to date has been on report card scores, the real and ongoing issue is in getting the healthcare system to look at itself to improve healthcare and services for the consumer. As an extension of this movement, for example, health plans are now beginning to measure provider performance and publicly report on the results. This is a dramatic and daring departure from report card results that are used for internal comparisons against established benchmarks (e.g., HEDIS), or more recently, plan-to-plan comparisons.

Consumer satisfaction continues to be a primary means for employers' assessment of health plan and provider performance. Consumer satisfaction with clinical and administrative services represents the kind of data most easily obtained and therefore featured in public reporting. The use of consumer satisfaction data as one component of HEDIS is an example. Employers have used these data to report to consumers the differences in plan performance and to have health plans improve satisfaction.

The development of another consumer satisfaction survey, the Consumer Assessment of Health Plans (CAHPS) study, was prompted by interest from purchasers such as Medicaid and Medicare. CAHPS is a health plan quality assessment tool developed by the Federal Agency for Health Care Policy and Research, and an important addition to the growth of effective, uniform consumer satisfaction measurement. These efforts have produced information that is comparable by plan: an evolutionary step in that never before has this been possible (i.e., plan comparisons, including those of NCQA, are against benchmarked standards). The CAHPS work also allows measurement of satisfaction to be extended to health plans other than HMOs, such as PPOs and indemnity plans.

Consumer satisfaction information results led Edison International to engage in quality improvement initiatives with health plans and performance requirements in plan contracting. Edison included the direct input from employees and retirees with consumer committees and focus groups. One result was that Edison worked with *Health Pages,* a consumer-focused health information publication, to develop an online provider directory compiled with all the health plans so that finding out which plan or plans each provider participated in would be made easy.

The Pacific Business Group on Health (PBGH) and the Medical Quality Commission co-sponsored a 1997 survey of consumer satisfaction at the healthcare provider group level. The release of these data resulted in medical groups looking at their own service and communication processes to improve their relationships with their patients. As a result, PBGH has helped produce information that is more meaningful for the consumer, and PBGH has made this information available to its members and the general public on its Web site.

PBGH's example illustrates a trend in employers serving as communications "intermediaries," translating raw quality health plan reports, for example, into consumer-friendly guides. In addition, employers are stepping up their demands of providers for more and better information for consumers.

Chevron, with the support of HealthNet (a large California HMO that is part of Foundation Health Systems), worked with a large medical group in northern California to address consumer concerns directly. California Health Decisions, a nonprofit, nonpartisan organization dedicated to involving the public in health decisions, conducted focus groups with employee members of this medical group to define issues and concerns with respect to quality of service and quality of care from the consumer perspective.

Edison International changed its communication approach with employees and retirees to reflect the way consumers of healthcare use health plan information. When Edison introduced new health plans to employees in 1994, the communications were focused on how to choose a health plan. As Edison staff members met with committees of consumers in 1995 and tracked consumer problems and complaints, executives began to understand that the consumer thought first about a particular physician or facility, then he or she considered the plan. Consumers did not understand the medical group organizational structure (particularly, provider referrals within a designated group of practitioners) and reimbursement systems in the California market. A subsequent restructuring of the company's directory and consumer communications materials resulted in increased understanding of how these systems work.

Promote Patients' Access to and Connections with Providers

Employers recognize the importance of the patient–provider relationship and are working to foster ways to strengthen it on the belief that, if consumers like their physicians, they will be more likely to trust and use the services available to improve their health. The Buyers Health Care Action Group (BHCAG) in Minneapolis, a group of 24 innovative employers, demonstrated its commitment to consumers by guiding them to select health-care systems at the provider level. That is, consumers select a provider group as their system of care. Performance by providers in both clinical and service quality is reported so that consumers can use this information when making choices about which provider to use.

One large medical group in southern California conducted an assessment of its patients who were age 80 and older to see whether it could improve self-help in chronic conditions and to learn how the patients viewed their relationships with their providers. After it received the assessment results, the group sponsored communication improvement training for their providers. This type of initiative is shown to improve patient satisfaction and correlates with lower patient visit costs, according to an Institute for Health Improvement project that is currently under way to improve office practices.

A program in development with GTE in Everett, Washington, based on experience from a pilot program conducted in southern California by Edison International, is designed to improve the patient–provider relationship. Using the Dartmouth COOP Clinical Improvement System, a system designed by physicians to address practical problems in a simple, flexible, and inexpensive manner, GTE will ask its employees to take the health assessment and share the results with their physicians. A local clinic is working closely with GTE on the project. Prior use of the assessment system has demonstrated improvements in health status from the health education aspects of the program. A high patient–clinician interaction score also was found to directly correlate with greater satisfaction with overall care and lower per-visit costs. The Institute is using the system for health improvement in its Idealized Design of Clinical Office Practice Project. GTE wants to measure improvement in quality of care, health status, and satisfaction for its employees and to provide more information for employees to use in decision making. GTE continues to lead in supporting its employees to be effective consumers.

Differentiating between plans is an increasing concern for employers because today, many providers contract with multiple plans. Edison employees participated in a consumer satisfaction survey in which the questions were designed to differentiate consumers' experiences with plans and providers. Edison shared the results with the plan administrators and the employees. Satisfaction with plan services differed significantly. For example, the ability of the plan representative to answer questions varied widely. Twenty-two percent of employees enrolled in one plan were satisfied with the plan representatives' abilities to answer questions, compared with 56% of employees enrolled in another plan. This information, coupled with other data reported to consumers, resulted in actions that led to a significant disenrollment in the plan that had the lowest level of satisfaction. These data demonstrate that even with providers' participation in multiple plans, there are differences in the level of service by each plan. Because the benefit design was the same for each plan, the issues were service and support for the consumer.

Anecdotal evidence shows that the level of complaints physicians have with health plans may have a correlation to the level of consumer dissatisfaction. One area of complaint for both physicians and patients is the complexity of referral processes. Employers are very interested in this level of data because more complaints by consumers translates to more cost for the employer in administrative and problem-solving resources. Higher levels of complaints may also affect the level of trust the consumer has with the health plan, provider, and health plan sponsor.

Increasingly, employers will be looking at a provider's ability to define and work in a team because more Americans need management for chronic and complex medical conditions. Reporting to consumers about the care management team will become increasingly important, especially when linked to chronic condition management and function. A care management team may include not only physicians but also health educators, nurse practitioners, physician assistants, and allied health professionals. The care management team members will vary for consumers with different chronic conditions and different needs.

Collaborative, Multidisciplinary, Community-Based Initiatives Toward Empowering Consumers and Promoting Health

Employers are partnering with their communities to build healthier communities. General Motors (GM), for example, demonstrates a significant investment in employee, dependent, and retiree education through the provision of extensive information on the health plans and hospitals for designated communities. Early results of these efforts by GM indicate that employees are moving to the plans that have higher quality ratings. GM extends its support to community-based efforts that involve the United Auto Workers in communities where GM has a large workforce. In Dayton, Ohio, Flint, Michigan, and Anderson, Indiana, GM supports health improvements for the community, in collaboration with government and local stakeholders. As an example, the collaborative community work in Flint identified the high volume of cardiac services with poor results. This led to the development of a broad-based task force to address the rate of cardiac catheterization. At the same time, education is provided communitywide to consumers about the facts of appropriate treatment.

Small Employers Expanding Access, Choice of Health Benefits

An issue that has received growing attention in the past decade is the fact that many small employers cannot afford to purchase health insurance for their employees. Consumer-Choice Health Purchasing Groups (CHPGs) have arisen in large part due to the urgent needs of the small business market. By pooling small employers' collective resources and purchasing benefits jointly, CHPGs provide workers and their families a choice of health plans that offer standardized benefits. The Institute for Health Policy Solutions, a nonprofit organization established in 1992 to identify, analyze, and develop strategies to solve healthcare system problems, supported the development of CHPGs.

The growth of CHPGs is indicative of the interest small employers have in addressing the varying healthcare needs of their employees. Small employers would not be able to offer multiple health plan options without the CHPG model. Varying state insurance regulations and health plans' willingness to provide coverage to small employers are two common issues in small employer markets. Currently, these purchasing groups are in California, Colorado, Connecticut, Florida, Illinois, Montana, New York, Ohio, Oregon, Texas, Utah, and Washington.

Other Tools Employers Are Using to Empower Consumers

Among the "tools" employers are embracing to promote consumer empowerment are education, self-help access through phone and Internet, work site support specific to certain conditions, and information to support decision making. Nurse help lines are used by innovative employers as a way to provide consumer-centered care and to promote linkages between the delivery system and physicians. Digital Equipment has worked with Harvard Pilgrim Health Care in Boston on an Internet-based, confidential health assessment survey that employees may take. The process links the individual's results to resources he or she may access through the health plan, including further information and education or follow-up. This approach is enhanced if the employee is a member of the part of the Harvard Pilgrim system that has an automated medical record system.

Health plan information on the Internet varies from stakeholders promoting their interests to consumers sharing their experiences to researchers sharing peer-reviewed results. An example of how employers are using the Internet is the availability of links provided on company Web sites. Company Web sites link employees to health plans and other resource sites such as the Centers for Disease Control and Prevention. It is important to recognize, however, that quality measures for Internet information will be necessary.

Investing in Evidence-Based Medicine

The Washington Business Group on Health, a nonprofit group representing major public and private employers who collectively purchase healthcare for more than 39 million employees in the United States, states in *The Health America Blueprint* that one of the principles that is a building block for healthcare delivery system reform is a commitment "to evidence-based health care and to fostering the flow of relevant information and ideas" (The Health America Blueprint, 1999). Promoting evidence-based care requires a change in attitude and expectation on the part of all participants in healthcare—from one of treatment, postfact, to one of prevention. A critical link to the successful implementation of evidence-based practice is information and education for consumers.

In the past, health plans have been designed to reimburse providers for services rather than to pay for what is appropriate based on the best evidence available. Today, employers understand that the involvement of the consumer in maintaining health has an effect beyond the direct cost of the health plan. Employers such as Union Pacific Railroad, which has a history of health promotion and wellness programs, are attempting to link their healthcare investments to employee productivity and functionality. Other employers have begun to measure their aggregate lost work time data and are looking for differences in the functional status of employees at the health plan or provider level.

In an era of downsizing and low unemployment, workplace productivity will continue to be a hot topic. Those issues that affect quality of life—and therefore stand to impact workplace performance—have become critical to health services and outcomes research and of intense interest to employers. Employers want to know now, more than ever, about ways to help keep employees healthy, and the impact of chronic illness on their workforce. For example, depression has been estimated to cost employers $23.8 billion in direct and indirect costs, such as lost workdays and compromised performance, according to a 1993 study reported in the *Journal of Clinical Psychiatry* (Greenberg et al., 1993). Because of this knowledge, employers are investing time and resources in disease management and care management initiatives in an effort to prevent illness by targeting those most at risk and managing the care of those who stand to benefit most.

Employers recognize that programs aimed at improving productivity have not been well coordinated, leading to high costs, unclear expectations regarding outcomes, and a low return on investments. Therefore, they are seeking approaches that integrate the major components of their health programs—employee health benefits, workers' compensation, disability management, and occupational health and safety. In integrating these components, employers aim to encompass the total cost of health as it impacts the worker and workplace to overcome program fragmentation. For example, employers are measuring their total health cost, including the direct expenditures for health benefit coverage with workers' compensation and lost work time. Texas Instruments and Kodak have work site influenza vaccine programs as a service for the employees and a benefit for the company. The cost for the program is offset by fewer lost workdays.

As employers begin to measure value in the workplace by looking at direct medical program costs, lost work time, accidents, and safety, they will seek more effective benefits design to produce the best outcomes, more integrated approaches to support employee needs through their work/family, and employee assistance programs.

CONCLUSION

Employers have moved along a continuum from providing healthcare for occupational health and safety to promoting health for employees. This movement has led to consumer-focused approaches by employers. The areas that demonstrate this consumer focus include demand for accountability, increased emphasis on information and education for consumers, drive for evidence-based care, and measurement based on value.

It is important to note that assessing value also requires a review of the incentives that drive behaviors within the healthcare system. For example, excluding coverage for the testing equipment for diabetic patients affects the ability of such patients to be compliant with blood sugar level monitoring. This may result in more costly care. Employers need to be open to realigning the incentives to produce the value.

Open access to health information via the Internet is influencing the rapid changes of how purchasers address the role of consumers. Access to information on the Internet can help consumers prepare for a discussion with the physician, decide whether they even need to see a physician, and find other health information at their convenience. The level of desired information can be selected by the consumer, from a general summary to a specific detail.

The consumer influence is pushing the purchasers to require more and better information at the provider level, more effective use of health resources in an integrated manner, and the science to support the rationale for services. As costs escalate, the needs are greater to educate consumers about choices in both quality and cost.

As information evolves, it will need to reflect the diversity of consumers, including how and when consumers use information. Much has been learned about what information is relevant to consumers and how to present such data. A remaining challenge is how to measure and incorporate the behavioral aspects that drive consumer actions and choices.

The work of purchasers will continue to support quality improvement for and on behalf of consumers and to build on the health of the corporate bottom line linked to the health of the workforce. All of the initiatives on the part of purchasers, as highlighted in this chapter, parallel the corporate America focus on product and service quality at the core business level. Businesses extended their own internal quality improvement initiatives to their suppliers of products and services to become more cost-effective, to increase quality, and to be globally competitive. American business did not comprehend that this was not happening systematically in the healthcare industry at the same time; healthcare had not made the infrastructure investments to be ready for the Age of Consumerism. An example is the fact that information at all provider levels is not uniformly available—even for correct office hours and whether new patients are being accepted, much less for satisfaction or outcome measures.

Consumers are already arming themselves with the information to understand their conditions and options for medical care. Expectations are for plans and providers to be prepared to support these consumers because the role and satisfaction of the consumer is a critical part of their success.

REFERENCES

Greenberg PE, et al. The economic burden of depression in 1990. *J Clin Psychiatr* 1993; 54(11):1–14.

Starr P. *The social transformation of American medicine.* New York: Basic Books, 1982.

The Health America Blueprint. *Building a consensus on reform.* Washington, DC: Washington Business Group on Health. 1999.

Wennberg JE, Gittelsohn A. Healthcare delivery in Maine I: patterns of use of common surgical procedures. *J Maine Med Assoc* 1975; 66(5):123–130, 149.

FOR FURTHER READING

Anstett P. New guide to health plans hits your computer today. *Detroit Free Press* October 5, 1998.

Bodenheimer T, Sullivan JD. How large employers are shaping the healthcare marketplace. *N Engl J Med* 1998; 338(14, 15).

Business & Health. The state of health care in America. 1999; 17(6 suppl A).

Future of public health. *Institutes of Medicine* 1988.

13
CHAPTER

Employer Groups (Purchasers) and the New Healthcare Consumer

Woodrow A. Myers, Jr., M.D., MBA

Diane L. Bechel, Dr.PH.

TUNING INTO THE "CONSUMER HEADSET"

In the early 1980s, Chrysler (now DaimlerChrysler), Ford, and General Motors, "The Autos," faced a new market reality—the voice of the consumer. Market research, JD Powers' ratings, "*Consumer Reports*" road tests, and focus group testing indicated that American cars were out of touch with the needs of "real people." Respondents no longer were content with the predominant style of the vehicles and wanted to know about performance and value for dollars spent. Foreign manufacturers were gaining market share in large part because they built vehicles that delivered on fuel efficiency and economy.

Ford turned its ship around, building driver and buyer expectations into its product line and streamlining the production process. Quality was now "Job One," and a true partnership with labor emerged. The needs and expectations of drivers became the sine qua non for the Company. In 1999, this tradition continues. Ford Motor Company's corporate vision is to be more than just the world's leading automotive company; it wants to become the world's leading automotive products and services *consumer* company.

Jack Nassar, Ford President and CEO, puts it this way, "Having a consumer focus also means having an intuitive—really visceral—feeling for the things that will surprise, delight, and excite." The year 1999 is marked as a year that Ford could replace General Motors as the world's largest corporation, with $156 billion in annual revenues. Ford may soon produce more vehicles than GM, as well: vehicle sales at Ford are projected to be 8.3 million by year's end, compared with GM's 8.2 million. This also marks a time of expanded global mergers—Ford with Volvo and Daimler-Benz with Chrysler.

At the core of this historical turning point in what could be considered the "rise of consumerism" and The Autos' receptiveness to it is the notion of giving consumers what they are seeking—comparisons they can use to make the decisions that are best for themselves and their families, and products and services designed with consumers' needs in mind. Underlying this ability to provide the data necessary for comparisons (displayed by the aforementioned market research companies) was The Autos' embracing of a continuous quality improvement framework—a commitment to better meet and exceed consumer expectations.

This chapter tells the story of one of The Autos, Ford Motor Company, and the lessons it learned and present success in having set, and achieved, a vision of quality that is built with consumers in mind.

THE INTERSECTION BETWEEN MANUFACTURING AND HEALTHCARE: WHERE THE CONSUMER FITS IN

What do healthcare and the auto industry have in common? The Autos are among the largest purchasers of healthcare insurance in the country, with their combined 1998 health benefit spending totaling $10 billion. Consider this fact along with the growing influence of the "new, empowered consumer" in healthcare, arguably a commodity much like any other, and the implications are formidable.

Although consumerism may be new to healthcare, manufacturers have long endeavored to understand, achieve, and exceed consumer expectations. Smart companies in all industries are increasingly consumer-focused, and with good reason. Recognizing the dignity and importance of the users of products and services is no longer an option, it is essential to firm survival. For example, a recent KPMG/Northwestern study showed that almost 75% of Americans agree that the healthcare industry is changing the way it operates because of consumer demands (KPMG, 1998). As baby boomers mature, and their technology-savvy children (the "echo boom") age, information-hungry consumers will demand new and better ways to evaluate their decisions.

In 1999, the almost $1 trillion American healthcare industry faces similar challenges. Technology brings a host of new, exciting possibilities—and sometimes exorbitant costs—too often without improving a patient's chances for a successful outcome. Medically unnecessary variations in hospital performance abound (Wennberg, 1999). Increasingly, purchasers of care, including healthcare consumers and their employers, want to understand why.

Traditionally, healthcare has been viewed by economists as a service that eluded the basic law of supply and demand. However, healthcare provider supply and competition have increased, information has become more accessible, and many patients have grown more comfortable in participating in treatment decisions. Both the healthcare and auto industries face prevailing challenges and trends. Among these challenges are excess capacity, dwindling administrative margins, an increasingly competitive marketplace, corporate mergers, streamlined production and delivery, and the quest for competitive advantage.

Uncharted seas lie ahead for both the healthcare and auto industries. In healthcare, hospital closures in many communities are all but certain. There are simply too many hospital beds, largely because the increased use of outpatient care has outpaced hospitals shedding inpatient capacity. Furthermore, no longer is the hospital the center of care, but rather one of many sites (e.g., freestanding outpatient surgical center, doctor's

TABLE 13–1

Ford Motor Healthcare Expenses: 1997–1998 Pharmacy Price and Utilization Changes

Drug	Utilization Change (2Q 97-4Q98)	Price Change (2Q 97-4Q98)	Total Change in Ford Costs (2Q 97-4Q98)
Prilosec	70%	12%	92%
Zocor	49%	11%	65%
Lipitor	425%	1%	431%

office, specialty clinic) that may be appropriate, depending on the patient's needs. Healthcare reimbursement systems no longer automatically fund capital expenses, research and development, or administrative luxuries. Processes and structures of care are under increased scrutiny to identify ways to improve quality and eliminate unnecessary costs.

In the auto industry, recessionary forces loom in the global economy. The profit margin on small cars remains low in the United States. At a time when environmental concerns are growing in importance, the more profitable small truck and sport utility market has become threatened. Lean production and a discerning customer base allow little room for error.

At the same time, healthcare costs face the potential to skyrocket again, due in large part to burgeoning pharmaceutical costs. During 1997 and 1998, both the price and use of Prilosec, Zocor, and Lipitor (Ford's cost "leaders" in its pharmaceutical expenses) increased markedly. Ford's expenditures for Prilosec, a gastroesophageal reflux drug, climbed from $2 million to $3.8 million (a 92% change). Zocor, a statin cholesterol-lowering drug, increased from $1.7 million to $2.8 million (a 65% increase), and Lipitor, a competitor to Zocor, blossomed from $443,000 to $2.4 million (a 431% change), as shown in Table 13–1.

The Ford Motor Company believes that understanding the "consumer headset"—what consumers need and want most—is vital to success in both the healthcare and consumer automotive sectors. In the Ford consumer automotive sector, purchase decisions are driven by package, price, quality, safety, value, and driving dynamics. In the healthcare sector, consumers have parallel needs—the right provider and the right treatment at a reasonable cost, care that meets acceptable standards, accountability from providers, and a healthcare system that is "patient-centered." Listening to the "consumer headset" of would-be patients (healthcare consumers) and of people receiving services (patients) is absolutely critical.

An "enlightened purchaser" framework is emerging among employers like Ford who value the "consumer headset" and the new healthcare consumer. These "enlightened purchasers" understand the needs of patients and the relationships between the following:

- Health status and productivity
- Employee and retiree satisfaction, corporate reputation, and attracting and retaining a talented workforce
- Informed, empowered, and knowledgeable workers and the quality of products and services

LISTENING TO THE PATIENT HEADSET: THE QUEST FOR PATIENT-CENTERED CARE

Reinventing the way that care is designed to focus on the customer's—not the providers—needs, preferences, and values is at the helm of a growing movement fostered by the consumer catalyst called "patient-centered care," which aims to do the following:

- Involve patients in treatment decisions.
- Increase patient communication with providers and patient understanding of what to expect from treatment plans, recovery, and after-care.
- Incorporate family members in care (Gerteis et al., 1993).

Cleary and McNeil demonstrated that "good communication with patients gives providers the information they need for accurate and effective treatment," and they showed that patient involvement in the healthcare process led to improved compliance, return for follow-up care, and better outcomes (Cleary & McNeil, 1998).

AUTO WORKERS: PROTOTYPES OF
THE NEW HEALTHCARE CONSUMER

Comprehensive healthcare benefits, low member cost-sharing, and comparatively generous compensation make automaker employees, retirees, and their families veritable prototypes of the new healthcare consumer.

Many new healthcare consumers want to participate in decisions about their care according to their own preferences, needs, and values. They are anxious to learn more and want credible, accurate information on which to base decisions. In fact, a national poll of 1,011 American households found that 83% would like to be better informed about how to evaluate quality of care from hospitals and physicians, and 72% reported that they would like more information to feel more confident about medical care decisions (National Coalition on Health Care, 1996).

However, healthcare is among the most personal and difficult areas of decision for most people. It affects not only the person receiving services, but his or her family, and often coworkers and friends. Information plays an important role in the partnership between purchasers, employees, retirees, and their families. Providing easily interpreted, impartial, accurate information on the performance of health plans, hospitals, and doctors allows patients to begin more actively participating in their care.

Unfortunately, until now, little information has been available to patients in terms that they can understand or measures that are meaningful to them. Equally disheartening, without credible, publicly available comparative measures, healthcare providers often lack the information and benchmarking incentive to deliver effective, efficient, patient-centered care.

New information and care technology allow enhanced methods of putting information together. To fulfill the new healthcare consumers' information needs and to engage healthcare consumers in their care, businesses, academic institutions, and provider communities must work together to use these tools to measure performance and to share results.

INFORMING CONSUMERS AND THE BOTTOM LINE

Communicating with patients is good medicine. It also improves the value of care because it discourages the use of expensive tests and treatments whose benefits are very small compared with their costs. Simply put, patients, physicians, and nurses must be informed about medical variation and the efficacy of medical interventions. When this occurs, it benefits not only patient health, but also the value of care (Phelps, 1992). Phelps and Parante (1990) found that "Even ignoring the obvious effects that biased rates of use (too much or too little care on average), the welfare gains from reduced variability exceed by one to two orders of magnitude the costs of producing and disseminating information about the proper methods of treating illness."

Information and communication benefits physicians as well. Good communication among physicians, nurses, and patients is a key factor in avoiding malpractice suits (Levinson et al., 1997). Levinson and colleagues found that when primary care physicians listen to their patients they reduce their risk for malpractice suits. Clearly, informing consumers and connecting them to useful information benefits patients, employers, and providers alike.

THE SYNERGISM OF JOINT STAKEHOLDER COLLABORATION

Health policy researchers have, especially in recent years, vastly improved the tools for measuring and monitoring care. Despite this, meaningful information is scarce in part because some providers do not believe that consumers need "report cards" on care, in part because some employers are content with using cost only as a way to gauge how hospital performance differs, and in part because although many want the finished information, few have the knowledge or resources to produce it.

Physicians, nurses, and other providers have many skills essential for informing and educating patients. Alone, providers, employers, or academicians face limitations in informing the new healthcare consumer. Together, their skills blend to produce more useful information for healthcare consumers.

Providers

Providers interact with patients on the frontline of healthcare delivery. Still, some providers may underestimate the ability of consumers to understand and interpret information. Sicker patients may be the most interested in information about their condition, yet a recent study of audiotapes of 1,300 patients found that the less healthy the patient was, the less physicians exhibited positive behavior during the office visit (yet they still showed concern for their patients and encouraged interaction) (Hall et al., 1996). As the time spent with physicians during an office visit grows shorter and more physicians report pressures to see more patients in less time, communicating the needed information in the time allotted becomes more challenging.

Employers

Employers design and communicate benefit options to employees. Yet, employer purchasers, acting alone to get information to healthcare consumers, similarly face a double-edged sword. Employees and retirees want comparative, easy-to-use information but may distrust employer-provided comparisons of quality and value, believing that employer "hidden agendas" distort the information. Furthermore, unbiased, accurate comparisons to national benchmarks that span different levels of providers in communities are almost nonexistent, requiring employers to catalyze measurement and the distribution of results (or be faced with no information to share with employees and retirees about the quality of their healthcare). At Ford, the partnership and strong working relationship with the United Auto Workers (UAW) permits active collaboration.

Healthcare Experts

University researchers and think tanks bring expertise in specific healthcare niches. They assess what has and has not worked in the past and look at the "big picture" of both direct and indirect effects of a proposed change. Both are critical to informing and improving future decisions, making the role of university researchers and think tanks vital. Yet, working alone, they too face significant obstacles. The pace and schedule of research often is much slower than in a business environment. Furthermore, laboratory conditions may be too removed from the "real world" to be representative. Research funds are increasingly scarce and distribution mechanisms generally are expensive. As a result, there is often a significant time lag for findings to complete the circle from pure research to use in an applied setting.

Healthcare Consumers

The employee and retiree base includes those who receive healthcare services and those who may someday need to receive care. At Ford, there are five major segments: (1) hourly retirees, (2) salary retirees, (3) hourly employees, (4) salary employees, and (5) dependents. Patients and consumers—the operative demand side of the market—want to participate and be more empowered in their care. Alone, patients and consumers must struggle through the healthcare system to ferret out information, a time-consuming and frustrating exercise. Without providers, employers, academicians, and consumers working together, often information is not distributed publicly.

Synergism among the Stakeholders

For all stakeholders, the field of consumer healthcare informatics—how to translate information and knowledge into usable tools for consumers—is relatively young. Enlightened employers involve all stakeholders, affiliate with experts and researchers, and importantly, collaborate with *patients and consumers* to guide efforts to design, implement, and monitor quality measurement and information initiatives. Joint efforts also increase credibility of findings to consumers and substantially reduce the potential for bias.

Internal and external efforts must be complementary and synergistic. They must create ways for patients and would-be patients to obtain the information that they want at the time when they want it. They must recognize that patients and healthcare consumers need a context to understand information, then present and disseminate the information in useful ways. They must do the following:

- Combine the best thinking of all stakeholders—patients, purchasers, providers, and plans.
- Be guided by impartial experts.
- Use rigorous, real-world methodologies to do the following:
  - Measure performance at the national level.
  - Vest improvement at the local level where structural and process changes need to occur.
  - Uphold clinical and statistical rigor, yet maintain feasibility and cost-effectiveness.
- Use the best of consumer-tested report design.
- Pursue a long-term vision.

Think about the information that would be available to you if you had to decide where to have heart surgery or which personal care physician you should select. Too often, the average consumer may have to rely on advice from friends, neighbors, and family members. Of the information that is available, it generally is not written or displayed in a consumer-friendly way, is not widely available, and often is produced by healthcare suppliers who stand to benefit from hospitals that buy their products and systems. Furthermore, such information is often deficient in adjusting for factors beyond a provider's control. For example, of the information available on the World Wide Web on healthcare topics, it is difficult to distinguish true information from well-designed marketing. Often, comparisons are local and do not use national benchmarks or national practice guidelines. As Brook contends, "Americans tolerate more variation in the performance of their healthcare system than they would ever put up with in the performance of an airline, a computer company, or even the manufacturer of their breakfast cereal" (Brook, 1998).

Public availability of good comparisons of hospital performance does more than inform healthcare consumers—it makes improvements in hospital care actionable and catalyzes an industry to compete on quality. In response to a recent Ford initiative to distribute provider comparisons to retirees and employees, for example, a large local healthcare provider implemented process and structure changes that resulted in quantifiable improvements in patient care.

FORD'S HEALTHCARE INITIATIVES

Ford's healthcare strategy, enabling informed decision making by employees and retirees, is manifested in programs that improve healthcare quality and eliminate inappropriate costs, focus on health status, and empower employees and retirees through information.

The remainder of this chapter describes three major information empowerment initiatives at Ford: (1) The Hospital Profiling Program, (2) The Coordinated Auto/UAW Reporting System (CARS) Consortium, and (3) The Quality Consortium.

The Hospital Profiling Program

There is no shortage of studies to demonstrate that consumers want information about hospital performance, and there is good reason to believe that consumers would actually use the information about hospitals in their area. First, healthcare consumers understand that unexplained variation in hospital performance exists, and they want to make informed choices when they seek care. For example, 79% of consumers in a national study believed that hospitals differed in the quality of care that they delivered (Inguanzo & Harju, 1985). In another study, 72% of those polled reported that they would like more information to feel more confident about medical care decisions (National Coalition on Health Care, 1996).

Ford employees and retirees are no different. They demand information they can use to make decisions important to their families and themselves. The Hospital Profiling Project supplies that information and aims to accomplish the following four key objectives that represent each of the major stakeholders within communities.

1. To provide accurate, meaningful, and reliable comparisons of cost and quality to purchaser employees, retirees, and their families that do the following:
   - Use sound scientific principles and national comparisons of hospital quality and cost outcomes, adjusting for differences among patient populations.
   - Are developed through a process that employees, retirees, and their families find credible and impartial.
   - Are easily interpreted by consumers.
2. To provide hospitals with information that can be used, in conjunction with other internal efforts, to improve the care received by patients
3. To enable employers to make choices that produce greater quality and value for their healthcare dollars
4. To develop more effective relationships between providers and purchasers

The indicators that are studied are listed in Table 13–2.

The Profile is a comparative consumer guide that shows hospital performance on whether patients report that they were told about danger signs to watch for after they were discharged, had results of their tests explained to them in a way that they could understand, and other key events in care. They also contain results on the mortality and complication rates at hospitals that are adjusted for patient factors that are beyond hospital control, as well as the cost of care.

The 1998 Hospital Profiles were distributed to more than 500,000 people in southeast Michigan. Results were shared with employees and retirees via two-color booklets that were mailed out to retirees and made available to employees by calling a toll-free hot-line. The report was also posted on an intranet and Internet (www.hiag.org) site. In 1999, the project was expanded through the formation of a partnership between Ford, General Motors, and DaimlerChrysler; the American Hospital Associa-

TABLE 13–2

Ford Motor Hospital Profiling Project: What Is Reported to Consumers

Profiling Component	Where Does It Come From?
"What Patients Say" section	Patient responses to surveys (Picker Institute inpatient surveys) on key events in care that consumers can reliably report on the following: ■ Respect ■ Coordination ■ Information and education ■ Family and friends ■ Physical comfort ■ Continuity ■ Emotional support
Risk-Adjusted Quality Outcomes section	Analysis of hospital discharge abstracts within specific, high volume disease categories on the following: ■ Unexpected death rates ■ Unexpected complications rates
Cost	Analysis of inpatient hospital insurance claims on the amount purchasers pay for care

tion; and local stakeholders in each region. In 1999, Profiles were produced for four additional areas: Atlanta, Indianapolis, Buffalo, and Cleveland (available at www.ford.com in the "Corporate Citizenship" section).

Sample pages of performance results for hospitals are listed in Figure 13–1 on page 322:

The Profiles demonstrate that the way patients were treated and the processes of care varied substantially.

- Eighteen percent of Detroit-area surgical patients and 29% of medical patients reported problems in coordination of care (doctors and nurses working as a team with patients).

- Twenty-four percent of obstetrical patients reported problems with emotional support offered by hospital staff (patients being able to discuss fears and anxieties), compared with 31% of medical patients (Southeast Michigan Employer and Purchaser Consortium, 1998).

F I G U R E   13–1

How Ford reports to employees and retirees on hospital performance on care quality. (Source: From the Southeast Michigan Hospital Profiles, 1998.)

Surgical Care... ...The Outcomes	Heart Surgery			
	Number of Cases	Length of Stay	Mortality	Complications
Teaching Hospitals				
Bi-County Community Hospital – Warren	33	★★	★★	★★
Bon Secours Hospital – Grosse Pointe	95	★★	★★	★★
Botsford General Hospital – Farmington Hills	98	★★	★★★	★★
DMC Grace Hospital – Detroit	72	★	★★★	★★
DMC Harper Hospital – Detroit*	1,237	★★	★	★★★
DMC Hutzel Hospital – Detroit	Not offered	—		
DMC Sinai Hospital – Detroit*	784	★★	★	★★★
Garden City Osteopathic Hospital	70	★	★★★	★★
Henry Ford Cottage Hospital of Grosse Pointe	Low volume	—		
Henry Ford Hospital – Detroit*	1,369	★★	★	★★★
Henry Ford Wyandotte Hospital	97	★★	★★	★★★
Mercy Hospital – Detroit	Low volume	—		
Mt. Clemens General Hospital	621	★★	★	★★★
North Oakland Medical Center – Pontiac	31	★★	Low volume	★★
Oakwood Hospital & Medical Center – Dearborne*	2,518	★★★	★★	★★★

Three stars: Better than expected
Two stars: Same as expected
One star: Worse than expected
Low Volume: Too few cases to analyze

Medical Care... ...What Patients Say	Indicators of Medical Care					
	Respect for Patients	Care Coordination	Information and Education	Comfort and Pain Management	Emotional Support	Involvement of Family and Friends
Teaching Hospitals						
Botsford General Hospital – Farmington Hills	★★	★★	★★	★★	★★	★★
DMC Harper Hospital – Detroit	Low volume					
DMC Hutzel Hospital – Detroit	★★	★★★	★★★	★★	★★	★★
DMC Sinai Hospital – Detroit	Low volume					
Henry Ford Hospital – Detroit	★	★	★★	★★	★★	★★
Mt. Clemens General Hospital	★★	★★	★	★★	★★	★★
North Oakland Medical Center – Pontiac	★	★★	★	★	★	★★
Oakwood Hospital & Medical Center – Dearborn	★★	★	★	★★	★	★★
Pontiac Osteopathic Hospital	★★	★★	★★	★★	★★	★★
Providence Hospital and Medical Center – Southfield	★★	★★	★★	★★	★★	★★

Three stars: Better than expected
Two stars: Same as expected
One star: Worse than expected
Low Volume: Too few cases to analyze

Expected Outcomes

Consistent with the four objectives of The Hospital Profiling Project, the project will contribute four kinds of expected outcomes, per four designated objectives (Figure 13–2): (1) inform consumers, (2) improve healthcare delivery, (3) inform purchaser decisions, and (4) create community dialog. As shown in Figure 13–2, different tool kits and applications are used to achieve each objective.

A large, random sample survey of report recipients and focus group evaluation of the 1998 pilot in Southeast Michigan demonstrated project feasibility and an overall positive response from employees and retirees. Key findings included the following:

- Well over three-quarters of evaluation survey respondents found the report to be useful or very useful.
- Fifty percent indicated that they used the results to better understand their health condition.
- Twenty-one percent participated in choosing a hospital for themselves or a family member.
- Fifty percent learned more about hospitals in their health plan.
- Fifteen percent learned more about effectively talking to their doctor.
- Nine percent actually used information in the Profiles to talk to their doctor.

Even more important was the effect that public distribution of the Profiles has had on catalyzing hospitals to implement process improvements to address areas where hospitals performed less well than they would have liked.

The Coordinated Autos/UAW Reporting System (CARS) Consortium

Before 1998, a spouse of a Ford employee who happened to work for General Motors would get two sets of information on how health plans they could choose from performed on key measures. Because different methodologies were used to evaluate performance by each company, the ratings were sometimes different, resulting in confusion.

Ford Motor hospital profiles: project goals, tools, and outcomes

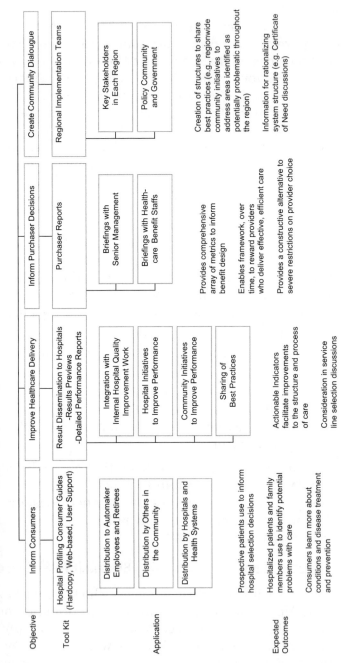

Therefore, since 1998, Ford, General Motors, DaimlerChrysler, and the UAW have worked together with other large organizations, including the Office of Personnel Management and HCFA, to develop a common health plan performance rating tool. This collaborative effort has become known as the Coordinated Autos/UAW Reporting System (CARS) Consortium. The goal of the Consortium is to ensure that the plans are fairly evaluated based on a nationally applied standard, to improve the usefulness of comparisons to employees and retirees, and to minimize burden to the health plans.

To lead the project and ensure that it benefited from the latest research on health plan quality, a team of experts from RAND, the Foundation for Accountability (FACCT), and National Committee for Quality Assurance (NCQA) was convened to work with employer staffs to design and coordinate a common method of health plan performance information.

Categories for communicating the outcomes of the evaluation were selected on the basis of research by FACCT regarding which categories were of interest to the intended audience. The categories chosen were as follows: NCQA accreditation status, access and service, consumer satisfaction, staying healthy, getting better, and living with illness. Measures were selected for each category based on available data sources. The measures included the member satisfaction survey component of the NCQA accreditation process, NCQA accreditation status, and Health Plan Employer Data and Information Set (HEDIS) results. When methodological issues arose, such as how to handle missing data; how to standardize scales; and how to weight and aggregate the individual measures, alternative options were identified and scenario analysis was used to assess how each option would impact results.

For reporting purposes, numerical scores were translated to "statistical stars" that identified performance within, above, and below two standard deviations of the mean, just like the Hospital Profiles. This makes it easier for employees and retirees to easily identify better (3 star) performers. Only HMO plans have been included in the report in the past. Over time, however, the project will expand to include all offered health plan benefit designs. Figure 13–3 is an example of a page from the 1998 report.

F I G U R E   13–3

How Ford reports to employees and retirees on health plan performance.
(Source: From Ford Open Enrollment Material, 1998.)

Plan Name	Consumer Rating of Care	NCQA Accreditation	Access to Care	Effectiveness of Care
Blue Care Network - Central	★ ★	★ ★ ★	★ ★	★ ★
Blue Care Network - SE MI	★	★ ★ ★	★ ★	★
Blue Care Network - East	★ ★	★ ★	★ ★	★ ★
Blue Care Network - Gr. Lakes	★ ★	★ ★ ★	★ ★	★ ★
Health Alliance Plan	★ ★	★ ★ ★	★ ★	★ ★ ★
M-Care	★ ★	★ ★	★ ★ ★ ★	★ ★
Medical Value Plan	■	★ ★	★ ★	★ ★
Omni Care	■	★ ★	★ ★	■
Care Choices - GR / Lansing / SE MI	★ ★ ★	★ ★	★ ★	★ ★

1Key: ★★★ Better than average   ★★ Average   ★ Needs Improvement   ■ Data not Submitted

The Healthcare Quality Consortium

How can you prepare for the long term in the midst of ever-present pressure for short-term results? Combining targeted initiatives with in-depth assessment and evaluations of patterns of performance lays the groundwork for informed business decision making. More than that, it allows for better and more creative solutions to real-world challenges.

Ford's Healthcare Quality Consortium is a unique and innovative way to merge the worlds of health services research and application of the research in the real world to optimize quality and value. The Consortium pairs premier academic and clinical researchers with real Ford healthcare issues. These experts strive to find creative solutions to important and complex problems and opportunities.

Funding the ongoing costs of an internal research staff is formidable, and it is unlikely that such a team could encompass the broad array of skills necessary to work with today's complex healthcare environment. The Healthcare Quality Consortium allows Ford to stretch resources with changing teams of experts and projects.

The Quality Consortium was created on the following fundamental beliefs:

- Good health is both an individual and a company asset.
- Quality can be defined, measured, and improved.
- Evaluation requires a high level of expertise and sophistication (often exceeding the level available within an organization).
- Talent is in high demand, which requires company–key supplier partnerships.

Quickly increasing pharmacy costs, inconsistent use of evidence-based medicine, and differences in the ways that patients receive care under workers' compensation and personal health benefits are challenges to Ford, and challenges to the healthcare industry at large. The Consortium endeavors to share discoveries of good solutions to problems so that care for *all* in our society can be improved.

The Consortium is a living, learning laboratory. It produces analyses, published articles, and pilots that test new approaches to old problems that benefit both Ford and the broader healthcare environment. Is this unusual for a Fortune 50 Company? Ford thinks it is essential—giving back to communities is a key part of its commitment to corporate citizenship.

The initiatives tackled by the Consortium are varied, but all have one thing in common: the potential for improving care. Current projects, for example, address the following issues:

- *Patterns of disease:* This study assesses the prevalence of hypertension in the Ford population to better understand the demographic factors and patient comorbid conditions. Findings can lay the groundwork for better designing programs to improve the health status and life quality of hypertensives.
- *Indemnity versus managed care performance:* This study tries to identify differences in readmission rates for

patients with congestive heart failure who are in HMOs relative to indemnity plans, and if there are differences, why they might exist.

- *Use of best practices:* Another study uses nationally developed guidelines for treatment of low back pain and compares them to how they differ from, or are similar to, expert clinical guidelines.

- *The whys of prescription drug costs:* Prescription drug costs have skyrocketed, but why? Are some drugs replacing invasive surgery successfully? Or are they being used as a complement to surgery? What influences patients' understanding of how and when to take the medication they were prescribed according to clinical instructions? By studying the critical factors in prescription drug cost increases, we hope to shed light on these important topics.

- *Episode of care analysis:* We all know that it is important to look at the experience of the whole patient—across settings of care and types of treatment—and not just isolated components of care. However, doing so is challenging because of the data required. This study looks at the level of postdischarge costs over time for patients who have received coronary artery bypass graft surgery. The goal is a better design of targeting strategies that improve care for cardiac patients.

The Consortium's potential is vast and will improve the potential for the following:

- *Health education:* Sharing information with members about preventing, effectively treating, and dealing with disease. Giving employees and retirees information that will help them become more informed about their conditions and better able to participate in care.

- *A catalyst for best practice delivery:* Sharing information with providers, employees, and retirees about comparative provider performance, and structuring ways to reward providers who deliver superior quality and value of care.

- *Informed decision making:* Basing health benefit design and administration decisions on real-world results.

THE CHALLENGE CONTINUES

Improving our present information-reporting efforts is an on-going process that involves the following.

- *Customizing the answers to "what, where, when, how, and why?":* What do consumers want to know about quality? From where do they prefer to receive information? When do they need information to make decisions? How does a consumer use the information? Why do they want the information?
- *Improving the display and design of reports:* Consumer healthcare informatics, the science and art of providing information about healthcare to consumers, is quickly evolving into its own domain. Even things as seemingly mundane as color choice, legend symbols on charts, type font and size, paper weight, and cover design have significant impacts on whether the contents of reports to consumers will be used.
- *Improved data quality and processing turnaround time:* Decreasing the time lag between the data on which the report is based and when measures are available is important. When timelier, more current results are available, they become more relevant to consumers, who know the healthcare system is rapidly changing.

Shoshanna Sofaer, Dr.Ph. (Sofaer, 1997), outlines the following "confidence marker" indicators that efforts are moving in the right direction:

- Consumers will feel greater confidence in the healthcare system.
- More consumers will be satisfied with their plans.
- More consumers who are dissatisfied with their current plans will shop for better ones.
- Plans and providers that perform well will increase their market share.

- Good-performing plans will be maintained or improved over time and bad-performing plans will either get better or go away.

The early 1980s exposed Ford to a period of great vulnerability from changes in market behavior and new competitors in its core business. In 1999, by embracing a continuous quality improvement framework and tuning into the "consumer headset," Ford emerged stronger than ever in their history. Success depends on working with new healthcare consumers to inform them and to design systems that are built with their health status improvement in mind. The new healthcare consumers, and the employer purchasers who represent them, will settle for nothing less.

REFERENCES

Brook RH. Managed care is not the problem, quality is. *JAMA* 1998; 278(19):1612–1614.

Cleary P, McNeil B. Patient satisfaction as an indicator of quality of care. *Inquiry* Spring 1998; 25:25–36.

Gerteis M, et al. *Through the patient's eyes*. San Francisco: Jossey-Bass, 1993.

Hall JH, et al. Patients' health as a predictor of physician and patient behavior in medical visits. *Medical Care* 1996; 34(12):1205–1218.

Inguanzo JM, Harju M. What makes consumers select a hospital? *Hospitals* 1985; 59:90–94.

KPMG Peat Marwick LLP and Northwestern University. *Consumerism in health care: new voices*. January 1998.

Levinson W, et al. Physician-patient communication: the relationship with malpractice claims among primary care physicians and surgeons. *JAMA* 1997;277(7):553–559.

National Coalition on Health Care. *How Americans perceive the health care system, national survey results*. Washington, DC: National Coalition on Health Care, December 18–22, 1996.

Phelps CE. Diffusion of information in medical care. *J Econ Perspec* 1992; 6(3):23–42.

Phelps CE, Parante S. Priority setting for medical technology and medical practice assessment. *Medical Care* 1990; 28(8):703–723.

Sofaer S. How will we know if we get it right? aims, benefits, and risks of consumer information initiatives. *Journal of Quality Improvement* 1997; 23(5):258-264.
Southeast Michigan Employer and Purchaser Consortium, *Southeast Michigan hospital profile: a consumer guide*, 1998.
Wennberg J. *The Dartmouth atlas*. Chicago: HealthForum, 1999.
www.hiag.org

Government Connections to the New Healthcare Consumer

J. Marvin Bentley, Ph.D.

INTRODUCTION

The new healthcare consumers are the knowledgeable and empowered citizens who play a significant role not only in evaluating and controlling their own personal and family healthcare, but also in determining the general direction of the entire healthcare system. To an even greater extent than in the past, government agencies seek to empower these citizens to become more savvy, market-oriented healthcare consumers. State and federal governments are redirecting their roles from traditional regulators of healthcare professionals and institutions toward activities that supply consumers with information on appropriate clinical treatments and guidelines, comparative treatment outcomes across physicians and hospitals, and information on the costs of these treatments. This information is released in government publications designed to help healthcare consumers make better choices among health plans and health providers and ultimately get better value for the dollars they spend on healthcare services.

Perhaps nowhere is the proliferation and dissemination of healthcare information by government agencies better exemplified than in the case of state health data agencies (HDAs). By a 1999 count, at least 40 states sponsor an agency that publishes data on some aspect of healthcare delivered within that state. These data may include the costs of the care provided, the size and financial status of hospitals or medical clinics, and in fewer cases, the outcomes from medical or surgical procedures. Some HDAs are designing programs that make traditionally published vital statistics more useful to health consumers, while others are working on consumer guides that are useful to patients with specific health needs, and still others are moving out in a new direction and publishing health outcome report cards that consumers may use to choose among competing health insurance plans and providers. Whatever the states' health data policies may be, it is clear that reaching the consumers of healthcare services with useful data and information is a key to applying this information successfully. With such dramatic growth in the links between government and healthcare consumers, the role of the new health consumer will undoubtedly continue to grow and may significantly change the path of healthcare delivery in the coming decade.

For the healthcare consumer, Internet access has dramatically increased the value and accessibility of government information on diseases and clinical guidelines. State and federal agencies are challenged to make the consumer's search for healthcare data user friendly and interactive. The combination of Internet access and a growing emphasis on the role of healthcare consumers as agents in reforming the healthcare delivery system is a critical link. It is rapidly changing the quality and kinds of clinical information governments make available and the kinds of questions that can be answered using these data.

Even with greater availability of information, many healthcare consumers still find it difficult to identify and obtain high-quality, cost-effective medical services. A story published in *The Philadelphia Inquirer* focuses on the angst that future healthcare consumers will likely feel when forced to select among health insurance plans and medical services in markets that are becoming increasingly competitive. The *Inquirer* story concerns a familiar, but complex, situation involving a public dispute between a hospital-based healthcare system and a market-dominant HMO. The issue concerns the degree of financial obligation of the HMO to the healthcare system for the services it provides to HMO enrollees. The public debate is quite predictable. The HMO offers to pay rates that are lower than last year's and the healthcare system counters that it cannot provide quality care at the rates the HMO is offering.

Such complicated financial conflicts force us to question whether and how healthcare consumers can have a significant impact on the decisions and offerings of insurance companies or healthcare providers in the present business environment. The ramifications of these public negotiations go well beyond the parties to the contested contract. They extend to the employers whose workers are enrolled in the HMO's health plans and to the concerns of these employees. As healthcare consumers, employees question whether their access to care and the quality of that care may change based solely on the results of business negotiations.

In the future, we are likely to find more complicated stories like this one, as the employers who sponsor and finance health plans, the medical providers and institutions that deliver care, and the health plans that insure and manage care all test new strategies that they hope will enable them to prosper in ever more competitive markets.

Such negotiations represent an economic battle between large companies whose primary interests and goals may be quite distinct from those of the patient populations they serve. It is hard to imagine circumstances in which the medical needs and preferences of healthcare consumers could become the driving force that determines the outcome of such business negotiations. The general public recognizes the need for cost-effective delivery of medical services and trusts that competition between buyers and sellers within free markets is the best way to reach this goal. At the same time, however, we assign a special kind of primary status to medical care and wish to guarantee all people access to medical services, whatever their ability to pay. Thus, while applauding the concept of competitive medical care, we are challenged by a conflict of values that restricts the options available to control the growing costs of medical care. This conflict of values is a major reason why both federal and state governments have begun to mandate a larger role for healthcare consumers in the organizations charged with improving the effectiveness and controlling the costs of medical care in the United States. Whether healthcare consumers are sufficiently educated and empowered to play a pivotal role in this task is a central consideration for state and federal governments. As a result, they have developed a number of programs and agencies to provide consumer healthcare data.

THE CRITICAL LINK: GOVERNMENT INFORMATION FOR THE CONSUMER

The medical needs and preferences of new healthcare consumers may vary widely depending on their current circumstances, past experiences, and preferences. Medical needs, which may be caused by acute, chronic, and preventable conditions, change as we age and may vary based on gender, occupation, ethnic background, and geographic location; health plans designed for families with young children will likely cover a different set of treatments than those covered by a plan for an older population. Therefore, to be effective, the information made available by government agencies must consider these and other factors, including costs, expected quality of care, and the "comfort level" the patient feels with his or her physician and health plan, to provide the types of data that patients need most.

State and federal governments publish three kinds of healthcare data or information for consumers: (1) vital statistics, (2) injury- or disease-specific information, and (3) medical report cards.

Vital Statistics

Vital statistics provide information on the general health and well-being of the population. Such information includes morbidity and mortality rates, in addition to data on the frequency of specific medical conditions listed as the principle cause of death. They also contain the rates at which certain acute and chronic medical conditions (e.g., diabetes, pneumonia) surface in the general population, the prevalence of health-risk behaviors (e.g., smoking, drug use, sexual activity) in the population, and data such as average birth weights. These rates can be especially useful to healthcare consumers when they are reported by gender, age, or ethnic or social groups because they alert people from diverse backgrounds to the specific medical conditions they are more likely to face.

Vital statistics reports have primarily been used by public health officials and others involved in setting health policy priorities. In fact, if you asked typical health consumers how they have used vital statistics to improve their personal health, they would probably feel pressed to make a connection. However, these government-provided vital health statistics are a critical resource for public and private organizations involved in community health assessments and planning. In their effort to improve the health of the entire community, these organizations publish lists of the key threats to community health, as well as consumer guides designed to help people use medical care more effectively. There are also the new "information" companies who construct "healthy communities" indices from government-published vital health statistics and publish lists such as the "Top 10 Healthiest Cities in America." It is likely that some, although certainly not all, healthcare consumers pay attention to these lists and, when possible, choose to live in more healthy communities. In effect, a private company gathers standard government-provided vital health statistics and adds value to healthcare consumers' experiences by converting this information into a convenient tool they can use to "shop" for a more healthful lifestyle. Such information may also stir interest and "healthy" competition among communities and local organizations.

Injury- or Disease-Specific Health Information

In contrast to the vital statistics that are published as averages or counts for entire populations, government-funded health data agencies provide a second type of health data that are relevant to the medical and social needs of individuals and families—injury- or disease-specific information. Not surprisingly, consumers are most likely to seek health information during events that trigger such a need.

Events that trigger high levels of healthcare consumer activity are either unexpected and sudden, requiring rapid acquisition of critical information, or constant and ongoing, requiring a continuing stream of information and decision making on the part of the healthcare user. The common denominator in both situations is the immediate need for clear, accurate, injury- or disease-specific information.

Putting Information to Use: Case Examples

In the following case examples, independent government publications can facilitate consumer decision making in any number of areas, including concerns about the nature of the disease in question, prognoses, and recommended treatment therapies.

A family caring for a relative with Alzheimer's disease may use this government-provided information to help them organize care for the patient. Alzheimer's is a chronic condition that requires continual care and is a financial and social burden on many families. At least three federal agencies provide information on the treatment and care of Alzheimer's patients: the Administration on Aging, the National Institute on Aging, and the Agency for Health Care Policy and Research. Their offerings include a patient and family guide: *Early Alzheimer's Disease* (AHCPR), an Alzheimer's disease education and referral center (NIA), and information on U.S. Alzheimer's organizations and chapters (AOA). These references provide information on the nature of the disease, the prognosis for Alzheimer's patients, and the types of medical and social support resources available to assist in the daily care of patients. They also provide timely results from clinical trials testing the efficacy of drugs and therapies proposed for the treatment of Alzheimer's patients.

A second example concerns healthcare consumers faced with organizing treatment for themselves or family members with medical conditions such as diabetes, hypertension, or congestive heart failure. Choosing between an indemnity health plan versus an HMO plan can be a special challenge. On one hand, healthcare consumers might be concerned that HMOs will inappropriately pressure their network physicians to treat these conditions conservatively. On the other hand, HMOs often set up disease management programs for these medical conditions and assign case managers who aggressively monitor the treatment of individual patients. By so doing, HMOs are trying to reduce the number of acute episodes that result in inpatient care. If successful, such HMO programs reduce the treatment costs of patients with special medical conditions and can also improve the quality of care these patients receive.

Medical Report Cards

Government agencies offer a third kind of health data in the form of "report cards." Report cards enable the healthcare consumer to compare the past performance of health institutions such as medical clinics, hospitals, and nursing homes; physicians; and health plans licensed as HMOs. These report cards include performance data for up to three areas: (1) the outcomes from treatments delivered by an institution or physician, (2) the costs of delivering these treatments, and (3) healthcare consumers' ratings of their experiences with healthcare providers or the HMO in which they are enrolled.

The "outcomes from treatments" data are designed as an indicator of the effectiveness of medical care delivered by a provider. In most reports, treatment effectiveness is measured by the percentage of cases that end in death. However, to make this measure comparable across hospitals and physicians, government agencies have to adjust the percentage of deaths to reflect the severity of illness for patients treated at different healthcare entities.

The "costs of treatment" data are designed to reflect the efficiency of providers in delivering medical care. Treatment efficiency is measured by total charges for a patient's treatment or the patient's length of stay (LOS) in the hospital.

The level of consumers' satisfaction with their healthcare providers or HMO plans is based on structured surveys of consumers enrolled in competing plans. Because the health needs of consumers are likely to vary, surveys of consumer satisfaction are adjusted to cover populations of consumers with special medical needs.

The first public-sponsored report card on healthcare outcomes was released by HCFA in the late 1980s. The report compared rates of in-hospital deaths for Medicare patients in hospitals licensed by Medicare. However, due in part to criticism leveled by hospitals noting that the rates of in-hospital deaths were not adjusted for differences across hospitals in case mix and severity of illness of patients, HCFA stopped publishing Medicare outcomes reports in the early 1990s.

In contrast, a number of state agencies have begun to publish report cards since 1990. However, although these states clearly regard report cards as an important policy tool for reforming healthcare markets and regulating HMOs, it is surprising how the reports differ across states. For example, Pennsylvania has published annual Hospital Effectiveness Reports since 1990, covering treatment outcomes and hospital charges for 57 DRGs; released an annual CABG report, which included patient outcomes by hospital and primary surgeon; and made available a Heart Attack report that shows outcomes by patients' health insurer or HMO. New York has focused entirely on a CABG outcomes report based exclusively on clinical outcomes reported by the hospital and primary surgeon. Minnesota has concentrated on reports that compare levels of consumer satisfaction across medical clinics and HMO plans.

States often choose to publish report cards because they believe the public release of comparative performance data will help them achieve two policy goals: (1) make healthcare providers and health plans more accountable and (2) help healthcare consumers get more value for the dollars that are spent on their health services. Both goals enjoy public support. Increased accountability is needed because of the growth of competition in markets for professional healthcare services and HMOs, which has made traditional policies for regulating healthcare delivery insufficient. Additional data comparing health outcomes are supported because healthcare consumers want and need more specific information to make choices in this less regulated and more competitive environment.

GOVERNMENT SUPPORT FOR THE NEW HEALTHCARE CONSUMER: EXAMPLES OF HEALTH INFORMATION SERVICES OFFERED BY FEDERAL AND STATE AGENCIES

A large number of federal and state agencies have been established with the primary goal of helping consumers make better choices regarding their personal health. State agencies, or HDAs (introduced at the beginning of this chapter), can be thought of as policy incubators that test concepts that may enhance public knowledge of healthcare, promote a more "market savvy" group of health consumers, and create new strategies for reforming healthcare delivery. The information they gather and make available to healthcare consumers varies significantly in content depending on the legislative mandates under which they operate. At present, HDAs are in the developmental stage. Although they are testing a variety of approaches, all of the HDAs focus on programs that make the organization and cost-effectiveness of medical services more transparent to healthcare consumers.

This section discusses the primary mission of these agencies, how they translate their objectives into a relationship with healthcare consumers, how they are generally organized and governed, and the details of some health information services they offer the public.

Six agencies have been selected to serve as an illustrative sample of the more than 40 state agencies and numerous federal programs now in operation. One federal program, the Agency for Health Care Policy and Research (AHCPR), and five state health data agencies, California's Office of Statewide Health Planning and Development (OSHPD), Pennsylvania's Health Care Cost Containment Council (PHC4), New York's Bureau of Hospital and Primary Care Services (NYBHPC), Missouri's Bureau of Health Resources Statistics (MBHRS), and Minnesota's Health Data Institute (MHDI) will serve as the basis for discussion.

AHCPR is noteworthy as the federal agency that sponsors research on the entire U.S. healthcare delivery system, including its organization and financing, clinical protocols, and the education of providers and consumers of healthcare. The five state HDA agencies were chosen to provide a balanced sample, showcasing the variety of programs that states nationwide are using to reach consumers.

Moreover, much has been previously written about both the state agencies and the AHCPR program; ample information exists that can be used to evaluate their impact on healthcare consumers. For purposes of this discussion, the state agencies have the added benefit of having been analyzed in the consumer-behavior and health-outcomes literature.

Federal Agency Reports: AHCPR

AHCPR was established in 1989 as part of the U.S. Department of Health and Human Services. The National Advisory Council for Health Care Policy, Research, and Evaluation provides advice to the executive director of AHCPR. Its mission is "to improve health care quality through research and education." AHCPR's chief tasks include producing and distributing information about healthcare services; providing information on the structure and governance of firms that deliver and manage the risks associated with healthcare, its costs, and effectiveness; and guiding the public's access to appropriate healthcare. The agency's goal for this effort is to enable society, its providers, purchasers, health insurance plans, and consumers to make better healthcare decisions.

Two AHCPR programs designed for healthcare consumers are the *Consumer Versions of Clinical Practice Guidelines* and *Consumer Assessment of Health Plans* (CAHPS), which is AHCPR's effort to measure "healthcare quality from the consumer perspective."

As part of its program to develop and distribute clinical practice guidelines, AHCPR publishes consumer versions, or what it calls "Patient and Family" guides, for 19 common diseases that require medical attention. The guide for early Alzheimer's disease is typical (*Early Alzheimer's Disease,* 1996). It is based on clinical practice guidelines established by a panel of experts on Alzheimer's and describes how the disease is diagnosed, what treatments are effective in managing the disease, and what steps should be taken to ease the burden of care and enhance the patient's quality of life. Finally, the guide lists private and public organizations that provide support for Alzheimer's patients and their families. In summary, the guide is for people concerned about the possibility of early Alzheimer's; it should help patients and families understand what physicians can do to diagnose and treat the disease; and, for those who require care, it can point them to organizations and support services that can help.

AHCPR has developed and now makes publicly available a product called *CAHPS Survey and Reporting Kit* (CAHPS, *1998*). This is a consumer-centered survey designed to measure the reactions of healthcare consumers to and their experiences with their health plans. Although organizations such as the National Committee for Quality Assurance (NCQA) collect data and set performance standards that can be used for plan-to-plan comparisons, CAHPS addresses the features of health plans and providers that are most important to consumers. For example, the CAHPS survey asks enrollees to rate their reactions to characteristics of health plans that consumers believe are important in selecting a plan. In addition, the flexibility of the CAHPS survey makes it relevant to healthcare consumers with special health needs. There is a core set of questions for all enrollees, but the survey can be modified by adding supplementary questions for consumers dealing with chronic conditions and mental health disorders. The survey can also be modified for enrollees in different kinds of health plans, including enrollees of various Medicare and Medicaid plans. Thus, consumers with special health needs can compare CAHPS responses of consumers with the same needs. Consumers enrolled in the same type of health plans can compare CAHPS responses across different plans of the same type and across different types of plans.

AHCPR expects a number of public and private health-related organizations to sponsor CAHPS surveys of targeted groups of healthcare consumers enrolled in health plans. For example, HCFA plans to use CAHPS to survey Medicare enrollees and publish the results from competing plans so that Medicare consumers can consider these data to make subsequent selections. State agencies that administer Medicaid programs may conduct CAHPS surveys and distribute the results to healthcare consumers in the open enrollment periods. Finally, companies that offer indemnity and managed care health plans may use CAHPS surveys to gauge consumer reaction to the policies that they offer.

AHCPR has worked hard to achieve a low administrative, low financial burden survey from the provider/plan perspective, which facilitates outcomes reporting. AHCPR will have indeed empowered healthcare consumers if CAHPS surveys are adopted on a large scale and sponsors report the results to healthcare consumers faced with selecting among competing health plans.

A Sample of Health Data Agencies Sponsored by State Governments: California's Office of Statewide Health Planning and Development (OSHPD)

In California, government healthcare data activities are centered within OSHPD and especially two divisions of that office: Health Policy and Planning (HPP) and Healthcare Information Division (HID). Although OSHPD is a government agency and part of California's Agency for Health and Human Services, the California Health Policy and Advisory Commission—a bi-partisan group of eleven commissioners who represent various health organizations in the state and are appointed by the governor and the legislature—advises OSHPD on matters regarding the gathering and public reporting of health outcomes data.

HPP sponsors programs that publish public reports on risk-adjusted outcomes from hospital care. A good example is the *Report on Heart Attack (1991–1993)*, which is a publication developed by the California Hospital Outcomes Project. The legislature required all state hospitals to participate in this project. The treatment outcomes were measured by the percentage of patients who died within 30 days after being treated in a hospital for a heart attack. The public report listed hospitals in three categories: (1) those experiencing significantly more deaths than expected, (2) those experiencing deaths within the range expected, and (3) those experiencing significantly fewer deaths than expected.

A second example is HPP's Coronary Artery Bypass Graft (CABG) Mortality Reporting Program. This program is supported jointly by a public–private partnership between OSHPD, the Pacific Business Group on Health (a large employer purchaser coalition in the state), and the California Society of Thoracic Surgeons. Hospital participation in this program is voluntary, and the focus is entirely on the outcomes of patients receiving CABG surgery. In the program's first public report, hospitals' performance will be based on the percent of CABG patients who die in the hospital. Hospitals will be labeled as having death rates that are significantly higher, expected, or lower than expected.

The mission of OSHPD's Healthcare Information Division (HID) is to act as a clearinghouse for information on the costs, access to, and quality of services delivered by licensed healthcare facilities in California. In that regard, HID coordinated the activities of the Managed Health Care Improvement Task Force, which delivered its recommendations for "Improving Managed Health Care in California" in December of 1997 (Managed Health Care Improvement Task Force, 1997). Many of these recommendations centered on health-outcomes information and its potential for empowering health consumers. In general, the Task Force suggested that the state develop new information on the quality of care, create performance information that was more relevant to consumers with special health needs, and take steps to encourage employers to expand the choices of health plans offered to employees. At this stage, it is unclear if these recommendations will surface as standardized public reports offering healthcare consumers information they can use to select among competing health plans and their network providers. Nevertheless, the Task Force recommendations clearly point to a larger role for state government in publishing more and better-defined performance information that healthcare consumers will need in the emerging healthcare markets.

Pennsylvania's Health Care Cost Containment Council (PHC4)

PHC4 was authorized by the Pennsylvania legislature in 1986. The legislative mandate for this 21-member, independent council was "to promote the public interest by encouraging the development of competitive health care services in which health care costs are contained and to assure that all citizens have reasonable access to quality health care." To further this end, the legislation charged the council to provide current, accurate data and information to purchasers and consumers of healthcare on both cost and quality of healthcare services, and to public officials for the purpose of determining health-related programs and policies and ensuring access to healthcare services. Eighteen of the nonpaid, part-time council members were appointed by the governor to represent key stakeholder groups affected by the legislation, including hospitals, the state medical society, managed care plans, Blue Cross and Blue Shield, and labor and business interests. Three government representatives on the council are the Secretary of Health, the State Commissioner of Insurance, and the Secretary of Public Welfare. The state treasurer allots public funds to the council to organize and hire the staff to carry out programs that it is elected to sponsor.

As a state-funded, independent council authorized to organize its own professional staff, PHC4 has been able to establish its own priorities and programs apart from the state bureaucracy. From the start, the council's chief priority has been its data files on inpatient hospital discharges, which include both administrative and clinical data on every patient discharged from an acute-care Pennsylvania hospital. For example, specific fields in each discharge record include total hospital charges, the patient's length of stay in the hospital, the ICD-9 codes identifying treatments delivered to the patient, and the patient's key clinical findings. This database has allowed PHC4 to publish a variety of Consumer Guides that compare the effectiveness and charges for treatment services across hospitals competing in a limited market area. Two of these reports are characteristic of the performance data PHC4 provides to healthcare consumers: the *Hospital Effectiveness Report* and the Annual CABG Surgery Outcomes Report.

In 1991, PHC4 published its first "report card"–type guide to hospital effectiveness in the state. The information contained in these Hospital Effectiveness Reports was taken from the council's files on inpatient hospital discharges described previously. Data from these discharge records were aggregated into 57 diagnostic-related groups (DRG) (treatment categories) within roughly 160 acute-care hospitals and presented as performance measures of each hospital's treatment effectiveness and cost in each of the 57 DRG categories. Each hospital was placed into one of nine market areas and regional reports compared hospitals within these market areas. The performance measures were "risk-adjusted, in-hospital deaths" for treatment effectiveness and "average total costs" for costs. For each of the 57 DRGs reported, the report drew attention to hospitals that experienced significantly greater or fewer deaths than expected or those with total charges that were significantly greater or less than the regional average. Even though the council warned healthcare consumers that these labels were based on statistical estimates and they should not use these labels as the sole factor in choosing a hospital, the Hospital Effectiveness Reports did signal hospitals and physicians that a new approach to accountability had been introduced.

In 1994, PHC4 introduced the *Pennsylvania's Guide to Coronary Artery Bypass Graft (CABG) Surgery*. The guide is designed as a source of information on CABG surgery outcomes across hospitals, cardiac surgeons, and health plans. Like its earlier reports, the CABG surgery guide includes risk-adjusted performance measures constructed from PHC4's inpatient discharge records and labels highly effective or ineffective hospitals on a similar scale. However, unlike earlier guides that reported on 57 DRG treatments, this guide centers on a single surgical treatment delivered by only 40 hospitals in the state. Moreover, in addition to the 40 hospitals offering CABG programs in Pennsylvania, the 1996 guide releases performance measures on the cardiac surgeons in charge of each CABG case and the health plans in which the CABG patients were enrolled. This meant that each of the 40 hospitals, roughly 220 cardiac surgeons, and 30-plus larger health plans that cover CABG patients were singled out if their patients experienced significantly greater or fewer in-hospital deaths than expected. Again, the guide cautions that these high and low performing labels are based on statistical estimates and recommends that healthcare consumers not base their choice of provider or health plan solely on these tags.

By extending performance information on CABG outcomes to health plans, PHC4 seemed to invite healthcare consumers, especially those with heart disease, to consider how health plans performed on CABG outcomes as a factor in choosing a health plan. The 1996 guide cautions the public that these data are in their infancy and explains that this is a first step in monitoring and reporting on the changing role of managed care organizations. Because these remarks were not directed to healthcare consumers but to the general public, this decision seems to reflect the council's effort to hold managed health plans to a higher level of accountability, rather than suggest that healthcare consumers use this information in selecting a health plan.

New York: Coronary Artery Bypass Surgery in New York State

In New York, the primary source of performance information on hospitals, physicians, and health plans is the New York State Department of Health. Various bureaus within the Department gather data on the characteristics of patients and their treatments for conditions such as trauma injury, heart disease, and cancer. These characteristics are analyzed carefully to determine whether they are risk factors affecting the outcomes of patients with these conditions. Other bureaus collect administrative and clinical data they use to evaluate the performance of managed healthcare plans. In either case, the Department has a history of cooperating with the hospitals and physicians in an effort to make clinical care more effective. They also work with health plans to make their finances and management more consistent with national standards and the needs of New York healthcare consumers. Thus, the New York strategy on performance measures contrasts with the Pennsylvania strategy, which is set and implemented by an independent council. PHC4 is not directly connected to the Department of Health and sees its mission as providing information more directly to healthcare consumers. Conversely, the New York State Department of Health's programs are viewed as improving outcomes through information provided primarily to the healthcare providers rather than to the public. There are arguable advantages, as well as shortcomings, to both systems.

This distinction is seen clearly in New York's report, *Coronary Artery Bypass Surgery in New York State*, first published in 1993. In the 1970s, the Department of Health, already interested in improving the care of patients with heart disease, established a State Cardiac Advisory Committee made up of distinguished physicians to oversee the Department's program in this area. Statisticians in the Department were able to identify risk factors that were significant predictors of patient outcomes. These risk factors were used in statistical models to predict rates of in-hospital deaths for the unique group of patients treated in a given hospital by a single cardiac surgeon. However, even though this tool enabled the department to monitor the effectiveness of CABG surgeries, there was no plan to make these results a public report card comparing the performances of hospitals and cardiac surgeons throughout New York.

This all changed when the press, arguing the public's right to know, received a court order forcing the Department of Health to release CABG results to the public. Thus, the Department was forced to communicate its performance information to healthcare consumers and purchasers who might use it as an aid in choosing among competing hospitals and surgeons (New York State Department of Health, 1998). However, the New York public reports on CABG continue to reflect the Department's chief priority to work in an interactive way with providers to improve the quality of care. The Cardiac Advisory Committee assists in interpreting the data and advises the Department regarding which hospitals and surgeons may need special attention. Finally, New York's CABG surgery reports do not include data that reflect the variations in the costs of CABG surgery across competing hospitals. Accordingly, the focus remains on treatment effectiveness and its improvement and not on empowering healthcare consumers with information that they might use to become more informed buyers of heart surgery. The New York approach, centered in the Department of Health and focused on interactive cooperation with healthcare providers, clearly places maximum effort on the provider accountability end of the scale.

The Missouri Department of Health

In Missouri, the primary source of performance information on healthcare providers has been the Bureau of Health Resources Statistics, now the Bureau of Health Care Performance Monitoring in the Department of Health. In 1992, the Missouri legislature passed a law that authorized the Health Department to gather patient data on the treatment outcomes and costs of services provided by hospitals and ambulatory surgical centers. The data collected under this statute became the centerpiece for a series of Buyer's Guides on specific healthcare services delivered in Missouri.

Missouri's first report card–type publication intended for healthcare consumers was the *Buyer's Guide: Obstetrical Services (OS)* (1994). In reality, this guide is the combination of an educational focus, aimed at expectant mothers perhaps in the market for maternity services for the first time, and a report card comparing performance measures across hospitals offering these services to a local market. The education piece is designed for the consumer of obstetrical services, discussing availability and characteristics of obstetrical procedures that are important indicators of the quality of maternity care. This section of the guide highlights that hospitals competing in the same regional markets often charge significantly different fees for the same procedures, and it suggests questions a healthcare consumer should ask about charges before choosing a provider. The quality indicators presented in the guide include results from a patient satisfaction survey, information on availability of appropriate obstetrical procedures offered by the hospital, and data that indicate how the hospitals manage patients with special needs, including cesarean deliveries and high-risk infants. There is also a section that describes how each of these indicators is related to quality care. Finally, the guide singles out hospitals with the lowest and highest charges within the different regional markets.

In 1997, the Missouri Department of Health published another Buyer's Guide on Hospital Emergency Services (HES) (*Buyer's Guide: Hospital Emergency Services,* 1997). A comparison between this guide and the first guide on obstetrical services provides a glimpse of how the Department's purpose for these guides, its interest in the costs of services, and the criteria it uses to judge the quality of care provided by hospitals may have changed between 1993 and 1997. Both guides clearly address healthcare consumers and follow the same general format, but there are striking differences. The first difference involves the important relationship between the Department and the hospitals reported in this guide. For the obstetrical guide, state law required hospitals to release information requested by the health department. However, for the *Buyer's Guide: Hospital Emergency Services*, hospitals voluntarily submitted information on their emergency services and a list of patients treated in their emergency service. In addition, the state's hospital association commended the state for ". . . urging Missourians to think about their use of health care services in advance of a medical emergency." In addition, the HES guide does not present data on hospital charges for emergency services, and the indicators that are presented are not labeled as quality indicators. Instead, the Department's purpose for this publication is to "give readers a better understanding of the level of emergency care their local hospitals have made a commitment to provide," and its hope is that "[the guide] may cause some hospitals to strengthen their commitment to emergency care . . . "

The changes observed between the first and last guide in Missouri's series raise an important question, "Do these differences signal changes in Missouri's relation with the healthcare providers that it regulates and/or its commitment to empowering consumers in the healthcare services markets?" Of course, managing the delivery of obstetrical services and emergency medical care are different matters to hospitals and judging the quality of these two distinct types of healthcare service presents dissimilar challenges for regulators. However, it remains possible that Missouri is leaning more on accountability as the incentive for healthcare providers to deliver more effective and less costly healthcare and trusting less in the ability of informed consumers to capture the benefits from report cards. The Missouri Department of Health released *Buyer's Guide: Managed Care Plans* in June of 1999.

The Minnesota Health Data Institute (MHDI)

The MHDI is a key healthcare data agency in Minnesota created by the state legislature in 1993. MHDI is a public–private partnership between the 21-member Board of Directors of the nonprofit Minnesota Institute for Community Health Information and the State Commissioner of Health. Members of the Board represent the Minnesota Consortium of Healthcare Purchasers, hospitals and healthcare providers, health plans, consumers, labor unions, and four state departments. MHDI is currently funded 70% from contributions by private stakeholders and 30% from public dollars. Its mission is "to design and implement an integrated, statewide health care data system to support the information needs of health care consumers, purchasers, providers, plans, policy makers, and researchers in measuring and improving the quality and efficiency of healthcare services in Minnesota" (http://www.mhdi.org). The Performance Measurement Program is one of two major programs supported by MHDI. Its mission is to develop and implement standard healthcare measurements of performance and to publicize this information so that consumers can help make the healthcare system more competitive.

Like healthcare data agencies in other states, MHDI releases report cards on healthcare providers and health plans that are addressed primarily to healthcare consumers. However, the consumer reports produced by MHDI are unique compared with those released in other states. For example, reports on CABG surgeries published by New York, California, and Pennsylvania are constructed from data contained in the records of inpatient discharges submitted by hospitals. Also, because of the limits of these data, these states measure the effectiveness of CABG surgery based on a single indicator—the rate of inpatient deaths. In contrast, the MHDI report cards are based primarily on the reactions of healthcare consumers to the health insurance plan in which they are enrolled and the clinics where they receive primary care. This means that the performance measures contained in MHDI reports are based on a broader set of characteristics that healthcare consumers have declared important in selecting a health insurance plan, hospital, or primary care provider (Minnesota Health Data Institute, 1998).

In its mission to help healthcare consumers make better decisions, MHDI has sponsored projects designed to elicit the kinds of information consumers think are important in comparisons of health plans and of healthcare providers. In 1995, MHDI distributed results from a statewide survey of Minnesota consumers on the reaction of enrollees to their health plans and medical care. The document was titled *You and Your Health Plan,* and it compared information on the performance of 46 health plans operating in Minnesota. Importantly, MHDI analyzed public reaction to this publication and learned that healthcare consumers thought the survey devoted too much to the health plans and not enough to the clinics and healthcare systems that were delivering primary care to enrollees in the managed care plans. Due in part to this finding, MHDI has focused more on the organizations providing the medical care—the primary care clinics, hospitals, and healthcare systems. MHDI is also partnering with organizations that have expertise in patient satisfaction surveys. For example, for the 1997 Medicaid and MinnesotaCare Managed Care Member Satisfaction Survey that MHDI did for the Minnesota Department of Human Services, the Institute used the AHCPR-sponsored CAHPS survey (Minnesota Health Data Institute, 1997). Likewise, MHDI's latest publication, *Vital Signs: A Guide to Health Care in the Northland,* was released in May of 1999. MHDI used the Picker Institute's Ambulatory Care Patient Satisfaction Survey to gather patient responses contained in this guide.

Of the state strategies covered in this chapter, Minnesota's stands out in several important respects. First, MHDI's decision to rely on patient satisfaction data is evidence of its commitment to healthcare consumers, whereas states that depend on hospital discharge records or information on ambulatory patient visits, at least in part, are committed to encouraging providers to improve their clinical outcomes.

Second, given the rate at which new kinds of health plans and providers are surfacing in today's healthcare system, it is important that report cards be flexible and relevant to the concerns consumers have with these emerging healthcare organizations. In this regard, report cards based on patient satisfaction surveys seem better than those linked to a narrow measure of treatment effectiveness.

Third, consumer interest in competing managed healthcare plans depends on a variety of factors related to the clinical care provided: its quality, the time it takes for enrollees to receive needed care, and how well enrollees understand the treatment they receive. Some healthcare consumers might find the MHDI-style report card more helpful in selecting a health plan, whereas other consumers, most likely those with serious chronic conditions or special needs, might prefer report cards that focus on treatment outcomes.

Finally, it is likely that in the long run, MHDI-type report cards will have greater regulatory value because they can be easily adapted and used nationally. MHDI had little difficulty adapting AHCPR's CAHPS survey for a Minnesota-based Medicaid population. The Institute also saved expenses and gained credibility by adapting the Picker Institute's Ambulatory Care Patient Satisfaction Survey for a consumer survey and report on healthcare systems in Minnesota and Wisconsin. In contrast, none of the health outcomes that states studied mentioned plans to use standardized protocols for collecting and reporting on treatment outcomes. This suggests that other states are more likely to adopt report cards based on patient satisfaction.

HOW WILL THE STATES AND FEDERAL GOVERNMENT SUPPORT FUTURE HEALTHCARE CONSUMERS?

This chapter has described how the relations between governments and the healthcare delivery system have changed over the past decade. The purpose was to characterize the drift of government policy away from traditional strategies in which states regulated the fees charged and set the standards for hospitals, health clinics, and health insurers to a new emphasis in which states concentrate on educating patients to become better users of healthcare services. To carry out this policy, states are providing healthcare consumers with information that they can use to select the health plan and healthcare providers that are likely to give the consumer the best value. The programs presented in this chapter demonstrate the kinds of strategies governments have implemented in making this transition.

Although it is too early to tell, it is important to question whether these programs will likely achieve the goals set by their government sponsors. In addition, studies have shown that state-sponsored report cards have led hospitals and physicians to improve the treatments they deliver (Chassin, Hannan, & DeBuono, 1996; Hannan et al., 1994; Longo et al., 1998). However, studies on the behavior of healthcare consumers have not suggested that report cards significantly improve the strategies that they use in searching for best buys (Chernew & Scanlon, 1998; Scanlon, Chernew, & Lave, 1997; Schneider & Epstein, 1996). Studies suggest that report cards do improve the subsequent performance of healthcare providers, but these same studies and others do not attribute the improvement to more informed and energized healthcare consumers. This suggests that increased levels of public accountability, which report cards impose on healthcare providers and not healthcare consumers, is the more likely cause of improvement in provider performance. For the report cards to change how healthcare consumers search for better values, consumers must face realistic choices among healthcare providers and plans. Consumer-focused information must be at a level of detail that fits the wide range of health conditions and preferences that exist in a group of healthcare consumers. In short, the kinds of public report cards that states have released are sufficient for accountability purposes but have not yet yielded more aggressive, informed, and selective consumers of health-related services that some government policy makers expected.

This should be a concern for the country and particularly for consumers of healthcare services. Government agencies are uniquely qualified to gather and distribute performance information on healthcare providers and plans. They can require that providers submit patient data that are used to construct performance information and can audit providers to ensure that these data are accurate. Moreover, people have a higher level of trust in government data because the states are neutral parties to private transactions that are linked to the report cards. If government agencies can capitalize on this advantage and release performance information that energizes healthcare consumers, the nation as a whole and consumers in particular should benefit from dynamic market competition created in the healthcare industry.

For this to happen, three policy-related changes must take place. First, employers have to offer more health plan choices to employees. This can happen if states encourage employers to form purchaser coalitions that offer a number of accredited health plan choices to larger groups of employees. States can also sponsor their own purchaser that welcomes smaller employee groups. Unless consumers have realistic choices among competing plans, publicly available performance information is of no value to them.

Second, states should adopt "reference" health plan contracts that are easily recognized and can be used as a reference when buyers and sellers negotiate the premiums and benefits on policies offered by managed care organizations. More important for consumers, reference contracts will mean that employers or purchaser coalitions can offer employees comparable cost and performance information on reference contracts available in a given market area. When costs and performance information are compared on standardized or reference contracts, healthcare consumers are more likely to study the comparative data and are more confident they are comparing information on comparable health plans.

Finally, the states that provide performance data will need to distribute these data to purchasers, healthcare systems, insurers, and consultants and rely less on standardized public reports that go directly to consumers. By wholesaling data services to intermediaries who, in turn, select out relevant patient cases or satisfaction records and format reports directed to smaller groups of consumers, states create greater value for the public dollars they invest in performance information. Although the larger public reports cover all providers in a market area, they generally do not focus on consumers interested in outcomes of patients with special needs or preferences. These more focused reports can be done best by private firms and providers who are closer to the consumers. Thus, by offering their valuable data at competitive prices, states encourage a distribution network of consultants and information companies that can release these data at a level of detail that make them more helpful to selected groups of healthcare consumers.

The policy changes called for herein are already being discussed in government agencies and legislatures. There is a good chance that they will materialize in some form in the near future. If indeed they do come to pass, both federal and state health data agencies will connect much more strongly with future healthcare consumers.

REFERENCES

Buyer's Guide: Hospital Emergency Services. Missouri Center for Health Statistics. Pub. No. 18.10. N.D.

Buyer's Guide: Obstetrical Services. Missouri Center for Health Statistics. Pub. No. 18.2. N.D.

Chassin MR, Hannan EL, DeBuono B. Benefits and hazards of reporting medical outcomes publicly. *N Engl J Med* 1996; 334(6):394–398.

Chernew M, Scanlon DP. Health plan report cards and insurance choice. *Inquiry* 1998; 35(1):9–23.

Consumer Assessment of Health Plans (CAHPS®): fact sheet. Agency for Health Care Policy and Research, Pub. No. 97-R079. Rockville, MD: December, 1998. http://www.ahcpr.gov/qual/cahpfact.htm

Coronary Artery Bypass Surgery in New York State 1994–1996. New York State Department of Health, October, 1998.

Early Alzheimer's disease: patient and family guide. Consumer Guide Number 19. Agency for Health Care Policy Research, Pub. No. 960704. Washington, DC: October 1996.

Hannan EL, et al. Improving the outcomes of coronary artery bypass surgery in New York State. *JAMA* 1994; 271:761–766. http://www.mhdi.org/mhdi/index.html, p. 1.

Longo DR, et al. Consumer reports in health care. *JAMA* 1998; 278(19):1579–1584.

Managed Health Care Improvement Task Force. *Improving Managed Health Care in California*. Executive Summary, Findings and Recommendations and Supporting

Documentation. http://www.oshpd.cahwnet.gov/hid/links/
manhct/report.htm.

Minnesota Health Data Institute. *1997 clinic survey pilot
project, consumer focus groups.* 1998.

Minnesota Health Data Institute. *1997 Medicaid and
MinnesotaCare managed care member satisfaction survey.* 1997.

Minnesota Health Data Institute. *Vital signs: a guide to health
care in the Northland.* 1999.

Minnesota Health Data Institute. *You and your health plan.
1995 statewide survey of Minnesota consumers.* 1995.

Scanlon DP, Chernew M, Lave JR. Consumer health plan choice:
current knowledge and future directions. *Ann Rev Public Health*
1997; 18:507–528.

Schneider EC, Epstein AM. Influence of cardiac-surgery
performance reports on referral practices and access to care: a
survey of cardiovascular specialists. *N Engl J Med* 1996;
335(4):251–256.

CHAPTER

Health System Initiatives: Responding to the New Healthcare Consumer

Philip A. Newbold

Diane S. Stover

INTRODUCTION

In thinking about the development of strategies that better serve a more empowered customer in healthcare, it is important to realize that we are in the midst of a fundamental shift in our orientation, mind-sets, mental models, and strategies. Over the past 40 to 50 years, we have developed one of the greatest "medical care" delivery systems oriented toward sickness, illness, and injury that has largely been "provider centric." Today, it is incumbent for healthcare systems to move to a "customer-centric" model that places the needs, demands, and wants of a more empowered customer at the center of all of our thinking. To maintain viability, healthcare systems need to take the consumer view very seriously and place the consumer at the center of key business decisions and organizations. This chapter discusses how healthcare systems are meeting this challenge through the development of innovative programs aimed at "keeping the consumer in mind." Exemplary initiatives of health systems nationally are highlighted.

BACKGROUND

To be effective in the future, it is vital that the healthcare industry use new models, new lenses in seeing the world, radically new thinking, and a fundamental shift away from many of the familiar and comfortable strategies of the past. One important tool in helping us change our way of thinking is to assume that the products, services, and approaches of the future will largely be reversals of assumptions of commonly held beliefs of the past. The consumer and retail industries provide examples to draw upon. Think back 20 to 25 years ago, when we wanted a pizza or to go see a movie. In both cases, we had to travel to where the pizza was being made and sold and to where the movie was being shown on a fixed theater screen. In expanding our notion of service delivery, to encompass a consumer-centered focus, we see the growth and development of whole new industries, that is, home delivery and movie video rental. Incidentally, rather than subtract or replace the switched business, both restaurants and movie theaters are increasing and broadening their customer bases rather than losing their traditional customer bases. This is also true in many aspects of our healthcare and medical care delivery systems.

A number of examples of changed thinking and assumption reversals are illustrative in designing new services, products, and programs for a more empowered consumer. The first of these is a shift away from a medical model orientation toward a health model orientation (Figure 15–1).

Following are several characteristics that define the medical model, which has served us so well over the past 40 to 50 years. The medical model is based on delivering medical services after the fact, that is, after disease, illness, or injury has already occurred. The health model reverses this and focuses on preventing illness and injury. The second defining characteristic of the medical model is the fact that it is set up so that patients can see certain providers who are available 24 hours a day, 7 days a week, like a hospital, or they have to work around office hours that are convenient for the physician. The health model reverses this assumption and says, "We will come to you to deliver services or prevent illness by being closer to you in neighborhoods, by being available with programs and services in congregations

FIGURE 15–1

Illustration of the shift in philosophies underlying healthcare delivery in the past few decades. These models have been held by consumers and clinicians alike.

Models		
From		**To**
Medical model	→	Health model
Medical care system	→	Lifestyle choices
Scarcity mind-set	→	Abundance mentality
Linear/Newtonian thinking	→	Organic/biological models
Physical disease	→	Holistic model
Characteristics		
Medical Model		**Health Model**
After the fact	→	Prevention
Patient comes to provider	→	Providers go to consumers
"Fix me"	→	"I can do it myself"
Knowledge of a few/language professions	→	Easy and wide access of information for everyone

and school sites, and by providing access into your home through the Internet, telephone triage systems, and mail-order delivery." The third characteristic of the medical model is that the patient comes to a provider with a "fix me" mind-set, and all of the power, knowledge, and control rests within the provider. The health model is more oriented toward the patient believing, "I can do it myself." The focus of power in this thinking rests largely in the domain of the empowered customer. Finally, the medical model has most of the technical knowledge concentrated in a few individuals with its own specific vocabulary and its own set of professional standards and guidelines. The health model makes access to information easily available and assumes that information needs to be widely available and easy to use for everybody.

The second major shift in thinking is oriented around the answer to the question, "Where does health come from?" If we refer to Figure 15–2, we see that the medical care delivery

F I G U R E   15–2

Only 10% of an individual's health status is directly related to the medical care delivery system.

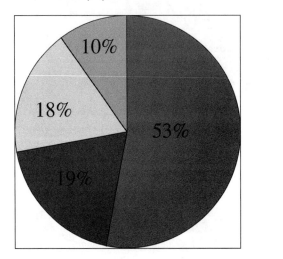

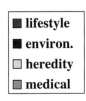

system is responsible for only approximately 10% of a person's health status.

The largest, and by far most important, segment is all about lifestyle–the choices that we make every day and how we conduct all aspects of our daily lives. These choices include the amount of daily exercise we engage in, the diet we keep, whether we smoke, whether we consume alcohol, the stress in our lives, and the choices we make for ourselves and for our loved ones nearly every moment. If we are going to empower customers to be more accountable for their own health and health status, clearly, the high leverage points and the new investments must be in and around improvements in lifestyle and the daily choices people make. The highest leverage points, of course, are those that impact children where we can begin to educate, role model, and provide positive choices that will encourage individuals to make lifestyle decisions that are healthy, that are responsible, and that will last a lifetime.

The third model or shift in thinking involves the moving from a scarcity mentality toward an abundance mentality. The scarcity approach is often focused within the medical care delivery system around technology, resources, and money. It assumes that only a limited amount of each is available to go around, and if one person or one organization has access or greater resources, somebody else will have less. This approach is based on a fixed-sum game and results in a win–lose approach. This model is very competitive and assumes that only a few resources are available to individuals, to organizations, and to the community; therefore, these very scarce resources must be allocated in competitive ways involving power, influence, and politics.

The abundance mind-set takes just the opposite approach. It assumes plenty of resources are available, in fact, almost an unlimited amount. This thinking is based on more of a reallocation model and assumes that assets and resources are plentiful only if we begin thinking in new ways. Most individuals, organizations, and communities are not aware of the assets, strengths, and resources that are available all around and in significant abundance. The abundance mentality is built around cooperation and collaboration as a way to develop an almost limitless supply of resources and affects everything from technology to all of the relationships that we share with our families, work groups, and neighbors in our communities. It is the sharing and the leveraging of existing strengths and resources that is the heart of the movement toward a more empowered consumer, a situation in which everyone can have available resources and greater strengths and possibilities (for further reading, see McKnight and Kretzman and Covey).

The fourth major shift is the moving away from a linear or Newtonian model of thinking toward a more biological or organic model. Change, it seems, is never very linear and simple, and most of our consumers exist in a web of relationships and connections that are very complex. Leland Kaiser, Ph.D., one of America's foremost health futurists, suggests that there are a few rules of quantum physics that are useful in moving away from this linear-Newtonian thinking. Dr. Kaiser suggests three important quantum rules for us to consider: (1) nothing stands alone, (2) everything is connected to everything else, and (3) when you change one thing, you begin to change everything. These laws of quantum physics suggest that we need to take more of an organic and living model approach to our thinking as we design a healthcare system that is more responsive to a more empowered consumer. We must therefore pay attention to the environments that people live within, the relationships among family members and workers, the design of habitats, and the interactive nature of much of the technology that is ever present in our future. This is why hospitals and healthcare systems need to be where relationships are developed and relationships are made, that is, in neighborhoods, schools, congregations, social and recreational settings—anywhere where people are making choices and engaging in behaviors that shape their future.

The fifth major change involves taking a more holistic view of the patient and the disease process. The old model suggests that it is the physical dimensions of disease that we must fix or treat as the primary role for the medical care delivery system. Our shift toward a more holistic view sees the physical dimensions as the center of much of disease, illness, and injury, but it also realizes that there is a ring of mental, emotional, and spiritual components that also must be considered. This model recognizes the connections, the interactions, and the many dimensions of individuals as they lead their lives, and the need to develop a more holistic approach toward programs and services. This is truly where the emerging complementary and integrative medicine of the East meets the traditional medical approach of the West.

HEALTH SYSTEMS MOVING FORWARD

The waves of change facing the healthcare industry are ubiquitous, and no one has remained unchanged. However, the impact of such change on business dynamics depends on the maturity of an individual market and myriad other issues. Although high-level assumptions about market trends and their impact on health systems is not the focus of this chapter, an awareness of their impact is important in prefacing this next section, which highlights examples of consumer-centric health system initiatives. The following collection of case studies features solutions to a variety of challenges and opportunities, initiatives spearheaded by Memorial Health System (MHS), as well as other systems throughout the country in an age of connected healthcare consumers. These programs are grouped according to some of the main themes in the healthcare system today: attending to facilitating access and the meeting of communities' basic psychosocial needs; cultural sensitivity that goes beyond recognition of diversity; grassroots-to-mainstream advocacy; on-site/point-of-service, barrier-free, "one-stop shopping" for healthcare services, especially preventive services, facilitated by the Internet, by savvy retail businesses; easy information access through new use of "old" technologies, such as the telephone; and the movement to reach and teach children about the benefits of health while they are young, with the aid of the latest in interactive education and entertainment.

First Things First

Two of the most basic concerns facing many families are things many people take for granted. The first program, Home Management Services, deals with empowering families with the skills necessary to manage day-to-day responsibilities. The second initiative highlights Kaiser Permanente's role in fostering an awareness of importance of cultural differences in patient–provider communication, building on the work of Noel Chrisman. Both initiatives emphasize the importance of the nuances of psychosocial issues and activities of daily living that can be overlooked in intervention development and that form the basic building blocks for personal empowerment.

Home Management Services

The Home Management Services (HMS) program, sponsored by MHS, grew out of an urgent need to provide female homemakers and mothers with the practical training and support they need to manage their homes, their families, and their personal lives. When home life is not well coordinated, many things, including healthcare, can suffer. Some women are not empowered and in desperate situations; for example, they may be single parents whose housing or child custody is in jeopardy, or they may have been abandoned by their husbands. Many feel as if they are swimming against the tide because their education is inadequate for suitable employment and they have insufficient finances to meet their needs. There are those who feel isolated and afraid and who lack the basic skills needed for successful management of the home. Others in the program may have a suitable income and have an education, but they may lack time management skills.

HMS, which serves hundreds of women and their families in northern Indiana and southern Michigan, provides a 12-week course in the fundamentals of managing our everyday lives. Individual follow-up is also offered. The course of instruction covers personal growth and development, household organization, nutrition and menu planning, management of household finances, and effective delegation. The program aims to help women find a renewed sense of purpose and hope in their lives, and it fosters home management and caregiving skills. Counselors/instructors take a rigorous 3-month course of instruction, and all are volunteers who want to do something concrete and who want to make a difference in the quality of family life in the area. HMS has an 85% attendance rate, and most women remain with the program for at least 1 year. Many of these women return to help so that others can take similar classes. This strategic alliance will be expanding to reach more families and interest corporate sponsors.

The Culture Connection

"Cultural competency" is a fairly new effort under way in health systems. The underlying premise is that unless a healthcare provider understands important cultural differences between patients, optimal care cannot be achieved. Noel Chrisman, Ph.D., of the University of Washington School of Nursing, has studied extensively effective cultural competencies in healthcare. Dr. Chrisman, who teaches medical teams around the country about the difference cultural awareness can make, finds that the following issues are often ignored, yet can have a serious impact on healthcare: dietary practices, food preparation preferences, religious practices, home remedies, illness behaviors, and family relationships. He believes that the key principles to effective cultural connections are (1) knowledge of the culture, (2) mutual respect based on knowledge, and (3) negotiation that is used when belief/ behavior conflicts arise between the patient and healthcare provider.

One health system that has operationalized this concept is the California Division of Kaiser Permanente. It has added a Director of Cultural Competence, Jean Gilbert, Ph.D., to enhance its care planning efforts. To date, her position is unique in the industry. She states that although most organizations emphasize diversity in terms of their workforce, the Kaiser program emphasizes skill building, knowledge, and "actions that are designed to better meet the needs of a diverse membership" (Chrisman, 1999). The Kaiser Cultural Competency program was seen as an important business strategy based on how ethnicity impacts member retention, medical compliance, and patient satisfaction. Dr. Gilbert is finalizing a series of Cultural Competency Manuals for all locations that may be available to other health systems in the future. The Kaiser effort also includes regular training sessions that feature a troupe of "care actors" who are hired to play various ethnically diverse roles. The care actors work with physicians, nurses, and other staff members to fine-tune competency development.

Advocacy in Action

The following program illustrates the power of advocacy: that in order for a clinical service or program to be effective, it must be serviced by the same clientele it wishes to reach. Women In Touch illustrates the growth and success of a grassroots commitment between healthcare organizations and energetic, committed leaders within the community.

Women In Touch
The Women In Touch (WIT) Learning History (www.quality-oflife.org/ich/wit/wit.htm) is a nationally recognized grassroots effort that has spread to many other communities in the country. WIT is a network of volunteers dedicated to improve breast cancer screening rates and lower breast cancer death rates for African-American women. Its mission is to empower

women in the community to take a more active role in meeting their health needs.

WIT's genesis is implicit in the alarming statistics regarding the prevalence and incidence of breast cancer among African-American women:

- Breast cancer is the second leading cause of cancer deaths for African-American women.
- Although the incidence of breast cancer in African-American women is lower than in white women, the death rate from breast cancer is disproportionately higher.
- Women in lower socioeconomic levels have a 10% to 15% lower survival rate from cancer than the average population. Of African-American females, 34% have an income below the poverty level.
- Health services research indicates that mammography screening among African-American women is underutilized and that they are underrepresented in clinical trials.

WIT began as a grassroots initiative. A meeting was called involving approximately 60 key female African-American community leaders to a dinner discussion to discuss community health issues and to form an African-American women's advisory panel. In several meetings that followed, the purpose and mission for WIT were clarified. Its goals are to do the following:

- Raise awareness of breast cancer in the African-American community
- Teach breast self-examination
- Assist in detecting breast cancer in its earliest stages
- Increase the rate of participation of African-American women in mammography screening
- Encourage participation in breast cancer prevention studies through education and risk assessment
- Educate the African-American community on pertinent high-risk health issues

Its concomitant objectives, per the goals just listed, were to do the following:

- Collaborate with the city's public health centers to recruit African-American physicians and nurses to provide better clinical direction and assist with access and follow-up care
- Establish a women's breast cancer outreach network
- Develop and implement culturally sensitive literature to complement the development of education and outreach programs
- Implement a marketing and advertising campaign, largely through word of mouth through many congregations and social clubs throughout the African-American community
- Create public service television commercials and visit local grocery stores, beauty shops, and congregations to promote early breast cancer screening and early detection
- Create a service to transport women to mammography screenings

In addition to the stigmas and fears many women feel about seeking help outside the home/reaching out to the health-care community, many tangible barriers also kept women from seeking WIT. Many women were not insured or were underinsured, so they assumed that seeking medical help would be futile. Some did not have a physician, and some had transportation, child care, and financial concerns that they consider more pressing to them than their own health. Over time, WIT has helped women find solutions to these obstacles.

Today, WIT screens more than 800 new women annually for breast cancer. WIT also sponsors three annual conferences with national speakers and wide community support. To date, they have performed nearly 50 education sessions and have trained approximately 200 volunteers.

According to Carl Ellison, Vice President, Community Affairs at Memorial Hospital in South Bend, Indiana, an African-American community leader and a WIT advocate, "WIT is not a 'recipe' type of program. . . . It has evolved slowly in order to reach its current level of success. From the start, volunteers were driven by their sense of ownership of the program and a recognition that there was no clear road map to follow" (Chrisman, 1999).

"WE WILL COME TO YOU"

One of the premises of empowering consumers of health services—helping them become more knowledgeable and accountable—is that services and access need to be closer to where people work, live, worship, and spend their leisure time. The Internet is revolutionizing consumer-centric services and eliminating access barriers, as illustrated with "HairNet" in the following section. Moreover, retail and mainstream businesses have taken the concept of "one-stop (health) shopping" to the penultimate, as exemplified by such consumer-friendly stores as Nordstrom's, which offers St. John's Wort–infused tortilla chips and on-site free mammography screening, to be discussed in the following section.

"HairNet"

"HairNet" is an innovative new approach that brings Web access to demographic groups that are underrepresented among computer users, including minority women. The free service is provided through a new project dubbed "HairNet," a joint effort between a hair salon and six community agencies, and Sisters Involving Sisters, a community group involved in efforts to empower low-income women. Free access to the World Wide Web is provided at a beauty shop and hair salon in South Bend, Indiana. Trainers are available at the salon about 30 hours a week to help teach newcomers how to hop aboard the information superhighway.

"One-Stop Shopping"

The upscale retail department store chain Nordstrom's is at the forefront of a trend in on-site healthcare services. Nordstrom's in the Chicago area offers a Mammography Screening Center, sponsored by Evanston Northwestern Healthcare. This is not a new concept per se, preceded by a perhaps familiar image of a community health nurse at the grocery store or other well-traveled site, administering blood pressure and cholesterol screenings. Increasingly, mammography and other diagnostic tests are becoming "portable." Among the benefits for the consumer are ease of access and, in the case of Nordstrom's and other retailers, an aesthetically pleasing environment.

INFORMATION IN ALL THE RIGHT PLACES

The following examples focus on new ways to offer easy access to crucial health information for adults and children, facilitated by new ways of harnessing old technology and thinking "outside the box."

The Nurse Call Center: Providing Easy Access to Health Information

A 1994 series of focus groups commissioned by the American Hospital Association included questions asking whom individuals trusted for health and medical information. The consumers were asked what they wanted if they could build a new healthcare system from scratch. The studies found that in group after group, people wanted someone they could call for advice. They rated nurses among those providers they would trust most. The nursing call center, today a service offered by many larger hospitals and health systems, was born. In most such centers, consumers have free, 24-hour access to a registered nurse who is able to discuss symptoms and guide patients to the most appropriate type of care. Says Donna Marshall, R.N., manager of MHS's call center, "Consumers are happy they can get quick answers without feeling guilty about bothering the doctor with what might be a stupid question. The physicians are thrilled to learn how few calls they need to receive at home once a nurse triage system is in place. This is truly a win-win situation" (Chrisman, 1999). In addition to the basic physician and program referral services, the nurses provide "After-Hours

Physician Office Triage Services" for the patients of 22 different primary care physician offices.

Stop in and Learn

An extension of the nurse call center that is developing around the country is a health resource center concept that includes easy access to nurses who offer one-on-one teaching and counseling. In North Carolina, the Wake Med Heart Center established a Guest Resource Center to make the most of what they call "teachable moments." This facility offers a comfortable club-like atmosphere and a library of books, teaching models, videos, and Internet computer stations. Visitors to the center can check out materials or relax in a recliner and learn more about their health.

Similarly, MHS is currently designing a Health Discoveries Center where patients and family members may visit to research a new diagnosis on their own or with the assistance of a registered nurse. This type of center also offers benefits for nearby physicians who can refer patients to the facility. Dissatisfaction with waiting times can be reduced when physicians support such a facility. At Memorial, physician offices will be encouraged to send patients to the Health Discoveries Center with a beeper. The patient can relax or do some research until they get a beep that says the doctor is ready to see them. Physicians can also feel better about time allotted to the patient education process for a new diagnosis by referring their patients to the center after an appointment. In addition to a book and video library on medical conditions and treatments, Internet terminals will be available for aided or unaided research. Nurses will also be available without an appointment for one-on-one education sessions using the nurse call center database as back-up.

Jump Starting a Healthful Life

Another exciting consumer connection at MHS in South Bend is the HealthWorks! Kids' Museum. The $3 million venture is founded on the fact that the choices children make early in their lives impact the length and quality of their lives. The facility is designed to help reach children with this message as early as possible and to do so in a fun and exciting environment. Although the concept of health education centers is not new, most of the centers around the country have basically been a classroom format with some audience participation and some hands-on projects. HealthWorks! Kids' Museum will make the most of interactive education and entertainment to help children make healthy choices throughout their lives. Children will explore how their bodies work and how to stay well when they visit larger-than-life suites on the brain and digestive system. They will have their choice of more than 30 other interactive exhibits that allow them to make choices, including a virtual reality bicycle ride. The 12,000 square foot facility is consistent with Memorial's mission of creating a healthy community and improving quality of life for families. After many focus groups with parents, teachers, school administrators, and children, the question went from, "What should be built?" to "How fast can it be ready?"

Although the facility is being launched for children in the South Bend region, the concept is being developed for expansion in communities around the country. The MHS team working on the museum is creating a "replication guide," which will include all of the key details and decisions that lead to the final facility. Other health systems interested in a similar facility can contact Memorial to share lessons learned in facility development and hopefully speed the process. Memorial's Web site, www.qualityoflife.org, can be visited to view the learning history. The vision of having a national network of similarly focused facilities relates to the potential for future innovation in health education. The shared learning and shared resources will allow each facility to maintain continuous improvement and enhancements.

CONCLUSION

The examples in this chapter support the belief that those health systems that are willing to embrace new ways to connect with their customers will increase their success by satisfying their existing patients through meeting them on their terms and listening to their wants and needs; by promoting health and wellness services throughout the community, fostering goodwill and alliance-building; and in striving to always put the customer first, by maximizing opportunities for attracting potential customers in an ever-competitive market.

The evolution of better-informed, more involved healthcare consumers is indeed a revolution that portends exciting developments in our healthcare delivery system of the twenty-first century. Healthcare systems willing to listen to their consumers will enhance their competitive advantage, but most importantly, healthier communities will be the outcome.

REFERENCES

American Hospital Association. *Capital communication strategies focus groups on attitudes toward hospitals.* 1994.

Covey S. *Seven habits of highly effective people: powerful lessons in personal change.* Fireside, 1990.

Crisman N. *Cultural competencies for effective health care.* Speech delivered at University of Washington, March 4, 1999.

McKnight JL, Kretzman JP. *Building communities from the inside out.* Northwestern University, 1993.

CHAPTER

The Healthwise Communities Project: Where Healthcare Is Practiced by All

Molly Mettler, M.S.W.

INTRODUCTION

This isn't your mother's healthcare system anymore. Expectations are higher, demands are greater, and roles are being recast. The patient, traditionally the recipient of healthcare, is being recognized as a primary provider and decision maker of healthcare. The physician, traditionally the provider of treatment and cure, is being asked to become more of a partner and to share in treatment decisions with the patient. And, almost miraculously, a tidal wave of health information is available to both patient and provider to help them in that partnership. The healthcare system is being rebuilt.

Three separate, but interrelated, profound changes are currently shaping the future roles of patients, physicians, and the delivery of care. The first change is the emergence of the "new consumer," whose role has shifted from patient to partner. The second fundamental change is how evidence-based guidelines are transforming the "art and science" of medicine. The third change is the influx of information related to healthcare that is now available to consumers on a scale unimaginable just a few years ago.

Healthcare organizations can harness and manage these fundamental changes in a positive and productive way by *making the patient the focal point of healthcare.* What are the practicalities needed for bringing the consumer fully into the center of healthcare? The model, the tools, and the research findings that are shared in this chapter are based on work done by the Robert Wood Johnson–funded *Healthwise Communities Project,* an unusual communitywide patient empowerment initiative. This population-based health improvement program was designed to help nearly 300,000 residents in four Idaho counties become the "most empowered, best informed medical consumers in the world" (Kemper, 1995).

Through Healthwise Communities, five new healthcare services were introduced to improve healthcare outcomes, lower healthcare costs, and improve satisfaction for everyone in the community. The project won support from consumers, providers, and payors alike. Winning the 1996 "Spirit of Innovation Award" from InterHealth and 3M Health Care, it has been hailed as a harbinger of the healthcare system of the future.

THE RISE OF THE NEW MEDICAL CONSUMER

Study after study signals the emergence of the "new medical consumer" and details how this cadre of informed, empowered, and technologically adept purchasers are shaping the healthcare system of the twenty-first century. Already, the purchasing patterns and habits of American consumers have transformed many U.S. retail and service industries. The informed and savvy consumer has many banking, investment, and retail services available from which to pick and choose. Healthcare has lagged behind these other industries, but it is expected that the new medical consumer's expectations and preferences will have a demonstrable impact on the service and delivery of medicine and healthcare. According to a 1998 report from the Institute for the Future, the new consumer differs in three primary ways from previous medical consumers (Kyrouz et al., 1998):

1. *Analytical sophistication:* The new consumers have had more college education. Consumers who have had even 1 year of college coursework make their choices more analytically than those who have had no college training. This applies to the choice of treatment and health plan.
2. *Disposable income:* The new consumers have enough disposable income that they are not limited by the least expensive healthcare options. This financial flexibility provides an opportunity for new consumers to apply their analytical skills in healthcare decisions.
3. *Experience with information technologies:* Analytical methods and money are of little value in making healthcare decisions without good information about the choices. The new consumers are more experienced with the use of information technologies such as the Internet because they use the technologies at work and home.

The authors of the study propose that consumers, as the drivers of the new consumer-focused healthcare, will indirectly influence a shift toward a more responsive, more consumer-focused healthcare system with choice (including choices of plans, providers, and treatment), control, customer service, branding, and information.

Another study, sponsored by The Health Forum and Arthur Andersen Health Care Practice, reported on research gathered from 12 focus groups of consumers who discussed their expectations vis-à-vis healthcare (Johnson et al., 1998). Some of the insights gleaned dovetail neatly with the previously mentioned study. The report found the following:

- The customer is taking charge. Empowerment is evident in all levels of consumer participation.
- Consumers are redefining choice. They are willing to change doctors, institutions, and health plans. They are also seeking choice in treatment and care options.
- Information is the central tool of empowerment. Consumers, particularly Baby Boomer women, are

gathering a substantial amount of information from both traditional and nontraditional sources.

Pushed by the first wave of Baby Boomers, the ranks of the new consumer have grown from 25% circa 1978 to 45% in 1998. This group will reach 52% by 2005, and they will have a significant and indelible impact on the way healthcare is delivered (Kyrouz, 1998).

It is important to remember, however, that consumers have always played a role in the delivery of healthcare. Rather than a startlingly new and unprecedented trend, what we see is the revival of age-old prerogatives.

CONSUMER PARTICIPATION IN HEALTHCARE DECISION MAKING: A BRIEF HISTORY

Laypeople have always played a role in healthcare decision making. Indeed, since the beginning of civilization, the majority of healthcare has been provided by the individual and the family. Ancient Greek and Babylonian texts record the importance of daily living patterns in maintaining health (Sigerist, 1951). Books on self-care are not a twentieth century phenomenon. In 1751, the Reverend John Wesley, founder of the Methodist Church, published a popular self-care book, *Primitive Physick*. The modern interest in self-care had a resurgence in the 1970s with such books as *Our Bodies, Ourselves,* published by the Boston Women's Health Book Collective in 1970, and *How to be Your Own Doctor Sometimes* (Sehnert, 1975).

Most of the healthcare in the United States continues to consist of what people do for themselves. Studies from North America, Europe, and Scandinavia confirm that 80% to 90% of symptoms are first treated at home, either by "watching and waiting," by using over-the-counter medicine or a cultural remedy that has been passed down, or by using information gathered from friends and loved ones, media, or books (Dean, 1983).

When we consider that 8 of 10 health problems are handled at home by laypersons without any intervention from a medical professional, we must recognize patients as the primary providers of their own care. Publishers have certainly recognized this; consumer healthcare books have become big business. Texts detailing common illnesses and injuries and what to do about them are available through bookstores, managed care organizations, Medicare and Medicaid, and employers' benefits departments. Employers and insurers are distributing self-care manuals in part to assist their employees and subscribers in providing good, sensible family care, and also to ensure the appropriate utilization of medical services.

THE RISE OF THE NEW SCIENCE OF EVIDENCE-BASED MEDICINE

Historically, within broad limits, each physician has been allowed to practice medicine as his or her training and experience suggested (prompting several to characterize medicine as more "art" than "science"). One result of highly individual patterns of practice is that a population of patients can receive widely differing treatment and achieve widely varying outcomes. The Dartmouth Atlas illustrates how the rates of certain surgeries can be twice as high in one community as in the next. For example, a male resident of Fort Worth, Texas, is 2.2 times as likely to get a radical prostatectomy than a man living in Houston. Conversely, there is a 40% lower rate of surgery for lower extremity bypass in Fort Worth than in Houston (Wennberg & Cooper, 1998).

Healthcare quality cannot be guaranteed or achieved in a system where medical treatment can be predicated more by geography than by the specific needs or preferences of the patient. Hopefully, the dissemination and practice of evidence-based medicine will help stabilize clinical variation. Painstaking research in the outcomes of medical treatments and interventions are leading to the construction of practice guidelines and clinical pathways that result in the best health outcomes for the most patients.

Slowly but surely, evidence-based medicine is making headway. Following the dictates of outcomes research, health plans, hospitals, and physician groups are spending millions of dollars to shift their doctors toward practice guidelines. However, it is possible that some physicians will be slow to adopt new guidelines, especially if they are seen as conflicting with the art of medicine. If some physicians cannot use their education, experience, and judgment to decide how they practice, they will reject efforts to force them into guidelines—no matter how good the science may be. The challenge is to shift the art of medicine to something that is more compatible with the *new* science—one that uses physician education, experience, and judgment to apply evidence-based guidelines to the special needs, values, and preferences of each patient. Through outcomes research and evidence-based medicine, the opportunity exists to reduce unnecessary practice variability and help physicians practice the best medicine. Furthermore, through patient empowerment and shared decision making, the opportunity exists to help consumers get the medical treatment that best suits their values and preferences. For art to meet science, three things need to be in place: (1) evidence-based practice guidelines, (2) physician expertise, and (3) an informed patient. These three things can be vastly aided by information technology that brings the best medicine to physician and patient alike.

MAKING THE MOST OF INFORMATION TECHNOLOGY

It is common to note that the Internet has transformed the world of health information: currently 36% of all adults who "surf" the Internet do so for health information (Miller & Reents, 1998). What the Internet does not lack is abundant information. What the Internet does lack is quality control over the existing information.

For laypeople, the challenge lies in obtaining and interpreting credible, unbiased, consumer-focused, evidence-based health information so that they, with their physicians, can participate in making medical decisions. Health plans and other providers have discovered that their Web sites serve more than a marketing role. Internet users, who are increasingly frustrated in their efforts to sort through dense and often conflicting information on the Web, now flock to personal and proprietary sites in an effort to find quality information. Consumers are clamoring for a "place at the table," and information technology is yet another factor helping consumers move from "patient" to "partner."

As healthcare professionals, we should be asking ourselves a number of questions: Why not broaden the role of "consumer–provider" to all aspects of medical care? What might be the impact in terms of quality, costs, and satisfaction if all consumers, regardless of insurance coverage, had access to the best consumer health information to help them in all aspects of their medical decision making (ranging from self-care for common problems to complete shared decision making for major and chronic health problems)? And, what can be called the "best"? These questions led to the formation and development of the Healthwise Communities Project.

HEALTHWISE COMMUNITIES: FROM PATIENT TO PARTNER

By making the patient a partner, we meet the new consumer's need for more information, choice, and control. By promoting the value of the physician's expertise in applying guidelines to each individual patient, we protect the physician's art while strengthening the doctor–patient bond. And by providing the new consumer with information about the new science and by involving consumers, deeply and thoroughly, in their own medical decision making, we can realize better outcomes, lower costs, and increased satisfaction.

This new vision reframes the traditional divide between "patient" and "provider." Rather than being pegged as a passive recipient of medical services, the new healthcare consumer is recognized as a capable and essential member of the healthcare team. When consumers are embraced as the primary providers of care for themselves and their families, they become partners in their care. In partnership with physicians, the new medical consumer provides appropriate home care, shares in medical decisions, and assumes partial responsibility for the outcomes. By working *together*, consumers and providers can have a significant impact on the cost and quality outcomes of healthcare.

Healthwise, Incorporated, a not-for-profit health education organization founded in 1975, began sowing the seeds for the

Healthwise Communities Project in the late 1980s by networking with local leaders and asking for their input for a communitywide health initiative. In 1995, Healthwise received a
$2.1 million grant from The Robert Wood Johnson Foundation,
on the condition that additional local funding could be obtained.
The financial and corporate commitment of Blue Cross of Idaho,
Regence Blue Shield of Idaho, and 17 other local sponsors made
it possible to offer the project's services to everyone living in
Ada, Boise, Elmore, and Valley Counties of southwestern Idaho
regardless of insurance coverage.

This coalition of local sponsors, which included the major
hospitals and employers in the region, shared a belief that informed and empowered consumers could make a change for the
better in healthcare. They hoped that the project would help
their employees, subscribers, patients, and all community residents do the following:

- Perform appropriate and high-quality self-care in the
  home.
- Use emergency and other medical services
  appropriately.
- Be informed about the outcomes of treatment options.
- Share in medical decision making with physicians.
- Ask for the care they really need; nothing more, nothing
  less.

The action plan for the project was simple and direct. The
first 6 months after receiving the initial grant from The Robert
Wood Johnson Foundation in September 1995 were spent
raising additional funds from local sponsors, assembling advisory boards of payors and providers, and doing outreach with
healthcare providers. The project went public in April of 1996
with the implementation of a populationwide medical self-care
venture (books sent to every home, a mass media campaign, and
workshops for consumers). Six months later, the second phase
was instituted. The focus was on building patient–provider partnerships and shared medical decision-making skills through the
provision of tools (a nurse call center, "information stations," and
a Web site), information (a comprehensive consumer health

information database and support [Information Therapy]), and provider workshops.

A BOOK IN EVERY HOME

The self-care phase began in April 1996, with the delivery of more than 125,000 *Healthwise Handbooks* to every residential mailbox in the four-county area. This basic medical self-care guide, first produced by Healthwise in 1976 and now in its fourteenth edition, helps consumers manage more than 180 common health problems. For each problem, simple guidelines help readers recognize symptoms of an illness and determine what they can do to treat it at home and when they should call or see a health professional (Kemper, 1997).

The books for the project were made available in both English and Spanish *(La Salud en Casa: Guia Practica de Healthwise)*. In addition, a special older adult version of the book, *Healthwise for Life* (Mettler & Kemper, 1998), was distributed at many senior centers and senior-citizen clubs. Provisions were made for individuals who did not get a book in the mail to either get a book from a public health clinic or, for a small fee, at a local pharmacy.

Studies done on the *Healthwise Handbook* and other self-care texts show that use of self-care guidelines does reduce doctor visits and emergency room (ER) visits (Kemper et al., 1992). However, the messages that accompanied the book, through the media campaign and in the consumer workshops, stressed that the information and project were *not* to keep people from going to see the doctor, but rather to bolster confidence and competence in trying self-care, as well as to get people to medical care sooner.

Use of the book was reinforced through self-care workshops, mass media, and provider outreach. Public health educators have conducted scores of workshops for consumers in clinics, work sites, churches, and community centers. In the 3 years since book distribution, more than 13,000 consumers have attended Healthwise self-care workshops and briefings. In addition, paid advertising; newspaper editorials; TV commentaries; a weekly newspaper column, "Being Healthwise"; and many public service announcements have all contributed to the high level of community awareness about the project and the use of the book. Within days of the book's release, personal stories came flooding into the project office. For instance, one man used the book to determine that his son's gas pains were not appendicitis, as he had first feared. He saved himself and his son a trip to the emergency room. A woman following the same guidelines determined that the abdominal pains her sister attributed to food poisoning might actually be appendicitis. She felt the symptoms did warrant an ER visit, which resulted in the successful and timely removal of an inflamed appendix.

THE HEALTHWISE KNOWLEDGEBASE: PUTTING CONSUMER HEALTH INFORMATION AT THE COMMUNITY'S FINGERTIPS

For major health problems such as chronic illness or recommendations for surgery, consumers need more information than any one book can provide. For example, Susan, a young Boise mother, needed to decide whether to try ear tubes as a treatment option for her son's chronic and persistent ear infections. Where could she go to find the information she needed to make an informed decision? Healthwise Communities sought to introduce and support shared medical decision making by closing the information gap that exists between patients and providers.

The consumer health information system that supported Idahoans in their fact gathering and decision making was the *Healthwise Knowledgebase,* an electronic consumer health database. By using the Knowledgebase, Susan could learn what the indications, risks, and outcomes are for ear tube insertion, and what her and her son's other options might include. With data on more than 450 health topics, 520 types of surgeries and treatments, and 500 support and self-help groups, this electronic database provides the information that the patient needs to participate on the provider team.

Beginning 6 months after the *Healthwise Handbooks* were distributed, everyone in the four-county area had free access to the Knowledgebase through three different means:

1. Via the *Healthwise Line,* a nurse advice line open toll free Monday through Friday from 7 AM to 7 PM. Staffed by specially trained nurses, the *Healthwise Line* was geared to offer, in addition to triage for health symptoms, coaching and counseling to help consumers sort through major healthcare decisions. More than 26,000 calls were taken during the course of the project, averaging about 70 calls daily. Two other hospital-based call centers operated in the community at the same time, sometimes leading to lighter-than-expected call volume and some consumer confusion. To ensure that all residents of the four-county area had access to the same information, Healthwise provided the two local hospital-based call centers with the Healthwise Knowledgebase for use by their nurses.

2. At *Healthwise Information Stations,* self-care resource centers located in libraries, clinics, hospitals, and work sites. Most of the information stations were outfitted with a computer, loaded with the Knowledgebase, and a printer so that the user could copy text from the database. All stations had a set of self-care and medical reference books for on-site research. There were 52 stations in the four-county area; these were located in each public library, in some of the project's sponsors' work sites, and in a series of primary care clinics. (Some of the remote mountain communities within the four counties had Healthwise Information Stations placed in a year-round resident's home and the accompanying reference books were made available to all neighbors.) The stations were used by more than 16,000 people.

3. Via the Internet at http://www.hcp.org. The project set up its own Web page so that anyone in the four-county area with Internet access and a project-provided PIN (personal identification number) could have free and easy access to the complete Healthwise Knowledgebase as well as other project information. Access was limited

to local residents so that some control could be exerted for evaluation purposes. Web use varied widely depending on advertising: between 5,000 and 12,000 users per month accessed the HCP Web site. The Knowledgebase is now available through several online channels worldwide.

PROJECT EVALUATION

The Oregon Health Sciences University (OHSU), funded by a separate grant from The Robert Wood Johnson Foundation, was charged with the evaluation of the entire project. OHSU used a series of randomized population surveys; in-depth analyses of insurer, employer, and HCFA claims data; direct analysis of hospital data for selected procedures; and trend analysis. Costs were monitored by both self-report and utilization/billing records from payors and providers. Satisfaction levels were determined by self-report through written or phone-based surveys with both patients and providers. The same methodologies were used both in the project area and in the two control group communities of Eugene, Oregon, and Billings, Montana.

Six Months into the Project

Did people use the book? Yes. Six months after the book distribution, OHSU conducted a randomized population survey ($N = 598$), and an Idaho-based independent researcher surveyed a random selection of employees from 13 of the project's sponsoring employers ($N = 608$) (Colby, 1996; OHSU, 1996).

- In the community research done by OHSU, 86% of households in the target area reported receiving the book. Of the employee population, 88% acknowledged that they received the book.
- Of those receiving the book, 69.8% of the general population reported that they or members of their households had used the book at least once. Of that group, 81.3% had used the book two or more times. Of

the employee population, 69% responded that they had used the book at least once.

- In a survey conducted by the State of Idaho, 64% of Medicaid recipients in the project area stated they had used the book at least once (State of Idaho, 1998).
- Within the first 6 months after receiving the handbook, 35% of the employee population stated that they had saved at least one doctor visit; 9% reported that they had saved at least one ER visit.

Twelve Months into the Project

A study conducted by Blue Cross of Idaho shows that per-member emergency room visits were reduced by 18% for Blue Cross of Idaho customers who lived within the Healthwise Communities test counties (Sternberg, 1998). This number is noteworthy in that it suggests that helping consumers access credible medical information had a positive impact on the healthcare utilization patterns of Idaho residents participating in the initiative. The study compared claims data from Ada, Elmore, Boise, and Valley Counties (communities participating in the initiative) to claims data from Canyon and Twin Falls Counties (communities not participating). It also examined utilization patterns before the start of the initiative and compared those patterns with utilization after the initiative started. The data show that ER visits were reduced in participating counties, whereas the number of per-member ER visits stayed virtually the same in the communities not covered by the services of the initiative.

Twenty-Two Months into the Project

Interim findings from OHSU 22 months into the project have shown some interesting results (OHSU, 1998). However, here's a caveat about the study results to date: these findings are preliminary and, except for the Blue Cross ER data, are all based on self-reported surveys. Although the response rate was good (46% to 60% in the three communities), and the questions were scientifically developed for objectivity, the final evaluation of the project will include an in-depth analysis of objective utilization and cost data. OHSU's final report is anticipated to be completed in the year 2000. The interim findings indicate the following:

- Of residents in the target area, 71% reported using a health or medical reference book (a 22% increase from baseline).
- Of those, 62% said the book saved a visit to the doctor within the previous 6 months.
- One-third said it saved an ER visit in the previous 6 months.

The use of nurse advice lines increased from 25% at baseline in Idaho to 29% after 22 months. About half of all nurse advice line callers reported that usage saved them a visit to the doctor. There was no significant difference among the communities in this regard. However, Montana nurse line users (one of two control groups) were more likely to report that using the nurse advice line saved them a visit to the ER.

The interim data showed that use of the computer for health-related or medical information also increased between baseline and 22 months. In Idaho, the usage increased from 8% to 20%. In Montana and Oregon, which showed a similar usage at baseline (8%), the increases were 13% and 17%, respectively. The differences were not significant.

PHYSICIAN INVOLVEMENT AND RESPONSE

A 15-member Provider Steering Committee composed of doctors, nurse practitioners, mental health professionals, hospital administrators, and other providers helped to guide the development and promotion of the project. Provider endorsement and buy-in was painstakingly acquired by working with this committee to keep every provider "in the loop":

- More than 25 project briefings were held at hospital staff meetings in the early days of the project, with attendance totaling 1,000 physicians and other hospital staff members.

- Six hundred and nineteen healthcare professionals (physicians comprising 13% of that total) completed the Healthwise Partnership Program, a CME/CNE clinic-based seminar for physicians, nurses, and office staff. The purpose of the program was to orient providers to the key role they play in reinforcing responsible self-care behaviors in their patients.

- More than 80 doctors participated in a Grand Rounds, and a special roundtable discussion, on shared medical decision making. Albert G. Mulley Jr., M.D., of Harvard Medical School and Massachusetts General Hospital (who is well known for his work in this area), presented both sessions.

Physician Response

Physicians across the nation are recognizing that their patients want more information than ever before. Unfortunately, physicians rarely have either the time or the in-office resources needed to respond to these requests. They also are reluctant to send patients to the Internet because of its lack of quality control. A solution is to write an "information prescription" to a source that is known to be evidence-based and medically credible.

The Healthwise Communities Project responded to the need for "prescription information." Information Therapy prescription pads allow physicians to quickly refer patients to the precise information that would most help the patients understand their treatment options. Patients can then either contact a nurse on the Healthwise Line or log onto the project's home page (http://www.hcp.org) and "point and click" directly to the section of information that the physician has prescribed.

Much work remains to be done to win physician support for Information Therapy and shared decision making. For many providers in Idaho and elsewhere, the doctor–patient relationship is considered sacred ground. Any attempt, however well intended, to insert any service or change in that relationship is viewed with suspicion. To win physician support, we followed three general guidelines: (1) demonstrate medical credibility, (2) use doctors to reach doctors, and (3) focus on benefits to providers.

Demonstrating Medical Credibility

Six months before the *Healthwise Handbook* was mailed to every household, every physician, nurse practitioner, and physician's assistant in the area (600+) received a copy of the book along with this message: "Every one of your patients is going to get this book. Please review it and suggest any changes that you think are needed." Having the opportunity to review materials before they went public helped area physicians trust the book.

To trust the accuracy and the objectivity of the 70 megabytes of information in the *Healthwise Knowledgebase,* physicians have had to be informed on the process of how the information is developed. Each *Knowledgebase* topic is the result of months of efforts by medical researchers, writers, editors, and expert physician reviewers to identify the evidence-based medical information on the subject and to organize it around decision points for the patient.

Hands-on use of the *Knowledgebase* by physicians helped as well. Primary care physicians had the option of trying the software on a 6-month trial basis. The clinics then had the option of keeping the software and adding it to their clinic's computer network free-of-charge during the grant period. Many of these clinics' physicians routinely gave prescription cards to their patients to check out certain information in the *Knowledgebase.* During the course of the project, more and more physicians trusted and used the information.

Focus on Physician Benefits

Although physicians in Idaho are interested in benefits of shared medical decision making for their patients, their practices are often too busy and demanding to add anything that they believe will take more time or effort to deliver, such as Information

Therapy. However, research consistently shows that patients who consider themselves informed about their options—working with doctors who listen to them—enjoy both better outcomes and greater satisfaction.

Steven Schneider, M.D., a family practice physician in Boise, Idaho, and Chairman of the Provider Steering Committee, spoke from experience. After installing a Healthwise Information Station in his clinic's waiting room and monitoring its use by his patients, he met directly with the area's primary care physicians to speak personally about how use of *Knowledgebase* had affected his practice and patients. His message was simple and direct: "This service will save you time and your patients will like it." This basic message, which speaks right to the daily concerns of practicing physicians, seems to have worked best for gaining physician support.

We continue to focus much attention on the provider community in the belief that in order to have a well-educated and empowered consumer population, one must have a supportive, empowering, and patient-centered medical community.

WHAT'S THE PAY-OFF?

One of the stated goals of the project was to reduce overall healthcare costs. Before the project began, savings from the handbook distribution alone were estimated to be at least $2 million per year, or $20 per family per year, saved by avoiding any unnecessary trip to a doctor's office or ER. This projection conforms to the consistent 3:1 minimum return on investment that has been regularly seen in medical self-care programs (Kemper et al., 1992). Twenty-two months after book distribution, 62% of the respondents who reported using a book reportedly saved a visit to a doctor's office, and 33% prevented an unnecessary visit to a hospital ER. Based on the test area's population, this translates into 46,000 saved doctor visits per year and 25,000 saved ER visits per year. Those avoided visits theoretically have produced total cost savings of more than $7.5 million per year or a 5.5:1 return on investment. (This is just on the book distribution alone.) Savings accrued from proper utilization as the result of residents accessing *Healthwise*

Knowledgebase by telephone or computer have not been assessed. Again, press time for this chapter precedes the project's final report. However, it is evident that people are using medical information resources, doing more self-care, avoiding unneeded medical visits, and seeing their doctor when needed.

Meanwhile, other communities have shown interest in replicating Healthwise Communities. The first iteration, Southern-style, is planned by Partners for a Healthy Community, a collaborative network of private and public funding based in Anderson, South Carolina. Targeting 150,000 families living in four counties in South Carolina and Georgia, Partners is seeking to realize the same vision as the Idaho project: to create communities in which residents will be empowered, well-informed medical consumers who do a better job of preventing or taking care of their health problems. The bold experiment continues.

LESSONS LEARNED

- *Launch all services at one time.* At the request of the evaluation team, we delayed the implementation of the call center until 6 months after the distribution of the books. The purpose was to better measure the separate impacts of the book and the call center. However, the delay diminished the power of the call center service.

  The distribution of the *Healthwise Handbook* to every household in the community created a huge wave of awareness and recognition. It is best to launch all aspects of the program simultaneously. However, because of the evaluation-requested delay, we were not able to promote the call center opening at the same time. We were never able to gain the same level of public attention in announcing the call center or Web service later. For replication projects, we strongly recommend the launch of the book, call center service, and Web site at one time. The book should be used as a doorway to both.

- *Do not duplicate services. Form alliances when possible.* The complete set of services outlined in the Healthwise

Communities proposal is good. It provides some level of health-related information as a resource to virtually every person in the community regardless of his or her income level, reading ability, or learning style. It is not necessary, however, that all the services be provided within the Healthwise Communities office. If community services that can be used to provide educational outreach or call center services already exist, it is better to engage actively with those services, contribute to their training if necessary, and include them in the project rather than duplicating any of their services.

- *Focus your advertising and promotion.* It is critical to spend some time and a portion of your advertising budget on defining the focus message and look of your project before implementation. Perhaps the best strategy is to tie this to the cover image and colors on your book. We learned that we needed to settle on a focus message to effectively reach the community. Adequate funds and preparation time budgeted for consulting, development, and dissemination of advertising are essential.

- *Line up continuation funding from the beginning.* Once project staff are deeply involved in the day-to-day management of the project, dedicating time to seek continuation funding becomes difficult. If the project is to become anything more than just a "3-year experiment," it is absolutely necessary that planning and campaigning for continuation funding be started from the moment the project is initially funded.

- *Don't do it all yourself.* Healthwise asked too much of ourselves and too little of our partnering sponsors. Although that approach may seem easier at first, it fails to develop the high level of involvement and buy-in needed to develop passionate champions of the program. Healthwise sponsors are appreciative, supportive, and enthusiastic about the project, but none have taken the next step to provide active leadership and championing in the community. We recommend that the planning and project leadership be significantly shared with the program sponsors. The sponsor role should go beyond passive review to active project direction.

THE BEST MEDICINE

This project demonstrated that a populationwide, educational approach can change the self-care practices and reduce the healthcare costs of an entire community. For the past several years, the U.S. government and insurance companies have tried a variety of strategies to contain healthcare costs. Hospital stays and charges have been capped for many government-paid healthcare procedures. Incentives have shifted reimbursement from specialists to generalists. Physicians have been placed in a "gatekeeper" role, which implies limiting access. Despite all of these interventions, the cost of healthcare has continued to rise. At the same time, a large percentage of the U.S. population is without healthcare coverage at all. Many of these uninsured people use the ER as their primary care clinic. In the absence of early preventive care, many of these people resort to the ER when their symptoms are advanced and more difficult to treat.

In this community, we did not restrict care. We did not limit the amount physicians or hospitals would be paid for their services. We did not limit any person's access in any way. We did not differentiate between people based on their ability to pay or their insurance coverage. We *did* give every single person in this community access to high-quality health-related information. That is all we did. As a result, significantly more people used that information to make better decisions about when they needed care and what type of care they needed. As a result of using this information, consumers made dramatic cuts in their use of ERs and doctor office visits. The implication is that if every home in the United States could be supplied with straightforward self-care and shared-care information, health-care costs would decrease. And this would be accomplished without penalizing any group or individual.

The *best* medicine is providing the medicine that is needed—nothing more, and certainly nothing less. In addition, the best resource for determining whether care is needed is the informed consumer working in partnership with a caring and competent physician. The *Healthwise Communities Project* helped reform a local healthcare system through community cooperation and participation by healthcare consumers. It features the following distinctive qualities:

- Instead of restricting supply, it manages demand.
- Instead of promoting competition, it relies on cooperation.
- Instead of building a better system, it builds a better patient.

The degree of the program's success in Idaho could determine whether it could serve as a national model for rebuilding the healthcare system for a more informed patient. By educating and empowering people, we can create communities where healthcare is practiced by all.

REFERENCES

Boston Women's Health Book Collective. *Our Bodies, Ourselves.* New York: Simon and Schuster, 1971.

Colby C. *Six-month follow-up survey with employer groups.* Boise, ID: Healthwise, Incorporated, Internal memo, 1996.

Dean K, et al. Self-care of common illnesses in Denmark. *Medical Care* 1983; 21:1012–1032.

Johnson K, et al. *Leadership for a healthy 21st century: creating value through relationships.* Chicago: American Hospital Association, 1998.

Kemper DW. *Healthwise communities project: where health care is practiced by all.* Princeton, NJ: A grant application submitted to The Robert Wood Johnson Foundation, 1995.

Kemper DW, Healthwise Staff. *Healthwise handbook: a self-care guide for you,* 14th ed. Boise, ID: Healthwise, Incorporated, 1999.

Kemper DW, et al. The effectiveness of medical self-care interventions: a focus on self-initiated responses to symptoms. *Patient Educ Counsel* 1992; 21:29–39.

Kyrouz EM, et al. *The twenty-first century health care consumer.* Menlo Park, CA: The Institute for the Future, 1998.

Mettler M, Kemper DW. *Healthwise for life: medical self-care for people age 50 and better,* 3rd ed. Boise, ID: Healthwise, Incorporated, 1998.

Miller TE, Reents S. *The health care industry in transition: the online mandate to change.* New York: Cyber Dialogue, 1998.

Oregon Health Sciences University. *Idaho community health survey follow-up.* Portland, OR: Oregon Health Sciences University, Internal memo, 1996.

Oregon Health Sciences University. *Idaho community health survey follow-up.* Portland, OR: Oregon Health Sciences University, Internal memo, 1998.

Sehnert KW. *How to be your own doctor sometimes.* New York: Grosset & Dunlap, 1975.

Sigerist HE. *History of medicine,* Vol. 1. Oxford, UK: Oxford University Press, 1951.

State of Idaho. *Healthwise communities project (Medicaid BRFS in Health District IV).* Boise, ID: State of Idaho, Internal memo, 1998.

Sternberg L. *Healthwise handbook impact study.* Boise, ID: Blue Cross of Idaho, Internal memo, 1998.

Wennberg JE, Cooper MM (eds). Quality of care: the use of ambulatory care. *The Dartmouth atlas of health care in the United States* Hanover: Center for Evaluative Clinical Studies/Dartmouth Medical School, 1998; 137.

Wesley J. *Primitive physick: or an easy and natural method of curing most diseases.* London, J. Palmar: 1751.

Williamson JD, Danaher K. *Self-care in health.* London: Croom Helm, 1978.

17 CHAPTER

Nursing: Linking Today's Consumer to a Changing System

Linda Stutz, RN, MBA

As healthcare providers, we are routinely reminded of the implications of escalating healthcare costs, increasing numbers of uninsured Americans, and the declining health status of the general population. Our industry is constantly seeking new ways to deliver quality healthcare services, to provide for appropriate use of services, and to control costs. To accomplish this task, we have implemented managed care, redesigned patient care, and downsized the work environment. Never before have times seemed more difficult for the healthcare industry. Yet, for consumers of healthcare, never before has the opportunity for "self-empowerment"—self-education and opportunities to be educated about options in healthcare—been so great. For the nursing professional, this transitional period—from a service-centered industry to a consumer-centered one—will significantly affect his or her future career choices, required skill sets, and places of employment. In fact, given the expected closure of hospitals, continued downsizings, and an increasing movement toward ambulatory care, a modest projection would be that

350,000 nurses presently employed by hospitals will be looking for work in nonhospital settings by the year 2000 (Lamm, 1996).

The good news for healthcare providers, nurses, consumers, and arguably, society as a whole is that despite managed care's earlier bad publicity, an evolutionary process that will transition managed care into the next generation of managed *healthcare* is occurring. Certainly, the complexities of population-based healthcare, the strong emphasis on primary and preventive care, and the current pressures on managed care systems are all focused on putting an end to a previously compartmentalized and silo-oriented system. Healthcare professionals, as well as consumers of healthcare, are forced to rethink their roles, functions, responsibilities, and culture in relation to a different set of expectations. Moving away from the safety of the hospital structure creates the opportunity for changing the content and processes of clinical work and for the negotiation of the new shared landscape.

Specifically, this chapter aims to do the following:

- Provide a brief history of the role of nursing, with its roots in and legacy of "patient-centered" care.
- Educate healthcare professionals about ways that nursing is rapidly evolving into a profession that is at once interdisciplinary, entrepreneurial, and dynamic, as it responds to the needs of society, specifically, consumers who are ever-sophisticated about their healthcare needs.
- Provide an overview of ways that nursing is serving as a critical link in the healthcare "landscape" of the new century.
- Serve as a "primer" for the nursing professional in listing those emerging roles forecast for tomorrow and beyond.

HISTORICAL BACKGROUND

It can be argued that nursing was founded on the tenets of prevention, health, and wellness, with Florence Nightingale's pioneering efforts in the war fields paving the way. Just as the

Hippocratic Oath of the physician promises "no harm," the nursing creed has always promoted a "patient-first" philosophy, establishing nurses as a primary link between the patient and the healthcare system. Historically, however, the nurse's role has not been recognized as such. Physician behavior and roles developed out of a "professional" model in which physicians affiliated with hospitals as an "extension" of their training programs thereby maintaining their autonomy, ascendant decision making, and final control over their work. At the same time, nursing became more of a "trade" as nurses trained exclusively within hospitals. In time, the hospital proved to be the only legitimate workplace out of which nurses could emerge. Therefore, nursing was seen as a support role to the physician; as the physician healed, the nurse cared and as the physician diagnosed and treated, the nurse cleaned and cared. As historic societal and professional barriers to women are increasingly surmounted, the nursing profession (founded by and traditionally dominated by women) has likewise evolved to embrace new roles for nurses and new modes of nursing practice.

Today, this evolutionary process is driven primarily by the changing marketplace and the advancing needs of the consumer. Nurses are uniquely qualified to facilitate this evolutionary process and ease the consumers' transition into a new age of healthcare. We are already beginning to see our healthcare industry embrace new technologies related to disease prevention, health promotion, demand management, and quality outcomes. No matter what terminology is used, the implications of all of these strategies include improving the health of our communities and increasing consumer responsibility for their own health-related behaviors. Before describing how nurses are accomplishing this evolutionary process for easing consumers' transition into a new age of healthcare, an overview of some of the forces impacting nursing is discussed.

CURRENT MARKET TRENDS SHAPING NURSING

Among the core drivers shaping the healthcare marketplace are growth in technology; consumer demand for information, including health outcomes of care; economic disincentives for

hospital inpatient beds; the aging of the Baby Boomer generation; and growth in consumer demand for complementary medicine. As a general consequence, the market is placing renewed
emphasis on a strong workforce of primary care providers that
include family physicians, general pediatricians, general in-
ternists, and advanced practice nurses (e.g., nurse practitioners, physician assistants, and certified midwives). The successful
nursing professional will have adapted his or her knowledge
and skill set with these forces in mind, with an eye toward
emerging trends.

The information technology explosion has accelerated our
ability to advance standards of treatment and disease management and has increased our ability to produce quality outcomes
through enhanced information systems. Consumer concomitant
demand for information as well as for increased convenience in
obtaining healthcare services is creating a new revolution in the
industry, especially as consumers begin to pay for an increasing
portion of their healthcare costs through increased deductibles,
co-payments, premiums, and other out-of-pocket expenses. Specifically, consumers spent $203 billion out of their own pockets on
healthcare in 1995 (Thorpe & The National Coalition on Health
Care, 1997). As a reference, this number equates to 18% of all
U.S. healthcare expenditures, a proportion larger than either
Medicare (17% U.S. total) or Medicaid (13%) (Thorpe & The
National Coalition on Health Care, 1997). At the same time, the
government is endeavoring to change the focus of health services
to make them more responsive to financial standards, which include remixing the Medicare payment formula for providers and
healthcare systems. For example, while the Balanced Budget
Acts (BBAs) are significantly reducing hospital reimbursement
by Medicare, they are also providing opportunities for consumers
(e.g., durable medical equipment and educational programs for
patients with diabetes are now covered).

Yet, despite many indications of a system that is becoming
more "consumer friendly," public opinion polls and surveys indicate that the consumer has been sorely neglected in the redesign
and transformation of the healthcare system. In a national
survey of 1,011 American households conducted by the National
Coalition on Health Care in December 1996, consumers revealed the following:

- A lack of confidence in the quality of healthcare
- A belief that the system is putting profits ahead of people and quality
- Fear that quality medical care is becoming unaffordable to the average American
- A desire for better information in order to evaluate quality and decisions about treatment

Compounding this complex picture is the fact that 77 million people in the United States, classified as part of the Baby Boomer generation, are set to retire in 2011 (McCarthy, 1996). The healthcare industry will be substantially affected as this large, college-educated population enters the phase of life where healthcare utilization is highest. To date, the Baby Boomer generation has turned each of its decades upside down as seen with education in the 1960s, housing in the 1970s, the workplace in the 1980s, the financial markets in the 1990s, and if history repeats itself, it will be healthcare in the 2000s (Herzlinger, 1997).

New models of care delivery are emerging as patient care is moving rapidly into community settings. The American Hospital Association (1993) reported that outpatient visits grew 73% between 1980 and 1992, and ambulatory surgery as a percentage of all surgeries is approximately 70%. In addition, financial pressures to control costs have resulted in an increase of care in physicians' offices, at home, and almost any place other than the acute inpatient unit of the hospital. The result is that chronic and acute care, as well as primary care, health promotion, and disease prevention, will now be provided in alternative settings for care delivery, such as ambulatory centers, birthing centers, subacute care facilities, hospice settings, residential homes, and halfway houses.

In addition, the United States is experiencing a sense of emerging spiritual renewal as individuals seek balance and purpose in their lives. Complementary medicine, once looked at askance by Western, allopathic medicine (although arguably embraced much earlier by the nursing profession) is gaining acceptance by the mainstream. Literally, with one-third of Americans interested in alternative approaches to healthcare, alternative medicine has quickly become a $12 billion out-of-pocket industry (Eisenberg, 1993). Preliminary research suggests that as more and more consumers become disgruntled and disillusioned with the results and/or lack of results from the medical profession, they are seeking other ways to approach their health and manage their illnesses. Consumers who are increasingly part of self-empowered "healthier" communities, once again, drive this trend.

THE IMPACT FOR NURSING

As the hospital increasingly becomes the detour rather than the center of the healthcare system, physicians, nurses, and consumers have been met with frustration, turf-battles, and opportunities to explore new roles and relationships. The factors having the greatest impact on nursing include the following:

- The balance between function, skill set, and role will be determined within the context of the circumstance and the needs of the population, as opposed to historically defined job titles and functional roles. With the skill mix within institutions shifting to include an increased number of unregulated healthcare providers, shortened lengths of stay, and more care activity occurring in the home, the focus of care delivery is changing. The question now becomes less "who" and more "what" is to be done in the name of optimal treatment. In turn, less focus should be placed on what should be done by a physician versus a nurse or another type of caregiver, and more focus should be placed on how all groups can assist patients and when patients should be allowed to assist themselves. This shifting of responsibility to patients and families has led to increased reliance on self-care. Indeed, the American Nurses Association (ANA) believes that "health care services provided by the most appropriate provider in the most appropriate setting can promote self-care consumer responsibility, ensure accessibility to health care and decrease the escalating costs of health care" (American Nurses Association Board of Directors, 1991).

- As a result of technical advances, complex and costly healthcare services can now be safely administered in the home. In the era of cost-containment, providers face an inordinate amount of pressure to discharge patients from the hospital quickly, in poorer states of health, and in more acute stages of illness. Therefore, it becomes critical for the staff nurse and other discharge planners to provide patients with the most accurate information about continued care at home.

- As the cost for nursing care increases, cost-conscious institutions will no longer be willing to pay nurses to perform care functions that do not necessarily require the skill set of a registered nurse. As a result, nurses are increasingly discovering new ways to manage the interface between consumer and health system outside the traditional hospital setting. For example, through health teaching, life maintenance, continuum services, health screenings, home care, and outreach services, nurses serve as the point of referral to the physician within settings such as the workplace, community centers, outpatient clinics, schools, and other specialty settings.

- The patient-centered model is a significantly different way of viewing healthcare than most traditional caregivers are accustomed. It means creating processes, which engage and invest the consumer in healthy behavior and lifestyle to reduce the risk for intervention later on. Healthcare providers and nurses must be willing to change their locus of control for their practice and enter a model for service that is culturally moderated and inclusive of other disciplines and the consumer.

- As evidence of primary care supervision becomes a criterion for payment of high-intensity specialty services, the need for advanced practice nurses (APN), who are increasingly carrying out primary care patient responsibilities instead of physicians, is heightened. Recently, the Pew Health Professions Commission recommended doubling the overall number of nurse practitioners, suggesting primary care nurse practitioners can satisfy the medical needs of 50% to 90% of the ambulatory patient population (Lamm, 1996). The Commission also suggested that within their area of competence, nurse practitioners, physician assistants, and certified midwives provide care whose quality is equivalent to that of care provided by physicians. With the shift of resources from acute care into primary care, prevention, and health maintenance, there are increasing numbers of APNs in the marketplace whose education and expertise are well matched for the new business at hand. Consequently, the emergence of nurse practitioner–owned or nurse practitioner–operated systems and primary care settings (with and without physician partners in the practice) is being seen. State legislatures have supported this movement by passing legislation that allows direct third-party reimbursement. Nudged by professional nursing groups and managed care companies, state regulatory boards have made prescriptive authority more available, thus allowing full use of the APN skills in managing the healthcare of populations. As the demand for these services continues to increase, it is clear that APNs will be required to undergo systematic review of their credentials and peer-review processes similar to that of physicians to ensure quality.

- Current efforts of organized nursing are directed toward the establishment of reimbursement formulas for the payment of nursing services and the promotion of models of care delivery and financing of nursing services that are relevant to consumer needs.

A DEARTH OF EDUCATION AND TRAINING OPPORTUNITIES FOR NURSES

There are significant opportunities for nurses to support programs and increase efficiencies of care simply by paying attention to these drivers in the current marketplace. However, if

TABLE 17-1

Comparison of the "Old" versus "New" Model of Nursing Practice

Old Model	New Model
Success is based on high hospital census.	Payor mix is more important than patient census.
Nurses are rewarded for working double shifts.	Nurses are rewarded for cognitive and critical-thinking skills to achieve outcomes.
FTEs are controlled to meet financial goals.	Cost per unit of service is controlled to meet goals.
Focus is on sick care and treatment.	Focus is on customer service.
Focus is on hospital care.	Focus is on caring for the patient in the right setting at the right time.

From Brock R. Head for business. *Hospitals & Health Networks*, December 5, 1996; 62–66.
FTE, Full-time equivalent.

nurses are to support the evolution to the new consumer and succeed in the new healthcare marketplace, they will need a basic understanding of the fundamentals of managed care as well as the business goals of healthcare organizations today. Programs designed to help nurses understand the overall business of healthcare are absent, and on-the-job experience and the rare training opportunity have been the main mode of preparation for the plethora of nontraditional niches. Although there is some growth in curricula and training programs for nurses, healthcare-related educational program directors, continuing medical education (CME) program developers and universities should pay attention to the differences between the old model of healthcare and the new model as new programs are developed. Table 17–1 compares these models (Brock, 1996):

In addition, health educators should help reinforce the fact that personal development is necessary to enhance an individual's talent. This is certainly true in the healthcare industry, where the ability to exert a positive influence is key to personal success. It is important to realize that the current healthcare situation is a result of how health professionals are presently thinking. Thus, personal approaches and skills must be shifted just as paradigms must be. Important new skills and cues for key behaviors include the following:

- *Repositioning skills:* In addition to clinical knowledge, nurses should be able to articulate an understanding for finance, human resource utilization, politics, and customer service. For example, nurses should be able to demonstrate how services provided on a patient care unit are associated with the costs of a care encounter, staffing, and service effectiveness.
- *Networking skills:* Nurses can learn new practice strategies by participating in professional benchmarking with colleagues; for example, conferring and collaborating with social workers to discuss child care options for a patient who will be immobile after discharge and with an occupational therapist about interventions and devices that could help a stroke victim regain manual dexterity while in the hospital.
- *Critical thinking skills:* Nurses should be encouraged to challenge the systems and practices that have become nonproductive. When viewed as a business, healthcare cannot afford to retain past practices that no longer work. For example, eliminating the unnecessary moving of patients from unit to unit keeps patients in familiar surroundings, prevents the loss of personal possessions, and avoids administrative confusion in the computer.
- *Risk-taking skills:* In challenging the system, nurses need to be able to act on ideas that improve care efficiencies. For example, one might consider the risk of moving admissions to the patient care unit.
- *Skills for anticipating customer service needs:* The best example of "great" customer service can be observed at local retail stores and restaurants. Once the nurse has experienced what customer service is all about, from the customer's point of view, these services can be applied within the healthcare environment as well. For example, perhaps healthcare organizations should bring services to patients instead of transporting patients to services.

The reason for developing all of these behaviors in the nurse is to influence the quality of patient care in its new forms. Other supporting disciplines and science bases that can offer training and educational programs for the evolving nurse include exercise physiology, nutrition or dietetics, bariatrics, clinical psychology, health education, health services administration, rehabilitation services, sports medicine, occupational health, preventive medicine, employer-based benefits management, alternative medicine and holistic healing, epidemiology, and sociology.

NEW ROLES FOR NURSES

Given the mandate for demonstrated, improved health outcomes, as well as tangible connection with the consumer, the career opportunities for nurses in the future are endless. In many cases, these opportunities will present a significant paradigm shift as healthcare professionals learn to deliver *healthcare* to consumers in multiple settings, in nontraditional ways, and working in multidisciplinary teams (with colleagues from the community, including social workers, youth workers, voluntary organizations, and sometimes housing officers and local planning authorities). The multidisciplinary dimension suggests that there will be many players in the future healthcare marketplace. In some contexts, the nurse will be the key player; in others, he or she will be one part of a larger team.

The new opportunities within the more traditional healthcare settings will include consultations, program development, telephone triage systems, community-based programs, network development, expansion of patient advocacy programs, and the designing and writing of health-related materials. From an administrative focus, nurses will have opportunities to develop effective cost-containment strategies and quality improvement and outcomes management programs, and to create continuing education and training programs for healthcare professionals. To that end, nurses will provide these services and/or products as independent contractors working from home, in partnership with others, or within established traditional organizations. With the expanding roles of advanced practice nurses, midwives, case managers, and the influx of various nurse-run clinics, further opportunities will exist to deliver primary care services to consumers within the respective communities.

As nurses move into the community, increasing numbers of holistic practitioners and more nontraditional roles will continue to be seen. For nursing professionals, holistic nursing gives them opportunities to apply the knowledge learned in nursing school, which is predicated on the interrelatedness of the body, mind, and spirit. As has often historically been the case, rather than the nurse dictating to the patient what they "should" do, this new breed of professional encourages the patient to assume responsibility for his or her own healthcare choices. In fact, some research suggests that people who are using nontraditional modalities are staying healthier; leading happier, more productive lives; and staying out of the hospitals (Hartwell, 1997). Their numbers are growing exponentially, as are the number of nurses who are exploring lucrative careers in holistic nursing.

Other new roles will include nurses designing office space for outpatient centers, developing computer software, operating nurse-run community fitness centers, performing forensic and criminal nursing, conducting military educational programs, assisting accounting and consulting firms that are redesigning healthcare systems, leading cruise seminars, and overseeing adult day-care centers. Specifically, data analysis and healthcare consulting firms are routinely looking for well-educated nurses who know how to improve systems and can help address the future needs of healthcare systems. As healthcare continues to expand into multiple settings while trying to provide a full continuum of care services, new partnerships between healthcare systems and healthcare-related vendors and manufacturers will emerge. As a result, vendors and manufacturers such as pharmaceutical and durable medical equipment companies will look to professionals such as nurses to facilitate program and opportunity development.

Table 17–2 lists the many examples of career directions and niches, broken down into categories, in traditional as well as nontraditional work sites. The list is not meant to be exclusive; rather, it should be used as a framework for developing other new and creative career opportunities.

Depending on the nurse's current area of expertise, the additional skills and knowledge required may be as simple as

TABLE 17–2

New and Emerging Career Opportunities in Nursing

Consulting and Program Development in the Following Areas:

Cost-containment strategies	Information technology
Outcomes management programs	Data analysis and outcomes research
Medicolegal	Sales and marketing
Facility design	Employer-based programs
Patient-centered care workflow design	Workers' compensation and disability
Hospital bill auditing	Home healthcare
Regulatory accreditation	Disease management
Policy and standards development	Nurse call center
Community health improvement	

Nurse-Run Clinics (free standing or within existing infrastructures)

Adult day-care centers	Women's health clinics
Skin and wound care clinics	Chronic disease clinics
Indigent care clinics	Pain control centers

Caregiver Roles

APNs and midwives	Personal counselors/trainers
Case managers	Space nursing
Holistic practitioners	Forensic nursing
School nursing	Military nursing
Parish nursing	Correctional facility nursing

Educators in the Following Areas:

Disease management support groups	Health improvement
Healthcare management training	Stress management
Managed care training	Relaxation therapies
Nurse practice development	Motivational workshops
Consumer self-care programs	Nutritional counseling

Multimedia Development

Web-based and CD-ROM training	Self-care books
Software for specific disease states	Health promotion materials
Children's books: healthy principles	Outcomes tracking software

reading a book or as complex as going back to school for another college degree. Given the virtually endless list of career options, healthcare educators and nursing program managers will need to stay focused on the changing marketplace if they are to continually support the needs of *their* customer, the nursing student.

CONCLUSION

For hospitals, physicians, and nurses who are not prepared for the competition of the new healthcare marketplace, managed care has become a great source of frustration. Today, payors control the process of governing treatment decisions, choice of medical institution and provider, hospital length of stay, admission, and reimbursement dollars. Providers are poorly prepared to define the high-cost traditional practices and utilization patterns because of the lack of data on long-term patient outcomes. Instead, payors rely primarily on cost and length-of-stay data to identify "best" provider services because this data is readily available. As healthcare providers and institutions struggle to compete in contracting relationships, they most often identify the frustration of not knowing their true costs of care. Increasing consumer involvement places additional pressure on organizations as they compete for the best patient satisfaction scores—yet another driver of plan enrollment. However, there is a "silver lining," not just for nursing, but for the consumer.

Central to managing risk and demonstrating outcomes are the concepts of disease and demand management, health management, performance measures, critical pathways, population-based health improvement systems, and evolving information systems that support these processes. In turn, the concept of health, wellness, and preventive care is central to the issues that link quality outcomes to the business of healthcare. Changing medical management strategies in managed care that are founded on the concept of prevention are beginning to show significant value, that is, demonstrating improved healthcare outcomes and cost-efficiencies. At the foundation of preventive care—a marker for which is appropriate self-care—and disease management strategies are education and counseling, two responsibilities that have always been synonymous with the profession of nursing. In fact, achievement of appropriate self-care is possibly the best proxy measure for the effectiveness of nursing practice (Moritz, 1998).

Today, the call is for a more coordinated and proactive approach to the provision of services, which includes early engagement and demand management approaches that change the way consumers and providers come together around care delivery. The hoped-for result is healthier patients, with less invasive and resource-intensive approaches to service. Managing health means managing populations and intersecting with health plan subscribers at multiple times and places throughout their lifetime. Following patients' care over time requires a redistribution of effort and resources and more strongly defined primary care approaches.

The increased emphasis on preventive primary care, the related move to community-based care, requirements for evidence-based practice, and shared provider–patient decision making all support the push for creating the empowered consumer. Nursing has a unique and critical role to play therein. Never before have so many opportunities existed for nurses to take a leadership position in the evolutionary process of the healthcare industry.

The transition to managed healthcare will mean many things to many people but the fundamental beliefs remain the same. Managed healthcare means doing the right thing for others and for ourselves, in the right way, at the right time, and in the right place. It means going back to basics and embracing the very reasons health professionals went into healthcare in the first place. Also, as it turns out, healthy people are good business.

REFERENCES

American Hospital Association. *Trendlines: ambulatory surgery.* 1993.

ANA Board of Directors, New Position Statement. *Referrals to the most appropriate provider: nursing's agenda for health care reform.* ANA: 1991.

Brock R. Head for business. *Hospitals & Health Networks* December 5, 1996; 62–66.

Eisenberg D. Unconventional medicine in the U.S. *N Engl J Med* 1993; 328(4):246–252.

Hartwell J. Exploring new frontiers in nursing. *Revolution: The Journal of Nurse Empowerment* 1997; winter:88–91.

Herzlinger R. *Market-driven health care.* Reading, MA: Addison Wesley, 1997.

Lamm R. The coming dislocation in the health professionals. *Healthcare Forum Journal* 1996; 58–62.

McCarthy R. Controlling costs for the new flood of retirees. *Business & Health* September, 1996; 56–64.

Moritz P. Demonstrating clinical impact with indicators sensitive to care and environmental context. *New Medicine* 1998; 98–101.

Thorpe K, The National Coalition on Health Care. *Changes in the growth in health care spending: implications for consumers.* Tulane University Medical Center, 1997.

18

CHAPTER

The Elderly as the New Consumer of Healthcare

Elizabeth White, M.D

Ann Danish, M.S.W.

INTRODUCTION

The new millennium portends formidable challenges, as well as opportunities, in successfully meeting the needs of our aging society. Culturally, socially, economically, and functionally, the older population in the United States (defined as 55+ years) is highly diverse. This heterogeneity, along with the growth in numbers and in the prevalence of elderly—aging Baby Boomers being well represented among this population—and a dearth of resources precludes easy approaches to ensuring their care and well-being. Yet, other forces are converging to make this era one of great possibility for the elderly: advances in medicine and healthcare, more choices that can enhance quality of life, a greater awareness on society's part of the elderly's rightful "place at the table," and of the elderly's growing clout as consumers.

Nonetheless, some disturbing trends indicate that the poor, less-educated elderly continue to be at greater risk for ill health and disability than those who are affluent and educated. It becomes clear that effective interventions, whether the focus is on prevention, stabilization of chronic illness to prevent disability, or acute care, must be developed with the unique characteristics of the respective elder population in mind.

In an aging society, the needs, preferences, and contributions of the elderly are powerful forces. As a "special interest group" and as consumers, the elderly have made great strides. As evidenced by the household name recognition of such concerted (and powerful) advocacy groups as the American Association of Retired Persons (AARP) and the Grey Panthers, the elderly are wielding their influence at all levels of society. Approaches to and implications of "healthcare consumerism" for our aging society is the focus of this chapter. Within this framework, key demographic changes in the United States are outlined; health implications of a diverse, aging population are discussed, as is study data on disability and other health-related issues relevant to an elder healthcare consumer; and finally, available research on how the elderly make choices about their healthcare is reviewed.

KEY DEMOGRAPHICS

The demographic characteristics of the 65-and-older population provide a context for examining current and future health-related issues. The elderly population in the United States has increased in absolute numbers and in proportion to the total population throughout the twentieth century. The "oldest old" (age 85 and older) (Neugarten, 1974) is the most rapidly increasing elderly subgroup. It is projected that as the Baby Boomer cohort ages, the number will increase to at least 90 million in 2050, or 5% of the total population at that time (www.census.gov/socdemo). The number of persons age 65 and older was estimated at 3.1 million in 1900 and at 34 million in 1998; it is expected to double by 2030, largely because of the impact of the Baby Boomer generation (the approximately 76 million people born between 1946 and 1964) (Administration on Aging, 1998b).

The proportion of elderly in the nation will increase within the next 30 years, from approximately 13% to somewhere around 20%. Simultaneously, life expectancy is also increasing. Although experts differ based on varying assumptions about fertility, mortality, and immigration, the Bureau of the Census' middle series projections released in 1996 suggest life expectancy at birth in the year 2050 will be 79.7 years for men, compared with 72.5 years in 1995; similarly, life expectancy for women in 2050 is predicted to be 84.3 years, compared with 79.3 in 1995 (Administration on Aging, 1998a).

Women outnumber men, particularly among the older population. Projections are that by 2050, there will be about 4 million more women over the age of 85 than men of the same age. This fact has profound practical implications for health and social service planning because women are the greatest users of healthcare resources and, particularly later in life, tend to live alone and have lower incomes. Older men are more likely than older women to be married. Almost half of older women in 1997 were widows (Administration on Aging, 1998b).

Another critical trend is the faster increase in the elderly population among minorities than among whites. The term *double jeopardy* has been used to convey the notion that the disadvantages of aging are compounded among minorities (Institute on Aging, 1997). The 1990 census indicated that 7.5% of the 65-and-older population were nonwhite, and it is projected that by 2025, 25% will be nonwhite (Institute on Aging, 1997). African-Americans are the largest group of nonwhite elderly. In 1990, about 12% of the U.S. African-American population were older than age 65, as were 5% of the Hispanic population, 6.3% of Asian/Pacific Islanders, and 6% of Native Americans (Morgan, 1998). It is anticipated that growth rate will be greatest among Hispanic and Asian populations (The Public Policy and Aging Report, 1998).

Economically, today's elderly are better off than previous generations as demonstrated by declining poverty rates and higher incomes. Of the elderly population, 3% have annual incomes exceeding $75,000. Yet, 10.5% live below the poverty threshold (The Public Policy and Aging Report, 1998). There is large disparity in financial well-being according to race and gender. Of those elderly living in poverty, almost 75% are women, particularly those living alone and minorities. However, real income of the elderly is expected to continue to rise (Zedlewski et al., 1990). It is suggested that in general, most

Baby Boomers will have higher incomes than current retirees because of such economic factors as wages rising faster than inflation, more women in the labor force, greater eligibility for pensions, and inherited wealth. However, certain subgroups, specifically the less educated, single parents, and nonhomeowners, are not expected to share the gains (Manchester, 1997). Living arrangements and family composition are varied and will continue to diversify.

Most (66%) noninstitutionalized older persons lived in a family setting in 1997. About 31% lived alone. Only approximately 4% of the total over-65 population lived in a nursing home, although the proportion increases greatly with advanced age (Administration on Aging, 1998b).

Educational background is related positively with income and health status. Of persons older than age 75, 55% have finished high school, as have more than two-thirds of those between the ages of 65 and 74. However, basic literacy is a problem for many elderly, especially for minorities. Twelve percent of African-Americans and 27% of Hispanics older than age 65 have less than 5 years of formal education (Kart, 1997). Future generations are projected to have a much higher level of secondary education. Of Americans aged 55 to 64, 76% have completed high school and beyond (Kart, 1997). Numerous studies have demonstrated clear links between years of education and disease/disability in old age. For example, the prevalence of six major chronic conditions (arthritis, hearing impairment, diabetes, heart disease, hypertension, and emphysema) is significantly less in those older than age 65 with a high school education (German & Shapiro, 1997).

DISABILITY PATTERNS IN THE ELDERLY

A central debate in the field of gerontology focuses on whether the advances in preventive and acute-care medicine will enhance what John Rowe (Rowe & Kahn, 1997) terms "successful aging," leading to compression of disability; in other words, as the aging populace expands, will the number of disabled elderly rise just as exponentially? Fries (Fries, 1989), the major proponent of the theory of compression of morbidity, believes that there is evidence to show that as fatal events, such as heart attacks and strokes, are postponed, nonfatal diseases causing major disability would also be postponed, leading to a compression of the time in a person's life that functional loss and illness is experienced. On the other side of the debate, Olshansky (Olshansky & Rudberg, 1997) maintains that as the death rate continues to fall, this only expands the time frame in which an individual may develop debilitating conditions.

Although the actual outcome of this debate will have significant consequences for public policy and management of healthcare resources for the elderly, Olshansky cautions that at this time, it is almost impossible to reach a definite conclusion about the state of compression of disability in future elderly cohorts. The elderly in the next 20 to 30 years will differ dramatically in age distribution and genetic diversity compared with the surviving cohorts of today, making it impossible to infer the future from current data.

Helping to shed light on the debate are recent results from National Health Interview Surveys. Conducted from 1982 to 1993, the study surveyed adults born between 1915 and 1959. The researchers found that although disability levels appear to be waning among the older cohorts, later-born cohorts are showing increases in other types of disability. Specifically, rates of cardiovascular disease in men and in women have been steadily decreasing, except in well-educated women. Arthritis has shown large decreases among later-born groups, whereas the prevalence of other chronic illnesses, such as asthma and orthopedic and muscular skeletal diseases, has increased (Reynolds, Crimmins, & Saito, 1998).

At the same time, these gains may be offset, according to the National Academy on Aging, by recent evidence suggesting that long-term care needs in the nonelderly have increased substantially. The main reason cited is higher survival rates of the severely ill and injured, resulting in permanent high-grade disabilities. In fact, of the 12.8 million Americans who need daily assistance, only 57% are 65 or older (Facts on Long Term Care, 1997).

The Canadian Study of Health and Aging (1990–1991), indicates that nearly twice as many cognitively intact seniors older than age 85 had functional disabilities, compared with those 65 to 84, and that increase in age was the only significant factor explaining decreases in instrumental activities of daily living in that age group. In the younger age group, chronic illness was significant in explaining the increase in functional disability. Thus, the study concludes that many disabilities occur in the very old, unrelated to chronic illness present (Hagan, Ebly, & Fung, 1999).

Results from the ongoing National Long Term Care Survey support the theory of compression of morbidity. Data from 1994 showed that 1.2 million fewer older people were disabled than would have been expected if the rates of disability observed in 1982 had remained. The actual number of older people with functional problems in 1994 was 7.1 million, not the expected 8.3 million. This is equivalent to 21.3% of the over-65 population being chronically disabled in 1994 compared with 24.9% at 1982 rates. Another heartening finding was that the rate of decline of disability has increased, suggesting fewer disabled individuals in the future.

IMPLICATIONS FOR LONG-TERM CARE SERVICES

The National Long Term Care Survey data suggested that disability among older people seemed less severe in more recent cohorts, as shown by a greater drop in the number of those age 85 and older who had more than three impairments of activities of daily living, commonly considered the cut off point for long-term care services (National Long Term Care Survey, 1999). These findings are similar to government data released in the Profile of Older Americans in 1998. In 1994 to 1995, 52.5% of the older population had at least one disability, with one-third reporting a severe, limiting disability. These disabilities increase significantly with increasing age.

Even if the average time spent living with disability should decrease, the overwhelming increase in absolute numbers of elderly most likely will necessitate a significant growth in need for long-term care services.

The Health and Retirement Study/Assets in Health Dynamics Among the Oldest Old study (Soldo et al., 1997) provides valuable, if not surprising, information on the health of older Americans. This study, begun in 1992 and sponsored by the NIA, Social Security Administration (SSA), Department of Labor, U.S. Department of Health and Human Services (DHHS), and the AARP, focuses on the relationship between changes in health, work, and financial security of Americans around retirement age. This study revealed some surprises. Although many of the elderly respondents report chronic health problems (most commonly high blood pressure, diabetes, cancer, bronchitis, emphysema, cardiovascular, congestive heart failure, and stroke), 33% of the older population report no chronic conditions of any sort.

Those elderly reporting poor health status have a higher number of chronic medical problems than those who report excellent health. Furthermore, elderly with poor health status spent six times as much as those reporting excellent health for out-of-pocket expenses for healthcare, spending an average of $30,000 annually. As is to be expected, those under the Medicare eligibility age of 65 have higher out-of-pocket expenses.

The study also found a strong relationship between health and wealth. Results indicated that the average income of households with both spouses in excellent health is quadruple that of households in which both are in poor health. This relationship holds true for net worth of a household by a factor of 10. The evidence seems to show that it is *health* that ultimately facilitates higher income, rather than wealth allowing better healthcare (which would, in turn, ensure better health).

IMPLICATIONS OF RESOURCE ALLOCATION/RATIONING FOR THE ELDERLY

The continuing debate in the United States on Medicare spending is proxy for the difficult question of resource allocation facing the industrialized countries with their ever-growing older populace (for an in-depth discussion of the Medicare debate, see *Health Affairs*. January/February, 1999, vol. 1). Binstock (1997) summarizes the issue well: in 1994, people older than age 65 accounted for about one-third of the annual U.S. healthcare cost (approximately $300 billion out of $900 billion). Government programs (Medicare and Medicaid, Veterans affairs) finance approximately two-thirds of these costs. Eight percent is funded by Medigap supplemental policies. The elderly pay for about 28% of the cost of their care out of their own pockets.

The cost for long-term care (e.g., adult day care, nursing home, nonmedical home care) is paid mostly out of pocket by families and recipients. In 1995, this amounted to about one-third of all expenditures, or $34.6 billion. Government programs financed about 57%, leaving the remainder to private insurance (Facts on Long Term Care, 1997). Long-term care insurance has begun to catch on; however, the benefit is cumulative, based on premium contributions over the course of one's lifetime.

At the time of this writing, evidence suggests that Medicare reimbursement cuts for hospitals and providers could result in more patients being referred into managed care HMOs, for example, Medicare Plus Choice/Physician-run Provider Service Organizations, a feature of Medicare Plus Choice that promised more physician control and cost-efficiencies. However, the early results of PSOs have not met original expectations. The impact of the aforementioned forces on elderly healthcare consumers could be felt in the following ways: on one hand, less access to specialist care and high-tech diagnostic tools; on the other hand, greater emphasis on primary and secondary prevention in the form of wellness programs that address physical, emotional, and spiritual needs. The trend toward releasing all but the sickest from the hospital will almost certainly continue, forcing the integration of nonacute services, such as skilled and nonskilled home care, assisted living and skilled nursing facilities with acute hospital care to finally forge a true continuum of care, so essential to the chronically ill. Finally, the emphasis on end of life planning will certainly continue, driven, unfortunately, in part by the debate on containing healthcare spending.

THE FACE OF DIVERSITY IN THE ELDERLY AND IMPLICATIONS FOR THEIR HEALTHCARE

The growing body of gerontologic research affirms that the major health issues of the elderly are those of chronic illness and disability caused both by pathology and by the aging process itself. However, because of the increasing diversity of coming cohorts, it will be important to understand the unique characteristics of the particular elderly group being served.

Therefore, future research must focus on this micro level, in the context of population-based studies. The Gerontological Society of America, in its handbook on aging and diversity, *Full-Color Aging: Facts, Goals and Recommendations for America's Diverse Elders,* calls for detailed studies that "evaluate and understand the roles played by local level factors in the lives of older persons* and their families" (Miles, 1999). The following section highlights demographic and health services research that explores the link between health, disability, and differences in ethnicity, social status, cohort, gender, and community.

It is well established that racial and ethnic minorities, as well as poor elderly, have earlier onset and higher prevalence of disabilities, crossing urban–rural lines (Wallace, 1997). In fact, African-Americans, in a north Florida study of 1,200 community-dwelling elderly, showed a greater likelihood of decline in health even when starting at a similar level as their Caucasian counterparts. Analysis of the data indicates that this is the result of lifelong differences in income and education (Peek, Coward, & Henretta, 1997).

Depression in the elderly is a serious problem that has been linked to chronic poor health and low socioeconomic status (Thoits, 1995). Although evidence of disparities in depression rates between ethnic groups is mixed, a well-designed study of African-Americans and Caucasians (aged 58 to 64) shows interesting differences in determinants of depression, indicating a need for targeted interventions. Fernandez et al. (1998) found that social network losses were significantly tied to depression in Caucasian men, not Caucasian women. African-American men's depressive symptoms were tied to work stressors, poor health, and retirement, whereas African-American women were

---

* In 1974, Bernice Neugarten was the first to distinguish between the "young-old" and the "old-old" and the related differences in health, socioeconomic status, dependency, living arrangements, and relationships. Those 75 years of age and older are generally considered to be higher users of health and social services because of the needs related to advanced age.

generally more likely to have an association between income and depression.

With adequate sampling of minority populations, large longitudinal studies such as the Health and Retirement Study (HRS) can provide useful information for healthcare planners. Clark et al.'s (1996) analysis of a 1992 sample from the HRS of African-American men and women ages 51 to 61 years showed significant gender differences in factors related to functional impairment. One-third of African-American men reported some problems with physical function, as did half of the women. Most of the factors associated with decline are potentially remediable or at least manageable: for men, these include alcohol abuse, smoking, obesity, cardiovascular disease, diabetes, and arthritis; for women, alcohol abuse, obesity, arthritis, and respiratory illness.

Several studies of the Hispanic population have not only provided significant information on health status but are models for the detailed research necessary to paint a comprehensive picture of the many different demographic subgroups of the elderly today. Black et al. (1998) looked at data from the Hispanic Established Populations for the Epidemiologic Study of the Elderly (EPESE) on rates of depression. Significantly, female immigrants were at higher risk, whereas male immigrants were at lower risk for depression than subjects born in the United States.

Sundquist and Winkleby (1999), using data from another national survey—the National Health and Nutrition Examination Survey II (NHANES II), demonstrate that risk for mortality from coronary heart disease (CHD) is highest in U.S.-born Spanish speakers of Mexican descent, followed by U.S.-born English speakers, trailed by Mexican-born individuals residing in the United States. This surprising variation in CHD mortality in a seemingly homogenous population (Mexican-Americans) underscores the importance of asking precise questions.

Angel and Angel's (1996) analysis of data from the HRS reveals that an increasing number of preretirement-age Hispanics in this country are at risk for lack of health insurance. In contrast, the number of uninsured, similarly aged non-Hispanic whites and blacks is decreasing. The implication is that many Hispanic elderly will continue to enter Medicare coverage in a poorer state of health because of a lack of adequate care in their fifties and sixties. For this group, supplemental insurance after age 65 will probably not be available, diminishing the care they will be able to get once covered by Medicare.

Finally, the U.S. government, in its initiative on Race and Health, presents dramatic statistics, compiled with goals, for cancer, cardiovascular disease, and diabetes in white and non-white populations (www.raceandhealth.hhs.gov). Mortality rates for cardiovascular disease and cancer, the two leading causes of death in the United States, are significantly higher for African-Americans. Other ethnic groups have isolated higher mortality rates for specific cancers, such as cervical cancer in Vietnamese women. Complications of diabetes, such as kidney failure and lower-limb amputation, are much higher in African-Americans and Native-Americans than in the Caucasian population. Of particular concern is the fact that rates of screening for cancer and cholesterol levels, two effective preventive measures, are unacceptably low in most minority populations. The U.S. government, through its initiative on Race and Health is attempting to address these disparities by establishing specific numeric goals for screening and secondary prevention (i.e., reduction of disease complications such as renal failure in diabetes) in the general population and certain subgroups at higher risk.

Considering what is known about the effects of ethnicity, education, and socioeconomic status, combined with across-the-board increases in life expectancy, we will most likely see compression and expansion of morbidity: the less well off and less educated, represented for the most part by minority groups, will continue to suffer in higher proportion from chronic diseases and subsequent early decline, whereas the growing, well-educated middle class will enter old age healthier than ever before, to enjoy independence late into their eighties.

THE OLDER CONSUMER OF HEALTHCARE

One of the hallmarks of healthcare for the elderly is prevention and management of chronic disease before the common end-point of functional decline is reached. Another is preservation of quality of life for the already-disabled individual and his or her caregiver(s). These goals are attained only through a long-term commitment by both the providers and those receiving care. Successful management of chronic illness or of wellness-oriented lifestyle changes is predicated on active involvement of the affected individual. Ideally, the older person (or caregiver) acts as full partner, or leader, in planning his or her healthcare. As Konrad (1998) states: "Strategies employed by people themselves to present or delay the onset of disease, or to minimize the impact of impairments on their functioning, assume an important role in the array of resources available to older persons as they face the challenges of aging in the 21st century."

USE OF FORMAL MEDICAL SERVICES

Symptom interpretation is a key to help-seeking behavior. Older persons already suffering from chronic medical problems are more likely to view new symptoms as serious and warranting medical attention than those who report feeling healthy. Similarly, those who live alone, have a low income, or have poor social supports tend to interpret unfamiliar symptoms as being more serious (Stoller, 1998).

The community-dwelling elderly average five to six doctor visits per year, but as Levanthal et al. (1995) point out, there is an optimal time delay for seeking professional care: too soon creates unnecessary costs and anxiety for the patient; too late can endanger the patient's health. Levanthal et al.'s research indicates that the older person tends to seek medical care more quickly than the middle-aged person for comparable problems. Centers for Disease Control and Prevention data on physician contacts per person in 1992 show that, except for children younger than 5 years of age, the average number of physician contacts increases with age (Kart, 1997). The elderly show greater use of a variety of healthcare services, including prescription medications, medical equipment and supplies, vision aids, and other providers such as physical therapists, podiatrists, optometrists, and psychologists. One serious gap is oral health. Dental problems increase with age, but according to the National Health Interview Survey, only about 43% of the elderly had seen a dentist within the past year, possibly because of poor insurance coverage (Kart, 1997).

Stoller (1982) found that the actual number of clinically relevant symptoms, as well as convenience and availability, predicted initial contact with a physician, whereas concern about health and function and insurance coverage determined the total volume of doctor visits.

USE OF LAY CARE

Not surprisingly, healthcare professionals tend to equate healthcare with the use of formal medical services. However, most people, the elderly included, never seek formal medical care for 75% to 90% of all episodes of illness (Defriese & Woomert, 1985). Older people do get more regular checkups and consultations for minor symptoms, but they are no more likely than those who are younger to see a doctor for serious complaints (Haug, 1981).

Stoller et al. (1993) analyzed health diaries detailing self-treatment strategies of older respondents. As expected, most managed their problems without using formal healthcare services. A common response was to take no action at all, particularly if the symptom was infrequent, caused little distress, and was interpreted as nonharmful. Symptoms such as muscle or joint pain that caused serious discomfort (and were therefore thought dangerous) or that interfered with activities were more likely to be treated with self-medication, either over-the-counter (OTC) or prescription drugs available in the home. Other popular interventions included physical modalities, such as hot water bottles, or folk remedies, such as herbal teas. A step-wise series of lay treatments were often used to rule out severity of a symptom.

The disabled and very ill older person typically relies on family members, particularly females, for caregiving. Edwardson et al. (1995) investigated the less-well-understood role of laypeople as "self-care consultants" to the well elderly in a survey of Minnesotans older than age 65. Of those surveyed, 55% reported that they discussed their symptoms with a friend or relative (usually female). The type of symptom, as well as marital status, also influenced consultation patterns. For example, men avoided discussing depressive feelings or nocturia with relatives. Married men most often consulted their wives exclusively, whereas married women preferred to speak with female relatives or friends. Widowed persons tended to discuss symptoms sparsely, if at all, usually with an adult child (Stoller, 1998). Advice ranged from do nothing (36%) to empathetic statements (12%) to modifying activity (15%) or seeking medical care (14%). Less than 10% of the time, specific interventions such as dietary changes were suggested. Interestingly, those who did consult with a layperson were more likely to seek professional medical care than those who did not.

Stoller (1998) points out that health discussions among laypeople demonstrate varying levels of intensity, from specific requests for advice and guidance to low-key, casual exchanges of information about symptoms and treatments. The very act of telling others one's health story can give reassurance by providing a realistic reference point, reinforcing current behavior, and offering validation of the experience.

Self-care consultation networks deserve recognition as being central to the older consumer by providing an easily accessible and supportive framework for the daily decision making required to successfully negotiate the life changes that go hand in hand with aging and chronic illness.

There will be natural concern among healthcare professionals that lay advice could prove dangerous to the health of the older person with complex medical problems. This is probably not the case, as suggested in research by Rakowski et al. (1990); in addition to more frequent doctor visits, Rakowski et al. show that individuals who actively seek health information from nonprofessionals tend to pursue other health-enhancing behaviors more frequently, such as regular exercise, use of seat belts, use of dental floss, and performance of regular breast examinations. Other studies (Kemper, Lorig, & Mettler, 1993; Rakowski et al., 1990) have found that lay advice is usually appropriate: the most serious symptoms, such as chest pain and shortness of breath, are recognized as such. Potentially dangerous advice is rare and is usually related to a treatment or medication being contraindicated in a specific situation, such as food–alcohol–drug interactions.

THE MEDIA, HEALTH INFORMATION, AND TELEMEDICINE

The older person also draws on familiar forms of the media for health information. Television is often cited as the number one source, followed by magazines, newspapers, radio, and even junk-mail (Freimuth, 1993; Gallop, 1997). With the exception of the library, these everyday sources will usually provide "incidental information," information randomly acquired and then integrated into an individual's understanding of his or her unique situation (Williamson, 1998).

The elderly, perhaps because they are often more isolated and have more leisure time than younger age groups, place a high priority on staying informed. Some elderly have voiced frustration with purposeful seeking of health information, finding that government or organizational pamphlets were either too general, too technical, or outdated. Particularly lacking seems to be comprehensive information on how to choose a health plan or understanding options for long-term care or the Medicare Choice program (Health Information for Older Adults, 1995).

Theoretically, the Internet is an ideal vehicle for imparting health information to the older consumer; both incidental and purposeful knowledge can be obtained with a click of the mouse—the World Wide Web is overflowing with health-related sites. (The American Association of Retired Persons [AARP] Web site has a comprehensive health page with links to useful and credible sites. See Table 18–1.) In addition, one can visit elder-only chat rooms and virtual communities, all from the comfort of one's own home. This medium has the potential to be a convenient and effective way to help the older consumer cope with health problems. Telemedicine has great potential for serving the elderly through the real-time linking of healthcare professionals with a home-bound, chronically ill client via a modem.

However, only a minority of those older than age 65 are actually using this technology. In the future, as the more computer savvy Baby Boomers age, the numbers will automatically increase, but it would be a missed opportunity to wait for that. Research has shown that the barriers to effective computer use in the current older cohorts can be tackled with excellent results. In 1997, the NIH and HCFA sponsored a project undertaken by

T A B L E 18–1

Health Page Links

Resources	Web Sites
Administration on Aging provides comprehensive statistics on older Americans	www.aoa.dhhs.gov
National Long Term Care Survey ongoing since 1982, looks at disability rates and need for long term care, through Duke University	www.nih.gov/nia
HRS/AHEAD Health and Retirement Study/Assets in Health Dynamics Among the Oldest Old ongoing since 1992, examines relationships between health and employment and retirement, through the University of Michigan	www.umich.edu/~hrswww
AARP Webplace American Association of Retired Persons nonprofit organization with more than 30 million members age 50 and older, providing advocacy, education and research in aging	www.aarp.org
AARP—Explore Health extensive health-related information with links to reputable medical Web sites and chat rooms	www.aarp.org/healthguide
AARP—Andrus Foundation funds gerontological research	www.andrus.org
Full-Color Aging: Facts, Goals and Recommendations for America's Diverse Elders (Ed. Miles P. The Gerontological Society of America, 1999. 1030 15th Street NW, Suite 250 Washington, DC 20005-1503; 202-842-1275) provides extensive annotated bibliography on minorities and aging	www.geron.org
Self-Care in Later Life, Research, Program and Policy Issues (Ed. Ory MG, DeFries GH. New York: Springer Publishing, 1998) provides extensive annotated bibliography on self-care in the elderly	(Book)

Setting Priorities for Retirement Years (SPRY) to assess older adults' motivation to use the Internet to obtain healthcare information. The project used a "train-the-trainer" approach for teaching older adults how to access and evaluate information on the Internet.

Results of the project indicate that training "had a positive impact on seniors' confidence in using computers and the Internet, in conducting consumer health information searches on line, and in sharing health care information with doctors, families and friends," according to NLM Director Donald A.B. Lindberg, M.D. Lindberg said, "Most importantly, we found that seniors can learn to use the Internet and don't want to be left behind on the information superhighway. Two-thirds of those who searched for health information on the Internet talked about it with their doctors, and more than half indicated they were more satisfied with their treatment as a result of their search" (NIH News Release, 1998).

As more health information specific to elder consumers is made available on the Internet, there is a clear need for training adapted to the learning pace and style of older adults. The American Society on Aging and Microsoft cooperated on research that shows a "digital divide," or gap between computer users and nonusers, that particularly affects older Americans. Although approximately 50% of Americans own and use computers, only 24% of individuals age 60 and older do. Many high-tech firms are now targeting the older market by distributing instructional videos, organizing training sessions, and creating senior-focused Web sites (Seniors Enticed to Join Web, 1999).

Czaja and Sharit (1998), in a study of attitudes toward computers as a function of age and experience, showed that older people may feel less comfortable but that they are just as interested in learning to use computers as younger people are. The researchers found that providing optimal support is critical to the success of computer-training programs for the older adult: providing a comfortable setting, using age-appropriate teaching methods, and minimizing frustration by ramping up level of difficulty slowly in the initial learning phase.

The veracity of health information found on the Internet remains a justifiable concern, not only for the elderly, but for all consumers. Consumers must become more discerning—guided by "Good Housekeeping"–type endorsements of quality approval, which are beginning to proliferate. The AARP has endorsed a number of medical Web sites and chat rooms, providing links to these through its own "Explore Health" Web site (Table 18–1).

Professionals must be willing to discuss patient's Internet discoveries and learn how to educate elders effectively on computer
and Web use. There is tremendous opportunity for planners and
providers to design and disseminate their own reliable online
health information.

AGING, DIVERSITY, AND HEALTH INFORMATION

As the older population grows in diversity, both consumers and
healthcare professionals will be coming face to face with people
of different backgrounds and beliefs. Consumers and providers
will do best by sharing the responsibility of creating, as Moody
(1998) calls it, a "dialogue across the cultures." The heterogeneity of older Americans profoundly influences how health
information is obtained and used. Basic literacy, which is associated with social characteristics such as poverty, being nonwhite, and having less schooling, can have major consequences
for personal health as well as for overall healthcare expenditures. Gazmarian et al. (1999) looked at 3,260 new Medicare enrollees across four states and found that 33% of English-
speaking and 53.9% of Spanish-speaking respondents had poor
health literacy, defined as the inability to read or comprehend
basic written healthcare instructions (such as for medications or
at discharge). Risk increased with increasing age regardless of
other factors. Other studies (Low Health Literacy Skills . . . ,
1999) show that adults of all ages with low health literacy use
substantially more hospital resources than those with higher-
level reading skills. These excess services resulted in an estimated increase of $73 billion to annual healthcare expenditures
in 1998. Thirty-eight percent, or $28.3 billion, of this was paid
for by Medicare. These numbers underscore the importance of
presenting and reinforcing health instructions and advice at a
level comprehensible to the given consumer. Applied research is
being conducted that will assist caregivers in the design of
better communication methods for the aging population (Morrow
et al., 1998).

Patterns of how cancer patients seek information illumi-
nate variations in behavior by age cohort. Despite similar circumstances at diagnosis, older women with early-stage breast

cancer show less interest than younger women in participating in treatment decisions and seeking more detailed information from healthcare providers. This may be partially a cohort effect or is possibly the result of less need to maintain a specific role, such as spouse, mother, or employee (Petrisek et al., 1997). In another study of patients aged 18 to 81, older people with cancer tended to seek less information from professional sources but pursued nonmedical establishment venues, such as the media and personal contacts, much more vigorously than their younger counterparts (Turk-Charles, 1997).

Traditions and behaviors specific to cultural and ethnic group also influence help- and information-seeking behavior in the elderly. Moon et al. (1998) found elderly Korean-Americans to be uninformed of the availability of long-term care and social services compared with whites. Cho (1998) believes that this is a reflection of the traditional Asian belief of the centrality of family; seeking outside help is often considered shameful, thus this type of information is ignored.

In the African-American culture, for example, the family and church are mainstays of support; health education efforts are often based in the parish, which provides practical and spiritual help during illness. Indeed, for many African-American men and women, a close and active relationship to God is a high priority (White, 1990) and can promote feelings of well-being in the chronically ill (Musick et al., 1998) or in family caregivers of cognitively impaired African-American elderly (Connell & Gibson, 1997).

Davis and Wykle (1998) summarize available research on health behaviors of aging African-Americans. They point out that African-American elders are by no means a monolithic block, but because of the common early experiences of segregation, and for many, rural southern life, there are observed and important differences. Many older African-Americans continue to rely on traditional medical healing practices rooted in the African, Caribbean, and Southern United States experience, whether due earlier to necessity (i.e., not being able to access the mainstream healthcare system) or through disenchantment with care perceived as inferior under segregation. The perception of insensitivity toward their culture, coupled with mistrust of establishment doctors and pride in their heritage, reinforces the use of folk medicine by African-American elders.

To further quote Moody (1998), ". . . Cultural differences become an occasion for communication and clarification, not a trump card that cuts off debate about right and wrong, as would be the case for simplistic versions of cultural relativism and, ironically, also with an abstract and impoverished notion of patient autonomy."

CONCLUSION

The overall graying of American society, coupled with the growing diversity of the aging population, will catalyze significant changes in healthcare finance and delivery systems over the next decades. Prevention and management of chronic diseases, with the goal of reducing known risk factors, thus maximizing functional independence and quality of life, will be central to the new healthcare environments.

Such health promotion models seek to impact older adults' health behavior by focusing on improving health practices and lifestyles, modifying unhealthy environments, and integrating cultural attitudes and health. Successful health promotion for the older consumer should encourage individual control and responsibility. Providers need to be sensitive to the many social and psychological factors that influence health information–seeking behaviors, such as cultural attitudes toward aging. Older cohorts may assume a more passive role and may be more cautious about using new technologies. The Baby Boomers may have different expectations, however. This generation has already had experience in demanding high-quality, sophisticated technology and access to complex, user-friendly information. It is likely that large numbers of this cohort will remain actively involved in healthcare decision making as they age (Blanchette & Valcons, 1998).

Minority elders are disproportionately affected by chronic disease, functional decline, and low health literacy. Language and cultural barriers to effective communication often exist, and full access to healthcare services is often limited.

Health planners will need to devote resources to understanding the specific group or community they wish to serve. An extensive and growing body of research is now available on the health profiles and behaviors of the elderly (see Table 18–1 for a list of elder-centered Web sites). Local factors can be addressed by including community members in the planning process.

Understanding health information–seeking behavior can lead to creative ways of educating the older consumer: tapping into lay consultation networks and using local television or traditional print media are some examples.

Technology can be a powerful tool for promoting healthful behaviors and managing chronic conditions. Enhancing coping ability in the face of chronic disease can be mitigated through Internet-based support groups and focused health information. Long-distance learning (e.g., self-care and healthcare consults—through telemedicine) are becoming a reality for many elderly, who often tend to live in underserved areas, live alone, or are shut-ins. Providers and planners will have a new role in systematically educating consumers in judging the reliability of health information sources, from Web sites to family and friends.

Consumers and providers will continue to move toward partnership in the ongoing management of lifestyle changes and chronic illness. This implies sensitivity to cultural-, ethnic-, and cohort-based differences in health beliefs.

With elders demanding a place at the consumer "table," the healthcare system of the twenty-first century may be more sensitive to the inescapable fact that we *all* are marching toward old age. Simply put, the system that we are counting on to take care of us tomorrow depends in large part on how much value we place on aging, and our elderly, today.

REFERENCES

Administration on Aging. *Aging into the 21st century*. Washington, DC: Administration on Aging, 1998a. www.aoa.dhhs.gov.

Administration on Aging. *Profiles of older Americans*. Washington, DC: Administration on Aging, 1998b. www.aoa.dhhs.gov.

Angel RJ, Angel JL. The extent of private and public health insurance coverage among adult Hispanics. *The Gerontologist* 1996; 36(3):332–340.

Binstock RH. Issues of resource allocation in an aging society. In: *Public health and aging.* Hicky, Speers, Prohaska: Johns Hopkins University Press, 1997: 53–74.

Black SA, et al. Correlates of depressive symptomatology among older community-dwelling Mexican American. *Hispanic EPESE J Gerontol* 1998; 53b(4):S198–S208.

Blanchette P, Valcons V. Health and aging among Baby Boomers. *Generations* 1998; XXII:78.

Cho PJ. Awareness and utilization. A comment. *The Gerontologist* 1998; 38(3):317–319.

Clark DO, et al. Physical function among retirement aged African American men and women. *The Gerontologist* 1996; 36(3):322–331.

Connell CM, Gibson GD. Racial, ethnic and cultural differences in dementia caregiving: review and analysis. *The Gerontologist* 1997; 37(3):355–364.

Czaja SJ, Sharit J. Age differences in attitudes toward computers. *J Gerontol Psychol Sci* 1998; 53b(5):329–340.

Davis L, Wykle ML. Self-care in minority and ethnic populations: the experience of older black Americans. In: *Self-care in later life.* New York: Springer, 1998: 170–179.

Defriese G, Woomert A. Self-care among the US Elderly. *Res Aging* 1985; 5(1):3–23.

Edwardson SR, et al. Symptom consultation in lay networks in an elderly population. *J Aging Health* 1995; 7(3):402–416.

Facts on Long Term Care. Washington, DC: The National Academy on Aging, 1997.

Fernandez ME, et al. Ethnicity, gender, and depressive symptoms in older workers. *The Gerontologist* 1998; 38(1):71–79.

Freimuth VS. Narrowing the cancer knowledge gap between whites and African Americans. Monographs. *J Natl Cancer Inst* 1993; 14:81–91.

Fries JF. The compression of morbidity: near or far? *Millbank Q* 1989; 67(2):208–223.

Gallop CJ. Health information-seeking behavior and older African American women. *Bull Medical Library Assoc* 1997; 85(2):141–146.

Gazmarian JA, et al. Health literacy among Medicare enrollees in a managed care organization. *JAMA* 1999; 281(6):545–551.

German PS, Shapiro S. Heterogeneity and multiple risk factors in aging populations: implications for research. In: *Public health and aging.* Hicky, Speers, Prohaska: Johns Hopkins University Press, 1997: 198–206.

Hagan D, Ebly E, Fung TS. Disease, disability, and age in cognitively intact seniors. results from the Canadian Study of Health and Aging. *J Gerontol* 1999; 54a(2):77–82.

Haug M (ed). *Elderly patients and their doctors.* New York: Springer, 1981.

Health information for older adults. Focus Group Report, 1995. Consumer Reactions to Information about Medicare Choice, 1995. www.spry.org/projdesc.htm.

Institute on Aging. *Caring for the elders: Geriatrics in ethnic communities.* Philadelphia: Temple University: 1997: 1.

Kart, CS. *The realities of aging.* Toledo, OH: University of Toledo, 1997.

Kemper D, Lorig K, Mettler M. The effectiveness of medical self-care interventions: a focus on self-initiated responses to symptoms. *Patient Educ Counsel* 1993; 21:29–39.

Konrad TR. The patterns of self-care among older adults in Western industrialized societies. In Ory MG, DeFriese GH: *Self-care in later life, research, program and policy issues.* New York: Springer, 1998: 1–2.

Levanthal EA, et al. Conservation of energy, uncertainty reduction, and swift utilization of medical care among the elderly. Study II. *Medical Care* 1995; 33(10):988–1000

Low health literacy skills increase annual health care expenditures by $73 billion. Fact Sheet. Washington, DC: National Academy on an Aging Society, 1999.

Manchester J. Aging Boomers and retirement: who is at risk? *Generations* 1997; XXI:19.

Miles TP (ed). *Full-color aging: fact, goals and recommendations for America's diverse elders.* Washington, DC: GSA, 1999.

Moody HR. Cross cultural geriatric ethnics: negotiating our differences. *Generations* 1998; XXII:32–39.

Moon A, et al. Awareness and utilization of community long term care services by elderly Korean and non-Hispanic white Americans. *The Gerontologist* 1998; 38(3):309–316.

Morgan DL. Facts and figures about the Baby Boom. *Generations* 1998; XXII:14.

Morrow DG, et al. Icons improve older and younger adults' comprehension of medication information. *J Gerontol Psychol Sci* 1998; 53b(4):240–254.

Musick MA, et al. Religious activity and depression among community dwelling elderly persons with cancer: the moderating effect of race. *J Gerontol Soc Sci* 1998; 53b(4):S218–S227.

National Long Term Care Survey. Press Release. April 18, 1999. Source: www.nih.gov/nia/news.

Neugarten BL. Age groups in American society and the rise of the young old. *Ann Soc Pol Sci* 1974; 415:187–198.

NIH News Release. December 4, 1998. www.spry.org.

Olshansky SJ, Rudberg MA. Postponing disability: identifying points of decline and potential intervention. In: *Public health and aging.* Hicky, Speers, Prohaska: Johns Hopkins University Press, 1997: 238–251.

Peek CW, Coward RT, Henretta JC. Differences by race in the decline of health over time. *J Gerontol Soc Sci* 1997; 52b(6):S336–S344.

Petrisek AC, et al. The treatment decision-making process: age differences in a sample of women recently diagnosed with non-recurrent, early stage breast cancer. *The Gerontologist* 1997; 37(5):598–608.

Rakowski W, et al. Information seeking about health in a community sample of adults: correlates and associations with other health related practices. *Health Educ Q* 1990; 17(4):379–393.

Reynolds S, Crimmins EM, Saito Y. Cohort differences in disability and disease presence. *The Gerontologist* 1998; 38(5):578–590.

Rowe JW, Kahn RL. Successful aging. *The Gerontologist* 1997; 37(4):433–440.

Seniors enticed to join Web. *The Philadelphia Inquirer* May 23, 1999.

Soldo BJ, et al. Asset and health dynamics among the oldest old: an overview of the AHEAD study. *J Gerontol* 1997; 52b(Special Issue):1–20.

Stoller EP. Dynamics and processes of self-care in old age. In: *Self-care in later life*. New York: Springer, 1998: 24–61.

Stoller EP. Patterns of physician utilization by the elderly: a multivariate analysis. *Med Care* 1982; XX(11):1080–1089.

Stoller EP, et al. January Self-care responses to symptoms by older people. A health diary study of illness behavior. *Med Care* 1993; 31(1):24–42.

Sundquist J, Winkleby MA. Cardiovascular risk factors in
Mexican American adults. A transcultural analysis of NHANES
III. 1988. *Am J Public Health* 1999; 89(5):994.
The Public Policy and Aging Report. February, 1998, p. 8.
Thoits PA. Stress, coping and social support processes: where
are we? What next? *J Health Soc Beh* 1995; (Extra Issues)
53–79.
Turk-Charles S. Age differences in information seeking among
cancer patients. *Int J Aging Hum Dev* 1997; 45(2):85–98.
U.S. Census Bureau. Sixty-five plus in the US.
www.census.gov/socdemo.
Wallace RB. Variability in disease manifestations in older
adults. In: *Public health and aging.* Hicky, Speers, Prohaska:
Johns Hopkins University Press, 1997: 75–86.
White SL. Promoting healthy diets and active lives to hard to
reach groups: market research study. *Public Health Rep* 1990;
105(3):224–231.
Williamson K. Discovered by chance: the role of incidental
information acquisition in an ecological model of information
use. *Library Information Science Research* 1998; 20(1):23–40.
Zedlewski S, et al. *The needs of the elderly in the 21st century.*
Washington, DC: Urban Institute Press, 1990: 73.

19 CHAPTER

Women's Health: Women as the (Not-so-New) Healthcare Consumer

Julianna S. Gonen, Ph.D.

INTRODUCTION

The 1990s have seen a number of changes in healthcare delivery in the United States—changes in how care is financed and delivered, as well as in how individuals interact with the healthcare system. These phenomena have occurred neither in a vacuum nor unrelated to one another. The evolution of healthcare delivery into managed care systems, combined with ever-increasing advances in medical and information technology, has served to activate individuals in their roles as healthcare consumers.

At the same time, women's health—a fairly broad term that comprises biological/medical and psychosocial dimensions—has become a prominent area of inquiry and action in scientific study, politics, and consumer activism. The last two decades have seen hard-fought recognition won on a broad scale of various long-standing inequities in women's health, from research to access. The historical exclusion of women from pharmacological research, for example, was remedied through changes in federal policy, and there is a growing (although by no means universal) awareness that gender-neutral medicine is no longer adequate. Although some of these changes have been led from within the scientific and medical establishments, they have also been spurred by consumer activism and the movement for women's equality.

Women's health includes conditions that are unique to women or some subgroups of women, more prevalent among women or some subgroups of women, more serious among women or some subgroups of women, associated with different risk factors for women, and amenable to interventions that may be different for women or some subgroups of women (Jacobs Institute of Women's Health). To understand how women's health fits into the current consumerism in healthcare, it is not only current trends and changes that are relevant. For although consumerism has reached new levels, women have in fact always been more active healthcare consumers than men, largely because of their social roles as family caregivers. It is a commonly cited belief that women make 70% to 80% of family healthcare decisions in the United States (Alpern, 1987; Callister, 1994; Center for Women Policy Studies, 1994; Christensen & Inguanzo, 1989; LaFleur & Taylor, 1996; Public Health Service, 1987). Their roles include making decisions about choosing health plans and physicians and making and keeping appointments for all members of the family. Thus, in some respects, "consumerism" has always characterized women's position within the healthcare system. In addition, women spend nearly two of every three healthcare dollars and purchase close to 60% of all prescription medications (CareData Reports, 1998).

This chapter explores women's health consumerism, first by providing some historical context within which to understand how women have historically functioned as patients and providers of care, and the role of women's healthcare activism in shaping the U.S. healthcare system. From there, the focus shifts to the individual consumer level to describe women's roles as family healthcare decision makers and the factors that drive that role. Recognition of this role by the healthcare system and various institutions' responses to that awareness is also explored. Finally, women's health is placed back into the broader context of the new healthcare consumerism.

ORGANIZED WOMEN'S HEALTH CONSUMERISM

Women's traditional role as family caretaker, which has by no means disappeared with the advent of greater numbers of women working outside the home, has meant that women have generally served as the manager of family healthcare needs. However, women's individual roles as primary healthcare managers and consumers is not a new phenomenon. In fact, a relatively organized women's health "megamovement" has existed for at least the past 150 years in the United States; indeed, women have been the perennial healthcare reformers (Weisman, 1998). Although the particular issues or agenda of the organized women's health movement may change over time, certain elements have remained relatively constant. These constants include a coincidence with other reform movements; leadership by white, middle-class women; and the use of organizational strategies to change healthcare. Weisman also cites several key themes that can be identified when studying women's health movements at different points in time. Perhaps most relevant to today's new healthcare consumer and readers of this book is that women have always demanded health information and education. Thus, women's healthcare consumerism in the 1990s has a substantial historical legacy. Other key themes include an ongoing effort by women to control fertility and childbearing and efforts by women to participate in the healthcare system as care providers. A brief look at the various stages of this movement will thus help the reader better understand women's health consumerism at the close of the twentieth century.

The Nineteenth and Early Twentieth Centuries

Although women's health issues have often constituted a central concern of the broader women's rights movement, the women's health movement must also be understood within the context of the overall state of medicine and public health, and indeed other reform movements. During the 1830s and 1840s, for example, the era of the Popular Health Movement, medicine was relatively unregulated and unorganized. Ladies physiological societies proliferated, as did women lay practitioners. The focus during this time was health education, self-help, and disease prevention (Weisman, 1998). Socially, women and men occupied distinctly separate spheres, with few women working outside the home in the paid labor force.

After the Civil War, a significant component of the women's health movement was a campaign against contraception and abortion. The former was seen as encouraging male promiscuity and exploitation of women, and the latter was opposed both on moral grounds and for professional turf reasons by the increasingly organized medical profession that opposed midwives and other lay practitioners providing care to women. During this era, women began to make initial inroads into medicine themselves. Elizabeth Blackwell became America's first female physician in 1849; her sister Emily followed suit shortly thereafter. The former opened the Women's Medical College in 1868, which, along with several other similar institutions, trained women in medicine until existing medical schools began accepting women at the turn of the century. At the same time, other reform movements were under way, including those for temperance and women's suffrage. The central focus within women's health was reproductive health, and subsequent generations of women's health reformers have struggled with expanding the conception of women's health beyond their reproductive roles.

During the Progressive Era (the late nineteenth and early twentieth centuries), the countermovement to *increase* access to birth control dominated, eventually resulting in the relaxation of prohibitive public policy around contraception. Reduction of maternal and infant mortality also became a dominant issue. This focus led not only to a significant expansion of maternal and child healthcare funded by the federal government but also to changes in physician practice to include preventive services such as prenatal care (Weisman, 1998). Thus, women's health reforms had both a substantial impact on a government health program that remains in effect today and on medical practice. This lesson is worth noting while exploring current women's health consumer activism.

The Modern Era

The next surge in women's health activism came when activism was defining the times—the 1960s. Perhaps more so than in the past, women's health was explicitly linked to the broader resurgent women's liberation movement. Reproduction was again a critical issue, but changing sexual mores meant more of a focus on access to birth control and, eventually, abortion. The advent of the oral contraceptive pill in the early 1960s was a critical element in this. Like the first organized women's health movement in the early to mid-1800s, self-help reemerged as a theme. Distrust of the medical establishment, particularly of unsafe or untested products and procedures, led to the establishment of women-controlled clinics and birth centers. There was also a movement to de-medicalize childbirth and loosen the hegemony of obstetricians.* Again, women's health activists influenced public policy in the healthcare arena, as they were successful in pushing greater government regulation of medical products and drugs. During this time, myriad women's health advocacy organizations were formed—some 250 identifiable organizations and approximately 2,000 informal groups and projects (Ruzek, 1998). In the meantime, women also began to enter the medical profession in increasing numbers. Thus, women would exert influence both from outside the system, as reform advocates, and from within, as practitioners.

In the 1980s and 1990s, attention to women's health continued to grow, and as the times changed, so too did the movement, with the addition of a more mainstream, professionalized layer. This in part resulted from the presence of more women in science and medicine, as well as in policy-making roles.

The recognition that women's historical exclusion from biomedical research has led to a dearth of knowledge of the effects of accepted therapies on women led to changes in policy at the federal level, first at the NIH and then at the FDA. These changes were championed largely by the Congressional Caucus

---

* Interestingly, a centerpiece of the backlash against managed healthcare in the mid-1990s was a controversy over shortened hospital stays for childbirth. The push for minimum mandatory lengths of stay, however, was championed more by professional provider groups (e.g., the American College of Obstetricians and Gynecologists) than by women's health consumer advocates.

for Women's Issues, established in 1977. No longer can federally funded research exclude women, and new drugs must include gender analysis to be approved by the FDA. By the late 1990s, all of the major health agencies of the federal government (in addition to those just named, the Centers for Disease Control and Prevention [CDC] and the Department of Health and Human Services [DHHS] overall) have established offices of women's health within their structures to promote attention to women's particular healthcare needs.

Although advances such as this share a similarity to past policy changes led by women in that their effect was an improvement in the health of women (and indeed everyone), the victories of the 1980s and 1990s also differ in an important respect. Unlike the efforts of Progressive Era women around maternal and child health, and of 1960s and 1970s activists around product safety, the reforms of the past two decades have been led largely by women leaders working *within* the government and the biomedical establishment, rather than outside of it. Indeed, the organized women's health movement of the 1990s has departed in significant ways from its predecessor. Lay leadership has given way to, but not entirely been replaced by, professionalism. Whereas safety was the galvanizing issue 20 to 30 years ago, the call today is for equity. The counterculture roots of earlier organizations, which caused them to eschew any associations with corporate or pharmaceutical entities, have been replaced by a willingness to accept capitalist largesse to promote organizational goals. And although the 1960s and 1970s saw an emphasis on lay control of health and healing, the push now is to establish women physicians and scientists as legitimate authorities (Ruzek, 1998). In addition, the term *women's health center* had in the past connoted a grassroots, community-based women-controlled clinic; such centers are now often found within institutional settings such as hospitals, which use them to market to women, the recognized majority of proactive healthcare consumers.

Consumer-Oriented Women's Health Organizations Today

The 1990s have seen a new cast of professional women's health leaders emerge, pressing for change within government and medicine. This does not mean, however, that consumer-driven reform efforts have fallen by the wayside. To the contrary, some of the grassroots-based organizations that had their genesis in the 1960s and 1970s remain active today, and they have been joined by a host of disease-specific advocacy groups that have proliferated.

Two of the more prominent general consumer-focused women's health organizations are the National Women's Health Network (NWHN) and the Boston Women's Health Book Collective, publisher of *Our Bodies, Ourselves*, the "grandmother" of consumer health publications. A classic from the grassroots women's health movement that has become a staple in many women's libraries, *Our Bodies, Ourselves* was first sold in newsprint in 1970. By 1996, it had sold nearly 4 million copies, including revised, foreign language, and special topic editions.

The Network, formed in the mid-1970s, retains much of that era's emphasis on remaining skeptical of the advice and treatment given to women by the government and the medical establishment. A sample of language from some of the organization's promotional material is illustrative:

> Some doctors—and even many pharmaceutical companies—may claim to know what's best for you. But you are the one who ultimately has to make that decision. To do this, you need to be informed. That's why the National Women's Health Network is such a valuable resource for women. The Network has been the one voice of truth in a sea of hyperbole about hormones and menopause—and many other issues affecting women. [The Network is] one of the only sources of information still independent of pharmaceutical companies and government influence and one of the few that truly can be trusted for information on women's health (NWHN fundraising solicitation letter, 1999).

These two consumer-oriented institutions of the women's health movement have allied themselves so that individuals joining the Network receive free copies of the Collective's publications as a member benefit. Other women's organizations whose agendas do not focus solely on healthcare, such as the National Partnership for Women and Families (formerly the Women's Legal Defense Fund) also devote considerable resources to advocating women's health issues. It is in fact telling to note that during the push for federal legislation to regulate managed healthcare (the push for "patients' rights") in 1998, the

Partnership was the designated informal leader of a broad coalition of both consumer and professional organizations advocating passage of a federal bill. Women's stake in a reformed healthcare system has meant that, once again, women are the perennial reform leaders.

In addition to these generalist organizations, other groups advocate for particular groups of women healthcare consumers. These include the Older Women's League (OWL), the National Asian Women's Health Organization (NAWHO), the National Black Women's Health Project, and the Lesbian Health Fund (LHF). White, middle-class women have long held hegemony in organized women's health activism, and these subgroup-specific organizations speak to the multiple inequities experienced when one is both female and a member of a minority group.

A third category of organized women's health consumer groups encompasses the disease-specific organizations, such as the National Breast Cancer Coalition (NBCC), the National Osteoporosis Foundation (NOF), and the recently formed Ovarian Cancer National Alliance. NBCC is an example of a subset of women's health activists that is extremely well organized and that has succeeded in raising the nation's consciousness around breast cancer to a striking degree. In fact, some argue that they have been almost too successful because many U.S. women have developed an exaggerated perception of their risk of breast cancer, while remaining dangerously ignorant of conditions that are responsible for comparatively greater morbidity and mortality among women, such as heart disease.

Women continue a long tradition of informal and formal organizing to express their preferences and influence the healthcare system. But certainly not all significant action takes place through organizations or groups. This volume is concerned with the growing phenomenon of consumerism in healthcare, and for reasons already described, women may indeed be the foremost practitioners of this trend. Thus, women's health consumerism at the individual level becomes the focus in the next section.

WOMEN AS INDIVIDUAL HEALTHCARE CONSUMERS

The evolving healthcare delivery system, the advent of women's health as a field of study, and the new consumer environment all warrant attention to the ways in which women as healthcare consumers access information about health and healthcare services, as well as attention to the types of information that influence women's interactions with the healthcare system. This section describes the kinds of information that women find credible and the types of information they seek and prefer.*

In the current era, the ability to assimilate information about healthcare is more possible, more critical, and more complex than ever before, largely because information is available more quickly and through more channels. "Women's strong desire for information about health products and services has created a nationwide industry in newsletters, pamphlets, and seminars from women's health centers, drug companies, and physicians" (Braus, 1997). Also, new forms of health plan and insurance arrangements proliferate. All of these trends, although exciting and full of promise for better-informed and healthier consumers, make the task of gathering and processing healthcare information monumental.

Profiles of Women as Healthcare Consumers

While all of these changes are taking place, women's roles as the primary caretakers and managers of their own and their families' health have not changed. Women tend to serve as the gatekeepers of their families' health and make most of the family healthcare decisions (Alpern, 1987; Callister, 1994; Center for Women Policy Studies, 1994; Christensen & Inguanzo, 1989; LaFleur & Taylor, 1996; Public Health Service, 1987). As stated in the *Women's Health Data Book*, "Women often take responsibility for the family's health, and it has been suggested that this role serves to enhance their interest in health. Women are also more likely than men to have a regular source of healthcare and a regular source of health information" (Horton, 1995). One study found that men were nearly three times more likely than women to be influenced to seek healthcare by a member of the opposite sex, and it concluded that women exert an important influence on the decisions of men to seek healthcare (Norcross et al., 1996). Other reports show that 26% of women but only 16%

---

* Portions of this section were derived from a white paper prepared for Merck & Co. in January 1998 entitled "Women's Health Care Decision Making: Lessons from the Literature."

of men are very interested in receiving materials regularly from healthcare providers, and more women (25%) than men (11%) regularly read about healthcare (American Hospital Association, 1990).

Recent survey data also bear this out. A 1996 survey by the Kaiser Family Foundation and the Agency for Health Care Policy and Research (AHCPR) asked respondents *who in the household makes most of the decisions related to healthcare*; more women (63%) than men (41%) reported making this decision alone. Another survey by CareData Reports, also in 1996, found that nearly all women respondents (95%) enrolled in a managed care organization had been responsible for deciding on a health plan for their families. The statistical portrait of the woman choosing the family health plan, which will cover at least two members of her family, revealed that she was 39 years old, slightly more likely to be married than single, believes herself to be very healthy, and has a household income of $43,000 per year; in addition, there is a one in four chance that she holds a college degree. When survey respondents were presented with reasons for choosing a health plan, women put more emphasis on affordability and on the option to continue with their current physician than did men and were more likely to use friends for advice (CareData Reports, 1998).

The tension between women's traditionally passive roles vis-à-vis healthcare providers, particularly physicians, and their responsibilities as the healthcare managers for themselves and their families makes the task of providing appropriate information to women complex. A recent Hastings Center Report editorial, for example, criticized the federal decision to reissue mammography guidelines for women aged 40 to 50 in 1997. The guidelines as first issued conceded that the evidence was mixed and did not take a firm stance on whether women in this age group should undergo regular mammographic examination. When this was assailed as failing women and jeopardizing their health, the panel reissued the guidelines with an affirmative recommendation. The editorial asserted that the "potentially offensive underlying message" in this reversal was that women cannot be given ambiguous information, even if that is the current state of the science, lest they become confused (Hastings

Center Report, 1997). As this example illustrates, although it is vital that women receive clear and accurate information to enable them to make informed healthcare decisions, this need should not be distorted in a paternalistic fashion by giving women simplistic information if a definitive answer simply does not yet exist. Women want answers, but they also want the truth.

The fact that women have generally been found to be the healthcare decision makers is not lost on the providers and institutions within the healthcare system that must market their services to consumers (e.g., Alpern, 1987). A recent study of women's health centers and marketing of services to women stated that the research supports marketing to women because they are the primary consumers and decision makers and that the logical conclusion is that if a woman is a satisfied patient of a hospital's women's health center, other family members will be likely to use the hospital when the need arises (LaFleur & Taylor, 1996).

Health plans also recognize women's important decision-making role, and they attempt to convey their proactive approaches to women's health to consumers. The American Association of Health Plans (AAHP), the national trade association for managed healthcare plans, recently published a series of consumer guides to best practices in women's health, highlighting programs of member plans in the areas of obstetrics and prenatal care, domestic violence, breast cancer, and hormone replacement and mid-life issues.

Where and How Do Women Receive Their Healthcare Information?

Consumers, and women in particular, have many avenues through which they may receive healthcare information that affects their interactions with the healthcare system. These avenues include the healthcare industry itself (e.g., individual providers and institutions, medical journals, health guides, health newsletters, pharmaceutical companies), employer-purchasers of healthcare (e.g., benefits managers, worksite health promotion programs, employee assistance programs), the government (e.g., Medicare and Medicaid programs, health departments, federal health agencies), the media (e.g., television, radio, the Internet, magazines, books), and social networks (e.g., friends, family, community). The relative credibility and type of information conveyed by each, and its influence on women's health consumerism, varies.

Credibility of Health Information Sources

The credibility of the information women receive is typically associated with who produced it and who endorses it. Information from interviews with more than 50 women in the United States and Canada, aged 16 to 77, elicited the sources of health information that they found credible. Books were found to be the most trusted source; consumers believed they had the most control over the information absorbed through books over any other source. Community health nurses also topped the list as one of the most credible information sources. They were followed by "specialists" and then doctors in general, dentists, and hospital nurses. Some interviewees said that they trusted their mothers as a source of health information; others did not. None indicated that they used fathers or brothers as information sources. Teachers, interestingly, ranked at the low end of the credibility scale (Crook, 1995).

The Kaiser/AHCPR survey mentioned earlier asked consumers to rate the believability of various sources of information about the quality of healthcare (Table 19–1). Friends and family topped the list, with 50% rating them as "very believable," followed by patient satisfaction surveys, which were at 34%. Individual doctors were rated in the top category by 29% of respondents, followed by employers at 19%. Independent organizations that evaluate health plans were rated very believable by 19% of respondents, and health plans themselves were close behind at 12%. Groups of doctors were not trusted nearly as much as individual doctors; only 9% rated them very believable. Government agencies and the media rounded out the bottom of the believability ranking, at 7% and 5%, respectively. Differences in responses between women and men were not terribly pronounced; the largest gender disparity emerged in the trust of doctors, as 26% of men ranked individual physicians in the top

TABLE 19–1

Believability of Information Sources on Quality of Healthcare (percentage reporting source as "very believable")

Information Source	All	Women	Men
Friends and family	50	50	49
Patient satisfaction surveys	34	36	32
Individual doctors	29	32	26
Employers	19	19	19
Independent organizations that evaluate plans	19	18	19
Health plans and health insurance companies	12	14	11
Groups of doctors like state medical societies	9	11	7
Government agencies	7	7	6
Newspapers, television, other media	5	5	4

Data source: Kaiser Family Foundation and Agency for Health Care Policy and Research, "Americans as Health Care Consumers: The Role of Quality Information," national survey of 2,006 adults conducted by Princeton Survey Research Associates, 1996.

category of believability, whereas 32% of women did so. Minor differences were found between women and men in believability of patient satisfaction surveys and groups of doctors (36% versus 32%, respectively).

The Kaiser/AHCPR survey also asked a similar but more focused question about how good selected sources would be in assessing the quality of health insurance plans. The gender differences were more pronounced on this question than on the general question about information source believability about healthcare quality generally; 74% of women but only 64% of men rated friends and family as good sources, and 46% of women and 36% of men ranked physicians as good sources. Employers were thought to be good sources by 40% of women and 33% of men. It was noted earlier that women have demonstrated considerable interest in information about healthcare plans, more so than men, therefore the more specific nature of this question may have served to elicit a greater gender disparity in responses.

As suggested by the Kaiser study, the information women find most credible varies; some rank media near the top, whereas others place it near the bottom. Furthermore, friends and family seem to consistently rate higher than the medical profession in terms of credibility. Perhaps more revealing is the particular *kinds* of information women seek.

Health Information Content

The degree to which women find a source of health information credible and trustworthy depends on the type of information being sought. That is, women will look to different sources for information on choosing health plans and providers, prevention, clinical aspects of disease, coping strategies, self-care, and information on expectations of the treatment experience. Physicians may be the preferred source for clinical information, but experiential information is more likely to be sought from a woman's social network.

Moreover, women's receptivity to healthcare information varies by education level, language spoken, and culture. Health education interventions must reflect the normative and symbolic reality of the focal audience, taking into account, among many considerations, the myriad factors that render women different and affect their receptivity to information, as well as their ability to act on it, including their present circumstances and prior experiences. Health education messages may fall short if such critical markers are not considered carefully. For example, with mammography, health education messages tend to be tailored on the assumption that women seek mammograms out of a sense of risk/fear of breast cancer. Yet the results of a study of older, low-income rural women found that risk may *not* be part of their decision-making process around receiving mammograms, which were provided free through the local health department (Holden, 1996). Sensitive targeting of women, taking into account their unique "systems," has been linked to positive behaviors in specific ethnic groups (Pierson, 1996)—an important implication for the development of public health campaigns. For example, Philadelphia's "Prevention of HIV in Women and Infants Demonstration Project," which targeted low-income African-American women in Philadelphia at risk for HIV, STDs and unplanned pregnancy, used special print materials involving role model stories to increase condom use by these women. These were "real-life" stories of women from the target audience who had successfully initiated or maintained condom use with their sexual partners. The materials' credibility was enhanced by references to the local community, culturally specific mores and norms, and the use of understandable language (Bond et al., 1997). Another study found that "culturally embedded" messages yielded the greatest increase in self-efficacy among African-American women, even in the face of barriers. The study also concluded that such culturally embedded messages can lead to enhanced behavioral outcomes.

Like culture, education also has a direct and important effect on how receptive consumers will be to information and how equipped they are to act on it. Lower reading ability, for example, has been correlated significantly with less mammography knowledge, which in turn depresses utilization. When developing targeted health education messages, researchers have recommended screening for reading level, which would identify the subset of low-income patients that would benefit from specialized educational efforts, particularly nonprint methods such as peer groups, stories, and videos (Davis et al., 1996). A study of misconceptions about gynecological cancers found that formal education correlated positively with correct responses to survey questions about cancer and concluded that individuals with the least formal education constitute an especially important target group for information (Carlsson & Strang, 1997). Another study found education to be one of the strongest factors correlated with use of Pap tests and mammography for women of all races (Edwards, 1995).

The 1996 Kaiser/AHCPR survey, in asking a number of questions relating to the *content* of information (versus *credibility*, see Table 19–1), revealed some noticeable gender differences regarding *how much various types of information revealed about the overall quality of a healthcare plan*. Women placed more emphasis on waiting time for appointments than did overall respondents, placing it above patient turnover resulting from dissatisfaction. Women also rated independent accreditation over physician turnover as a quality indicator. For women, patients' own quality ratings were ranked higher than patient reports regarding physician listening and explaining. Some of the most pronounced differences between women and men were in the weight accorded to independent accreditation (14% difference), patients' quality ratings (10%), percentage of plan members receiving screenings (9%), health improvement programs offered (8%), and ease of specialist access (7%). Again, this question focused on health plans, an area in which women have had to become proactive information seekers and navigators, which may explain the more pronounced gender differences in how various types of information are rated.

The Growth in Marketing to Women by Managed Care Organizations   As health insurance increasingly evolves into organized, prepaid managed care plans, these plans, particularly those in competitive markets, aggressively market to consumers to gain enrollment. Managed care organizations view women as the family healthcare decision makers and target their outreach marketing specifically to women. For the consumer, navigating this information for "comparison shopping" for both quality of service and access to services can be challenging. A national survey for Towers Perrin conducted by Louis Harris and Associates revealed significant differences between men and women in terms of their information needs when selecting a health plan (Isaacs, 1997). Women were found to be the more knowledgeable and astute health plan consumers because they read the plan materials and needed more detailed and pertinent information than men did. This was not considered surprising because women use the healthcare system more than men, managing the care for their families and visiting physicians when they are healthy as well as when they are sick. Specific findings were that women were more familiar with the content of their health plans; women say they need a lot more information about their choices in health plans, including the specialists in the plan, medical information on illnesses and conditions, and medications; and women focus significantly more on critical issues in choosing health plans, such as the quality of the doctors and the reputations of physicians and hospitals. The study concluded that the healthcare industry needs to give consumers, particularly women, better information about health plans.

Other surveys and focus groups have found that the factors women look to when choosing a health plan are as follows (in descending order of importance): whether a plan includes a preferred physician (the primary care physician and/or OB/GYN), the level of inpatient coverage, the inclusion of a preferred hospital, the plan's reputation, cost aspects (premiums, co-payments, lifetime caps), the scope of services covered, the ability to self-refer to a specialist, and the inclusion of dental and mental health benefits. Women have also indicated that they would be more likely to select a health plan if it included a women's health center (Stone, 1996).

Recognizing women's proactive approach to healthcare, health plans use numerous forms of information to attempt to influence women. The strategies that they use, in descending order of effectiveness (in the health plans' view), include the following: newsletters in the mail, direct mail, cross-marketing through physicians, media (e.g., television, newspaper, radio), open houses, billboards, and information distributed through employers (Stone, 1996).

Respondents to the 1996 Kaiser/AHCPR survey were also asked whether they had actually *used* information they had seen comparing health plans in making any decisions; one-third said that they had, and no gender differences emerged. They were then asked how much influence various sources of information would have on their choice if they *had* to choose a new health plan. The sources cited as most influential by women and men mirrored separately the overall responses, with only moderate differences in how many cited a source as very influential. The largest gender differences occurred in the top two sources: individual physicians (a 5% gender difference) and friends and family (a 6% gender difference). The same question about these same sources of information was asked of respondents if they had to choose a *hospital;* the same three sources—individual physicians, friends and family, and patient satisfaction surveys—came out on top, but gender differences were even less evident.

The survey also asked consumers to rank two principal information sources against one another; specifically, "Whose recommendation would affect their choice of a health plan if they *had* to choose between two plans—their friends' or that of experts?" For health plans, respondents were more likely to choose the one recommended by friends (52%) over the one rated highly by experts (43%). This difference was more pronounced for men (54% chose friends and 43% chose experts) than it was for women, who split 51% to 44% in favor of friends. For hospitals, those surveyed were asked, if they *had* to choose between two different hospitals, whether they would choose the one they had used for many years or a different hospital that was rated much higher. Here the disparity was much greater; 72% would select the familiar hospital and only 25% the highly rated one. This breakdown was approximately the same for men and women.

These survey responses appear to suggest that personal familiarity with the source of information may have more influence on consumer behavior than expert status. Individual physicians topped the lists when they were a response option, but when general "experts" go up against consumers' social networks, the latter are cited as more influential.

"Effectiveness" of Information: Physicians and Nurses Wield Influence
The aforementioned notwithstanding, literature on the effectiveness of various types of information in influencing women's healthcare-seeking behavior reveals that physicians, not surprisingly, wield considerable influence, as do nurses. For example, several studies confirm the importance of physicians as information sources, positively influencing mammography use (Coll et al., 1989; Fox & Stein, 1991; Grady et al., 1992; Sutton & Donner, 1992). Not only does physician advice positively influence adherence to mammography screening guidelines, women themselves indicate that they want their physicians to provide reminders to schedule mammograms (Horton, Cruess, & Romans, 1996). Other components of women's "information environment," such as family and friends, can also be important in influencing mammography use, but physician influence is still found to be the primary determinant (Pearlman, Rakowski, & Ehrich, 1995). One recent study found that the most important predictor of women's ever using hormone replacement therapy was a healthcare provider recommendation (Walsh et al., 1997).

Physicians can influence not only women's decisions regarding whether to receive certain services (e.g., mammography), but they can also be a critical source of information for women who are already in the system with a diagnosis and need to know how to proceed further with treatment. For example, in one examination of how women reached their decision for surgical treatment of breast cancer, subjects overwhelmingly listed the physician as the most important source of information used to make their surgical treatment decisions (Bisel, 1996).

At least one study (Degner et al., 1997), however, has found a substantial discrepancy between women's preferred and attained levels of involvement in making decisions about treatment. This discrepancy points to one critical problem with physicians serving as women's primary motivating information source regarding their healthcare choices: because of socialization around both women's roles and the authority and deference given physicians, women may often feel that they lack autonomy in making decisions about their own health. One retrospective study of the characteristics of decisions by women who had undergone elective hysterectomies found that nearly half did not in fact *make* a decision to have a hysterectomy. Nearly the same number believed they had no choice or were not given alternatives, and several indicated that their physicians had made the decision (Harris, 1993). It has been suggested that among the factors that create the conditions for shared decision making, as opposed to unilateral physician direction of the course of care, are decreasing asymmetry in the relationship between provider and patient and teaching patients about their problems (Andrist, 1993). This same study found that "women's prior experiences with physicians raised their consciousness about the kind of care they wanted—and moved them from silence to action in seeking care in which they could participate in decisions." The drawbacks to relying on physicians and nurses to impart information thus include the risk of undue influence and a lessening of women's autonomy and access barriers that prevent many women from even encountering this effective source of health information.

Popular Literature as a Source of Information

Popular magazines are cited as highly used sources of healthcare information for women. However, several studies cast a degree of doubt upon the quality of information that these sources are imparting. A content analysis of a sample of breast cancer and breast cancer screening messages in women's magazines from 1982 to 1992—conducted "because magazines are a primary means for the dissemination of breast cancer screening messages and are used by many women as sources of information on health issues"—found that the media constructs the breast cancer experience as a battle between technology and cancer, with women virtually absent. The magazines sampled in this analysis also portrayed women as incapable, frustrated consumers of healthcare or as passive victims. The study argues that the mediated coverage of breast cancer actually discourages adherence to screening guidelines by creating contradictions between risk, screening, and treatment information (Olive, 1996).

Although the information and prescriptive messages contained in magazines will not necessarily lead directly to women making the prescribed decisions, they do contribute to the context of whatever decisions are made. Such messages also will likely affect the pursuit of additional information; research has shown that information available in popular media seems to affect doctor–patient encounters, prompting women to ask particular questions based on information received outside the medical visit.

Thus, a complex picture of women's healthcare information-seeking behavior emerges. As the literature suggests, it would be too limiting to conclude that any one information source will suffice to impart any and all health information to women. In some instances, it may be the physician who will most effectively convey the message; at other times, a trusted friend or a health advocacy organization will be better heard. Most critically, to be received and valued, health messages and information must match the educational level and cultural context of the intended recipient. If information cannot be understood, it will have little effect on healthcare choices.

CONCLUSION

This review has attempted to draw out the lessons from the available literature and identify areas in which additional inquiry is needed. Specifically, it has examined the *sources* of women's healthcare information, the content and "format" of this information, and the effect that psychosocial, cultural, and educational factors have on women's access to information. Measuring the actual influence of various types of information is difficult, as tantalizing as these questions are. Numerous factors affect individual choices and behavior, making it difficult to trace an action or decision to one precise information source. Nonetheless, there is a growing body of literature that attempts to discern what kinds of information are more likely to have some effect on women's health decisions.

Among the important findings of this emerging body of work are the following:

- Women generally seek more health information than do men.
- Women are not well served by messages that oversimplify important health information; information should be clear and accessible, but not simplified to the point of being rendered meaningless.
- Although women tend to look to popular magazines for health information, some studies suggest that this should be done with caution because the messages may be misleading.
- Health information must be presented to women in a way that accounts for their cultural context, including ethnicity, educational level, income, and prior experiences.
- Physicians continue to serve an important informational role for women, but more emphasis is now being placed on ensuring that reliance on physicians does not compromise women's own personal autonomy in healthcare decision making.
- Lack of access to the healthcare system naturally limits the availability of healthcare professionals as information sources.
- Women's social networks are often as strong an influence as healthcare professionals; education, income, and literacy level often serve as intervening factors mediating which proves a greater influence on women's healthcare decisions.

This emerging picture paints a clear message: women are discerning and increasingly "empowered" consumers. Their decision-making processes are complex and are affected by both medical and nonmedical factors, including cultural, educational, and psychosocial influences unique to their life experiences. In addition, the information they seek is as varied as the reasons for their search. Thus, mapping out women's information sources and assessing their relative influence is likewise a complex task. It is nonetheless a critical one, which may then inform future efforts to communicate vital health information to women, as they navigate the increasingly complex healthcare landscape for themselves and their families. It stands to reason that better-informed healthcare consumers will ultimately be healthier, thereby increasing their own quality of life while reducing the costs of healthcare. Armed with information, consumers, and particularly women (who are the primary seekers and users of information, as they always have been), can better participate in the ongoing dialog over the future of the American healthcare system.

REFERENCES

Alpern BA. *Reaching women—the way to go in marketing healthcare services*. Chicago: Pluribus Press, 1987.

American Hospital Association. *Why women's health?* December, 1990.

Andrist LC. *A model of women-centered practice: shared decision-making between breast cancer surgeons and patients* (PhD Dissertation). Waltham, MA: Brandeis University, 1993.

Bisel DJ. *Knowledge, sources used and factors considered in the surgical treatment decisions of women with breast cancer* (MSN Thesis). Allendale, MI: Grand Valley State University, 1996.

Bond L, et al. Developing non-traditional print media for HIV prevention: role model stories for young urban women. *Am J Public Health* 1997; 87(2):289–290.

Braus P. *Marketing healthcare to women: meeting new demands for products and services*. Ithaca, NY: American Demographic Books, 1997.

Callister LC. Finding a fit: choice of a healthcare provider by childbearing women. *Clin Consult Obstet Gyn* 1994; 6:4.

CareData Reports. *In her own words: a report on survey results—women in managed care.* New York: CareData Reports, 1998.

Carlsson ME, Strang PM. Facts, misconceptions, and myths about cancer. *Gynecologic Oncology* 1997; 65:46–53.

Center for Women Policy Studies. *Women's health decision making: a review of the literature.* Washington, DC: CWPS, 1994.

Christensen M, Inguanzo JM. Smart consumers present a marketing challenge. *Hospitals* 1989; 16:42–47.

Coll PP, et al. Effects of age, education, and physician advice on utilization of screening mammography. *J Am Geriatr Soc* 1989; 37:957.

Crook M. *My body—women speak out about their health care.* New York: Plenum, 1995.

Davis TC, et al. Knowledge and attitude on screening mammography among low-literate, low-income women. *Cancer* 1996; 78(9):1912–1920.

Degner LF, et al. Information needs and decisional preferences in women with breast cancer. *JAMA* 1997; 277(18):1485–1492.

Edwards JN. *Nonfinancial barriers to women's use of cancer screening services* (PhD Dissertation). Ann Arbor, MI: University of Michigan, 1995.

Fox SA, Stein JA. The effect of physician-patient communication on mammography utilization by different ethnic groups. *Med Care* 1991; 29:1065.

Grady KE, et al. The importance of physician encouragement in breast cancer screening of older women. *Prev Med* 1992; 21:766.

Harris CM. *Women's decision making about having an elective hysterectomy* (MS Thesis). Columbus, OH: Ohio State University, 1993.

Hastings Center Report. *Complicating the mammography message.* 1997; 27:2.

Holden DJ. *The impact of perceived risk on low income, rural, postmenopausal women's decisions to get mammograms* (PhD Dissertation). Raleigh, NC: North Carolina State University, 1996.

Horton JA (ed). *The women's health data book—a profile of women's health in the United States,* 2nd ed. Washington, DC: Jacobs Institute of Women's Health, 1995.

Horton JA, Cruess DF, Romans MC. Compliance with mammography screening guidelines: 1995 mammography attitudes and usage study report. *Women's Health Issues* 1996; 6:5.

Isaacs SL. Men's and women's information needs when selecting a health plan: results of a national survey. *JAMWA* 1997; 52:2.

LaFleur EK, Taylor SL. Women's health centers and specialized services. *J Health Care Marketing* 1996; 16:3.

Norcross WA, et al. The influence of women on the healthcare-seeking behavior of men. *J Fam Pract* 1996; 43(5):475–480.

Olive TE. *Cultural and collective stories of health and illness: an analysis of women's stories and media representations of breast cancer* (PhD Dissertation). Tampa: University of South Florida, 1996.

Pearlman DN, Rakowski W, Ehrich B. The information environment of women and mammography screening: assessing reciprocity in social relationships. *J Women's Health* 1995; 4:5.

Pierson RM. *The benefits of culturally embedded health messages: targeting African-American women* (PhD Dissertation). Stanford, CT: Stanford University, 1996.

Public Health Service. *Report of the Public Health Service Task Force on Women's Health Issues,* Vol. II. Washington, DC: US Department of Health and Human Services, 1987.

Ruzek CB. *The History and Future of Women's Health.* Presentation at U.S. Public Health Service Office on Women's Health program, June 11, 1998.

Stone C. *Create an effective marketing strategy that will attract women to choose you at annual enrollment time.* Presentation at IQPC conference on Women's Health and Managed Care, Philadelphia, July 1996.

Sutton SM, Donner LD. Insights into the physician's role in mammography utilization among older women. *Women's Health Issues.* 1992; 2:275.

Walsh JME, et al. Postmenopausal hormone therapy: factors influencing women's decision making. *Menopause* 1997; 4:1.

Weisman CS. *Women's health care: activist traditions and institutional change.* Baltimore: The Johns Hopkins University Press, 1998.

20

Consumer Advocacy and Mental Health: Public Attitudes and Private Battles

Felicia Gevirtz, MSPH

INTRODUCTION

The prevailing attitude for most of the twentieth century that "the doctor knows best" has been challenged by users of health-care services over the past several years. The shift in the mental health arena is also moving away from this notion of the individual as a weak and helpless patient and moving toward more patient empowerment. "Consumer empowerment is a political movement that, among many goals, seeks to diminish the stigma and discrimination experienced by many people with severe and persistent psychiatric disorders" (Corrigan, 1997).

The purpose of this chapter is to educate readers about the struggles and successes encountered by individuals, families, and groups whose lives have been touched by mental illness. Specifically, this chapter describes the growing mental health advocacy movement and its role in furthering acceptance and respect for those affected by mental illness—family members, the medical community, and society in general.

This chapter begins with a brief history of mental illness, including treatment of the mentally ill and the societal burden of the illness. Next, the forces shaping the mental health consumer movement and the role of reforms are traced, beginning with postdeinstitutionalization in the early 1960s through today. The positive impact of the scientific advancements and technology, of the media and mass communications (e.g., the Internet, or information superhighway), and of new treatment models (e.g., managed care, community health centers) on the consumer movement are addressed.

The next section discusses federal and private initiatives aimed at improving quality of and access to care for the mentally ill. Following this, ongoing challenges and special considerations, such as confidentiality, consent, advance directives, and special patient populations (the elderly and children), are examined. Finally, appropriate treatment endpoints and quality outcomes are emphasized.

BACKGROUND

Research suggests that up to 20% of Americans suffer from some sort of mental illness, with a 14% community point prevalence for mental health problems (Byrne, 1999). Thus, about one in seven persons is impacted by at least one of the most common psychiatric conditions at some point. However, these figures are probably understated because many people are concerned about the social consequences associated with having a mental illness and thus remain untreated.

The toll of mental illness on patients, families, and society as a whole is considerable. In fact, the economic consequences of mental illness and other behavioral disorders exceed $148 billion annually (Rupp, Gause, & Regier, 1998). Much of these costs could be avoided by early and aggressive treatment of all individuals identified as having a mental illness. This group includes individuals, many of whom are elderly, who have a mental health condition, especially depression, alongside other physical conditions and illnesses. Although the mental and physical health conditions should be separated, with each illness being treated, mental health treatment is often ignored. In addition, untreated mental health conditions can actually result in physical consequences (Carlin, 1998; Dinan, 1999).

In the past, people with mental illness were subject to inhumane treatment because society believed that these individuals were to blame for their condition. Society has traditionally viewed people with mental illness as outcasts (Corrigan & Garman, 1997) and believed that these "crazy" people belonged away from society in a hospital, where they could be heavily sedated. Professionals who treated these people even believed that mental illness was caused by environmental factors, such as parental influence (Frese, 1998). Therefore, countless numbers of people with a mental illness who blamed themselves for their condition lived in despair and refused to get help, not wanting to be labeled as crazy or as an outcast, or worse yet, become hospitalized. Some were hospitalized, and the least fortunate committed suicide.

Negative public attitudes have continually plagued and negatively impacted mental healthcare. The myriad of stereotypes about mental illness has hindered the advancement of research (Byrne, 1999) and the consumer movement in mental health. The experience of mental health consumers has been dominated by such negative public perception. As a result, many mental health consumers have developed negative beliefs about their own self-worth, including the following:

- A sense of powerlessness because of the need for treatment
- Difficulties "qualifying" for housing
- Lack of work opportunities
- Social isolation
- Treatment resistance because of previously negative experiences when they were considered "noncompliant" (Corrigan & Garman, 1997)

EARLY EFFORTS TOWARD MENTAL HEALTH ADVOCACY

Changing Public Attitudes—The Early Efforts

Despite the negative mental illness "image," efforts surrounding mental health reform and consumer awareness began nearly a century ago. The earliest efforts directed toward consumer advocacy began in 1909, by Clifford Beers, who established the National Mental Health Association (NMHA). (For a complete list of the largest mental health advocacy groups, as well as other sources for more information, see Table 20–1.) However, the consumer advocacy movement remained relatively stagnant for nearly 50 years, until several events, both positive and negative, influenced many people with mental illnesses to form advocacy groups. Successful advocacy groups did not really begin until the mid to late 1960s, shortly after many institutions housing mental health patients were closed down, forcing a massive patient migration from the hospitals into the community or, in

T A B L E   20–1

Informational Sources

Nationally Recognized Consumer Help Groups

National Mental Health Association	www.nmha.org	800-969-NMHA
National Alliance for the Mentally Ill	www.nami.org	800-950-NAMI
National Institute of Mental Health	www.nih.nimh.gov	

Additional Sites of Interest

www.mhsource.com
www.mentalwellness.com
www.apa.org
www.psych.org
www.psychweb.com

General Health Web Sites with Mental Health Subsections

www.webmd.com
www.medscape.com
www.healthatoz.com
www.mwsearch.com

some cases, into the streets. In 1963, the Community Mental Health Construction Act was passed to help create community centers to assist recently released patients to integrate into the community and continue receiving treatment. Almost 15 years later, President Carter established the President's Commission on Mental Health. The goal of this 20-member panel was to identify the mental health needs and provide the President with recommendations for improvement based on these suggestions.

The Community Support Program (CSP) was then developed to help former psychiatric inpatients integrate into the community (Frese, 1998; McLean, 1995). Several community support programs were developed in local communities to help adults with serious mental disorders. By 1984, the goal of the CSP and the community support centers was clear: to provide "consumer empowerment" through consumer and community sponsored alternatives (McLean, 1995). By 1985, the federal government began funding community support programs to help former inpatients adjust to community living.

Posthospitalization Advocacy Groups

During the two decades following deinstitutionalization, former patients who had somewhat recovered, angered about the abuse and treatment they received during their hospitalization, began sharing stories of abuse (Frese, 1998) with each other. Horror stories were told about their "treatment," which often included restraints, patient neglect, corporeal punishment, lobotomies, heavy sedation with harmful drugs, and electroconvulsive therapy (ECT). These former patients, realizing that many forms of treatment were nothing more than efforts to "purge patients of ill humors," began to form advocacy groups.

Unfortunately, these advocates split into two groups, based on their beliefs about forced treatment for certain patients, including the use of ECT under extreme circumstances. Activists who began to refer to themselves as "survivors" called for an end to involuntary treatment and for the abolition of all forms of ECT. The survivors opposed treatment under any circumstances, whereas the "consumers" took a more moderate position on forced treatment. Survivors saw themselves as victims of oppression and advocated the right to *choose* treatment. They believed that forced treatment should not be accepted under any circumstances (Frese, 1998).

On the other hand, "consumers" feel "empowered" to make their own healthcare decisions and want to be treated with respect (Andreasen, 1995). Consumers generally collect information about their condition(s) from media sources, recommendations or advice from friends and relatives, and active consumer research, including information obtained through the Internet. However, consumers also make joint decisions with their healthcare providers.

In addition to group efforts to expose personal horror stories, several former patients began writing about their illness and the way they had been treated by their family, their friends, and medical personnel, including psychiatrists. Formerly hospitalized patients and other mental health consumers began publishing books, justifying and outlining the development of consumer/survivor groups. One of the earliest books, *On Our Own: Patient Controlled Alternatives to the Mental Health System,* was written by Judi Chamberlin in 1978. In her book, Chamberlin outlined how to coordinate a consumer advocacy movement and the rationale for doing so. Shortly after her book was published, three former patients who became leaders in the consumer advocacy movement published a more detailed, step-by-step book on how to effectively run consumer advocacy groups.

Family Members as Their Own Advocates

In the late 1970s, while former patients were organizing to protest the inhumane treatment of many patients, family members of the mentally ill began organizing their own advocacy movement to protest the common belief that the parents, especially mothers, were to blame for the development of schizophrenia and other illnesses. This group also advocated improved treatment for those with a mental disorder. In 1979, more than 250 family members, mostly parents, met in Madison, Wisconsin, to organize the family advocacy group, which is known as the National Alliance for the Mentally Ill (NAMI) (Frese, 1998).

Shortly after the development of NAMI, scientists had discovered the biological basis of mental disorders. This evidence helped NAMI educate the public that it was not poor parenting that caused these disorders, but rather a biological disorder. In less than two decades, NAMI membership grew to more than 165,000. In addition to their original goals, NAMI is also advocating that the term *neurobiologic disorders* (NBD) be used instead of mental illness because it more accurately reflects the true development of the disorders (Frese, 1998).

The division among the mental health advocates may have delayed an organized consumer movement, but the former patients, family members, and other mental health consumers continued to advocate mental health reform. The most successful personal and group advocacy efforts really evolved over the past 15 years. In fact, over the past decade, advocacy efforts have developed not only through organized group efforts but also through advances in science and participation from the media and many healthcare companies.

THE BIOLOGY OF MENTAL DISORDERS AND THE NEW MENTAL HEALTH REVOLUTION (LATE 1980s TO PRESENT)

During the same time, biologists had developed a theory that psychoses were caused by neurochemical imbalances. This evidence was met with mixed reviews. Many survivors remained opposed to forced treatment, whereas family members, relieved that they were no longer blamed for their child's illness, sometimes favored the psychiatrist's recommendation for treatment, even if the patient opposed treatment. On the other hand, as the technology improved and scientists were able to explore the brain in more depth, the field of neuroscience grew increasingly popular. In addition, this research suggests that because the underlying cause of mental health disorders may be no different than the underlying cause of many physical disorders, the appropriate pharmacological treatment should also be able to cure or minimize the mental health disorders.

Prozac

The introduction of the antidepressant Prozac by Eli Lilly in 1988 was a landmark event for patients suffering from depression. Patients with a long history of depression began reporting a renewed sense of confidence once they started taking Prozac. The remarkable responses prompted one psychiatrist to label Prozac as "cosmetic pharmacology." Almost overnight, healthcare providers quickly became aware of the advantages of Prozac over the traditional antidepressants and subscribed more than 650,000 prescriptions per month (Kramer, 1994). Other pharmaceutical companies began introducing similar drugs.

The Decade of the Brain

The advances in neuroscience made possible by new technology encouraged the government to pass legislation to stimulate further research. In 1990, President Bush enacted into law the 1989 Congressional bill, which declared 1990–2000 to be the "Decade of the Brain." The legislation was designed to maximize human potential by simultaneously studying the brain and the nervous system through basic research and then using this information to develop new technologies. During this period, new evidence continued to support the earlier theories in human behavior and mental disorders that biological and potentially genetic factors play a role in the development of schizophrenia, bipolar disorder, major depression, obsessive–compulsive disorder, and panic disorders.

The National Institute of Mental Health also declared the 1990s as the Decade of the Brain. Mental health consumers viewed this declaration with mixed opinions. Some believed that psychiatrists were no longer interested in their patients' subjective experiences. Others, however, saw this campaign as the opportunity to voice their experiences through personal accounts (McLean, 1995). At the same time, media attention to many of these issues increased the public's interest in mental health. All of these events helped empower consumers and give them a sense of purpose.

Self-Treatment and Alternative Therapies

In addition to the development of several new drugs over the past decade, alternative therapies have become a popular option for many consumers. This popularity is not only the result of several commercials and other media events describing the benefits of alternative therapy, but such types of therapy are available over the counter, without medical consultation. Herbal products have been introduced as "natural alternatives" for the treatment of certain psychiatric conditions, especially depression. Products such as St. John's Wort have become familiar household terms for many Americans. These products are commercially advertised as cheap, safe, over-the-counter alternatives to more expensive prescriptions.

The widespread use of these alternative products suggests that many consumers are treating themselves instead of receiving medical help or using these products in conjunction with whatever therapy their healthcare provider has recommended. Some of the most common herbal remedies used to treat psychiatric symptoms include the following (Wong, Smith, & Boon, 1998):

- Black Cohosh
- Ginkgo
- Lemon Balm
- St. John's Wort
- German Chamomile
- Hops
- Passion Flower
- Valerian
- Evening Primrose
- Kava
- Skullcap

There is some evidence that the use of particular herbal products actually mimics psychiatric symptoms (Emmanuel, Jones, & Lydiard, 1998). For example, a 40-year-old woman was diagnosed with a mood disorder and treated with fluoxetine. It was discovered several months later that the woman had been self-medicating with an herbal weight loss product and that her manic symptoms were actually caused by the herbal product she was taking (Emmanuel, Jones, & Lydiard, 1998). Products containing ma-huang (ephedra) or chromium picolinate as well as the herbal remedies Ginseng and Yohimbe may actually cause psychiatric symptoms (Emmanuel, Jones, & Lydiard, 1998; Wong, 1998). There is also evidence that other herbs, including Capsicum, Chaste Tree, and Siberian Ginseng, have central nervous system (CNS) side effects (Wong, 1998).

To diagnose and treat patients accurately, providers should question patients carefully about *all* medications they are taking, including over-the-counter and herbal products. Because there is no conclusive evidence that any of these products are superior to the conventional treatments (Wong, 1998), providers should also advise their patients against self-medicating, especially with products known to cause CNS-related adverse events and with products that have not been tested carefully for safety and efficacy.

THE MEDIA

The Media's Contribution: Friend or Foe

The media is a powerful tool that can significantly influence public opinion, depending on how a particular event or story is portrayed. Stories surrounding scientific breakthroughs and new treatments for mental health disorders have been covered in the media. The media's coverage of Prozac is a great example. The media became "obsessed" with Prozac after hearing rumors about the new drug. Prozac has been both hailed by the media as a wonder drug and condemned by the media as a dangerous pill that increases the risk of suicide for some people. The proof linking mental health disorders to chemical imbalances and the simultaneous introduction of Prozac brought new confidence to many mental health consumers. For the first time, these consumers were able to use many forms of the media as their allies.

The media should be credited for lifting many of the stereotypes and negative beliefs held by many individuals. However, publicity relating to mental health issues has not all been positive. For example, on several occasions, the media has mentioned that the alleged suspect in a crime had been taking

FIGURE 20-1

The Media and Mental Health

Positive Influence	Negative Influence
▪ Reduced stigma	▪ Alleged scandals in community-provided mental healthcare
▪ Exposed the scientific evidence about the causes of these illnesses	▪ Claimed Prozac related to suicidal tendencies

medications under psychiatric care. After such a report, the public may either create a link between taking the medication and committing the crime or claim the medication does not work, which is why the crime was committed. Yet details such as the length of care and medication use, which impact the effectiveness of interventions, are not included in the report. Other media reports have criticized community treatment programs for mental illness, claiming they are ineffective (Tyrer, 1998). Such reports can add to or justify the existing stigmas that some people have about individuals with a mental illness. When negative media exposure "confirms" popular discriminatory beliefs, it becomes a set-back to the mental health advocacy movement (Figure 20–1).

Through repeated stories discussing the link between many mental health illnesses and biological or genetic factors, the media has been able to eliminate some of the negative stereotypes about mental health illness that have prevailed. The media has played a crucial role in the success of Prozac, other CNS drugs, and herbal remedies, both through media coverage and through direct-to-consumer (DTC) advertising.

Regardless of the "trend of the day," the media's prolonged attention to Prozac was significant and helped glamorize the drug, making the topic more acceptable to talk about socially and on a more intimate level. For many long-time sufferers of depression, Prozac helped them finally feel like they were in control of themselves. This new feeling of vitality and the media's positive exposure to Prozac helped several well-known people publicly admit they had been suffering from depression. Going public has given long-time sufferers a new sense of freedom, has helped ease some negative stereotypes, and has encouraged some people who may not have otherwise gone to the doctor to seek help. This new sense of empowerment also has encouraged other, less-well-known people to write autobiographical books about their struggles and successes.

Direct-to-Consumer Advertising

Recently, healthcare and pharmaceutical companies have used different media channels to promote their products and educate the public about certain illnesses and disorders. These campaigns, often known as DTC advertising, have both empowered some consumers and helped decrease the general stigma. These campaigns can be either disease specific or treatment specific. Some campaigns have even discussed the signs, symptoms, and treatment options for people with a particular disease or illness without providing specific reference to their company's particular product. More often, however, pharmaceutical companies have product-specific campaigns. Some of these campaigns are well known in the media and are advertised on television, on the radio, on the Internet, and in physician offices. Many pharmaceutical companies now sponsor advertisements and/or disease-specific chat rooms on the Internet.

Healthcare companies (again, mostly pharmaceutical firms) have also initiated disease-specific consumer programs. (These programs are not traditional "disease management" programs. They do not provide integrated healthcare coverage, nor do they require physician participation.) Several companies are currently marketing their own depression-specific consumer programs. These programs provide materials and other forms of support to the individual. Some programs even offer these consumers reward points for sticking with their medication. Programs for other mental illnesses are also available.

Advocacy and Understanding through Personal Accounts and Other Publications

After the introduction of Prozac, publications describing personal experiences and struggles related to mental illness written by both consumers and providers began appearing in the popular press. As previously mentioned, this was not the first time such stories had been told. Yet, this may have been the first time that such types of books were widely read not only by patients and their families but also by the general public. *Listening to Prozac,* by Peter Kramer (1994), was among the first books published about patient responses to Prozac and is probably the most well-known publication written by a psychiatrist over the past decade. A number of autobiographies, including *Prozac Nation* (Wurtzel, 1994), *Prozac Diaries* (Slater, 1998), and *An Unquiet Mind* (Jamison, 1995) provided powerful accounts of personal struggles.

These accounts candidly discuss the suffering and anguish of mental illness in a way that cannot be understood by simply reading a textbook (Gask, 1997). They also are a way to try to help others understand why some patients attempt suicide and why some patients find it difficult to accept pharmacological treatment, believing that it makes them "weaker" than others for not being able to manage on their own. Regardless of what emotions or feelings the contents of these books evoke, many consumers feel a sense of empowerment after reading such personal accounts from people who have shared experiences that may be similar to their own.

THE MENTAL HEALTHCARE MARKETPLACE

Managed Care and Mental Health

Remarkable changes in science and medicine have changed both the treatment options and the perceptions of mental health. At the same time, the rise in managed care, combined with the overall reduction in available dollars for healthcare, has interfered with the delivery of mental healthcare for many people who do not receive healthcare in the public sector (Scallet, 1996). Within managed care, mental health (or, "behavioral health") care has been the easiest target area for budget cuts. As one author points out, "mental health care is the unwanted stepchild of most managed care systems" (Burns, 1998). Managed care has reduced the length of inpatient hospitalization days and the number of outpatient psychotherapy visits allowed per enrollee

(Pomerantz, 1999a), increased co-payments, and established higher deductibles (Scallet, 1996). There are three main reasons why many people are still unable to receive proper treatment. First, under the managed care gatekeeper model, many plans have either very limited or no mental healthcare benefits. In some managed care plans, consumers are treated exclusively by their primary care provider. Some plans limit the number of specialty visits per year. Some plans even use the gatekeeper model to prevent patients from getting the right treatment for depression (Burns, 1998).

Second, many plans often have restricted pharmacy benefits and will reimburse an individual only for a select list of medications. The choice of medications used to treat specific mental disorders is sometimes very limited, which may limit effective patient treatment.

Finally, managed care plans often lack adequate screening tools to even detect depression and other illnesses, leaving many people without treatment.

With the exception of certain governmental and large employer groups, many managed care plans do not offer their clients extensive or any mental healthcare coverage. Some plans require that patients get a referral from their primary doctor before seeing a psychiatrist or other trained mental healthcare worker. This is just one of many reasons patients sometimes seek treatment from their primary care provider, if they even seek treatment at all. Yet, primary care providers may not counsel patients because it is too time intensive for the rate of return under managed care reimbursement. Primary care providers often just prescribe medications, sometimes without even scheduling a follow-up visit with these patients.

Seamless Continuum of Care? Managed Care's Approaches to Mental Health Coverage through Carve-Outs

Managed care companies use three methods to provide mental health coverage. The "carve-in" option is where mental health benefits are covered as part of the overall health benefit (Guralnik, 1996; Scheffler, 1999). Managed care companies also sometimes use mental health "carve-outs" to deal with this special-needs population. In a carve-out model, the mental health benefits are provided by a behavioral health organization. Consumers can often go directly to a specialist without a referral from their primary care provider. Under this model, however, mental and physical health benefits are not coordinated. In addition, many consumers receive psychotherapy from a nonpsychiatrist and are referred to a psychiatrist when they need medication (Pomerantz, 1999b).

The benefits of carve-ins versus carve-outs are still open for debate (Tischler & Astrachan, 1996). The complex nature of many mental illnesses and the strong relationship between mental health and physical health (Kettl, 1998) suggest that the ideal model of care would integrate mental and physical health-care services. Collaborating to provide the most appropriate care not only could be beneficial to the consumers but could help reduce overall costs of medical care (Burns, 1997). A few organizations have attempted to integrate these services. They have created a collaborative model in which they use a comprehensive questionnaire to screen for physical and mental complaints. If the score indicates that the patient requires mental health-care, a behavioral specialist will work with the primary care provider to provide appropriate treatment (Burns, 1997). It is too soon to tell the true value of such programs.

Community Treatment Centers

In addition to the different healthcare treatment models already described, community treatment centers remain a valuable resource and an excellent alternative to institutionalization for many mental healthcare consumers. These centers provide both support and treatment for many patients in their own community. The success of these models is attributed to the joint federal–state efforts (often through Medicaid funding) to provide a flexible variety of services that support the changing needs of a potentially very expensive population (Scallet, 1996).

In an excellent article by Anthony Lehman, Lehman (1998) suggests five major community-based care intervention categories with substantial efficacy for persons with schizophrenia. These interventions, which are also appropriate for other psychiatric conditions, include pharmacotherapies, psychological treatments, family interventions, vocational rehabilitation, and case management/assertive community treatment.

RECENT PUBLIC AND PRIVATE CAMPAIGNS TO IMPROVE ACCESS, TREATMENT, AND OUTCOMES

Federal Initiatives

In the past decade, a few major legislative acts have been enacted to provide people with severe mental health disorders better employment and insurance protections. Other federally sponsored initiatives include evidence-based guidelines and treatment algorithms. Table 20–2 (on pages 480–481) is a summary of the components of major federal initiatives that pertain to mental health issues.

Employer Groups

Employers' direct and indirect costs of psychiatric conditions in the workplace equate to billions of dollars per year in lost productivity and absenteeism. In 1989, the New York Business Group on Health conducted a nationwide survey of companies to assess healthcare utilization. Nearly three-fourths of respondents reported that mental health problems are fairly to very common in their workplace (Russell, Patterson, & Baker, 1998). Yet, as mentioned, employer-sponsored mental health insurance is not common. It is essential for consumer groups to spread the word to employers about the cost-to-benefit ratio of employer-sponsored mental health insurance. A growing awareness of both the severity of these conditions as well as an awareness of the number of employees affected by such conditions has resulted in several employer-sponsored programs, as well as some group business initiatives.

THE ONGOING PLAGUE: ISSUES OF CONFIDENTIALITY, CONSENT, AND SPECIAL POPULATIONS

What Consumers Need from Providers

Although many consumers actively participate in their healthcare treatment, independently research treatment options, and feel empowered to make their own decisions, these and other consumers also still need help and support from providers. Not all consumers realize that they even have a mental illness when they enter the healthcare system. Consumers with milder mental health illnesses often enter the healthcare system complaining of mild malaise and end up with a diagnosis of depression or anxiety. Providers are responsible for providing comfort and education. Often, those with depression or other mental health disorders have feelings of loneliness and isolation regardless of whether they knew about their illness before the time of diagnosis. Therefore, providers need to explain to patients that they are not alone, that treatment is available, and that they are not crazy.

The relationship between the provider and patient is very important, especially when patients discuss and/or seek treatment for what they believe is a sensitive topic, such as their mental health disorder(s). As patient advocates, physicians should do their best to minimize patient burden and ensure intensive, quality care.

Providers should provide patients with all of the necessary information about their condition and treatment options and should allow patients to make their own decisions. Healthcare consumers need information about their particular disease, treatment options, and the importance of medication compliance. Providers must be empathetic to their patients and must explain how their disease may impact their professional and personal lives. Finally, when patients do make an informed decision, providers need to be supportive and respectful of their treatment decisions; they should not be insensitive and paternalistic.

Patient Confidentiality: Issues and Considerations

There are several reasons why the issue of confidentiality is particularly important for patients who seek mental health treatment. First, there is the ongoing stigma often associated with seeking mental health treatment. Second, patients must trust their provider in order to disclose sensitive and very personal information that may be necessary to receive adequate treatment. Although healthcare professionals are expected to adhere to an ethical code of confidentiality, many people fear that their privacy

T A B L E 20-2

Federally Sponsored Initiatives Supporting Mental Health Advocacy

Name	Year	Brief Description	Important Information for Mental Health Consumers	Remaining Issues	For More Information
Americans with Disabilities Act	1990	Prohibits discrimination on the basis of disability in employment, programs, etc. Protects consumers with psychiatric disabilities.	Title I of the ADA requires that consumers must disclose the existence of their disability to their employer in order to fall within its protections. Employers cannot ask questions about mental health history during an interview. Employers must keep all information about the psychiatric disability confidential.	Supreme Court to rule on whether Title II of the ADA has been violated in Georgia, where individuals with mental disabilities were treated in an institution rather than IN the community, despite the recommendation by the treating professionals http://www.usdoj.gov/crt/ada /octdec98.htm.	http://www.usdoj.gov/crt/ada/ adahom1.htm.

Name	Year	Brief Description	Important Information for Mental Health Consumers	Remaining Issues	For More Information
Mental Health Parity Act	1996	Equates aggregate lifetime limits and annual limits for mental health and other medical or surgical benefits.	The principle beneficiaries will be consumers with the most severe, persisting, and disabling forms of mental illness. The law covers mental illness, but not treatment of substance abuse or chemical dependency.	Applies only to employers that offer mental health benefits, but does not mandate such coverage. Does not provide coverage under Medicare/Medicaid. Employers with fewer than 50 employees are exempt.	http://www.nami.org/update/parity96.htm. http://www.nimh.nih.gov/research/prtyrpt/parity.pdf.
Mental Health Equitable Treatment Act	1999	Ends insurance discrimination against people with serious brain disorders; provides full insurance parity.	Prohibits unequal restrictions on annual lifetime mental health benefits, inpatient hospital days, outpatient visits, and out-of-pocket expenses for patients with the most "severe biologically based mental illness," as determined by medical science and defined in *DSM-IV*.	Includes a small business exemption for employers with 25 or fewer employees, BUT Removes the current provision that exempts employers who demonstrate that their premium costs rose more than 1% due to the parity.	www.nami.org/update/990416.html.

is not being protected (Petrila, 1999). The federal government has designed some laws to protect confidentiality of healthcare information and mental healthcare information in particular, but in reality, these laws provide very little protection. As a result of consumer pressure and growing public concern, Congress is in the process of creating a national standard of protection regarding healthcare information (Petrila, 1999).

The Confidentiality of Pharmaceutical and Medical Claims

The growth of managed care has created the need for organized pharmacy and medical information systems. These information systems contain patient level data about prescription use and perhaps other medically related information. Data on individual patients, including their diagnosis and treatment plan, are no longer protected.

Pharmaceutical manufacturers have expressed interest in acquiring the data from these databases for their own marketing use. When this occurs, patient confidentiality may be violated. This is a particularly sensitive issue for mental healthcare consumers. Consumers may even choose not to fill a prescription as a result, fearing that their employer may obtain these medical records. Unfortunately, the current state of the law does not provide adequate protection of confidentiality. In addition, there is little protection against the release of data to third parties from a federally funded project, under the Freedom of Information Act (FOIA) (Kohl, 1999). In 1998, more than 300 bills regarding medical records were considered by the states (Grinfield, 1999). Only Maine was able to pass a comprehensive package, yet the enactment of this law has been delayed. Clearly, these issues have yet to be resolved.

Direct-to-Consumer Mailings

Many consumers feel empowered because of the knowledge they gain through DTC advertising. Yet, what consumers may not realize is that healthcare companies are also engaging in another, more subtle form of DTC advertising: information is being sent directly to consumers who have been identified as having a particular disease or illness, without the knowledge or consent of the patient. How? Most of this information is abstracted from either medical or pharmaceutical claims. The pharmacy benefit manager, provider, or managed care company then initiates these mailings to try to educate consumers, in hopes of creating some cost savings. Yet, the use of these private records can be detrimental: sometimes, patients who are taking a drug for one condition are labeled as taking it for another condition based on the pharmacy record alone. This situation is particularly complicated for mental healthcare consumers.

Informed Consent

Mental illness may impair a person's decision-making ability. There has been a great deal of debate about whether individuals diagnosed with a mental illness are competent enough to provide voluntary informed consent for their treatment plan or participation in a clinical trial. Obtaining informed consent that is not coerced and truly reflects the patient's values can be a challenge. In addition, some physicians choose not to discuss treatment options with patients because they believe that they are acting on the patient's behalf. These physicians believe that their patients lack the ability to competently make their own treatment decisions.

The debate about informed consent for treatment has been addressed by both family members through the NAMI and mental health consumer groups. NAMI members often believe that they need to pursue treatment for their loved ones who either are in denial of their illness or are unable to help themselves. The position among mental health consumers is not as clear.

Three groups of subjects require special protection from research: pregnant women, children, and prisoners. Although two U.S. commissions declared that persons with mental illness should be regarded as a vulnerable population, protection of this group is determined by the local Institutional Review Boards (Stagno & Agioch, 1997). Yet, a review article by Shamoo and Keay (1996) noted that the authors of 15 of 41 studies involving the withdrawal of psychopharmacological agents did not report obtaining informed consent from their patients, and only one study mentioned that subjects understood their right to discontinue the trial at any time. Substitutes for immediate decision making, such as the use of advance directives are sometimes used. However, advance directives rarely discuss the patient's willingness to participate in research when unable to give competent consent (Helmchen, 1998).

Advance Directives

In the past decade, the use of advance directives has become a popular method to honor consumer preferences when they are unable to give consent (Frese, 1998). Consumers can use this as a tool so that their opinions can be respected when they are in an acute psychiatric episode and are not competent to give consent for treatment. While in remission, consumers can express what services they desire and what services they specifically oppose, thereby preventing forced treatment. The documents will also allow providers to treat patients who may otherwise refuse treatment in an acute phase. Consumers may realize they are incompetent to make a competent decision during an acute episode.

The Elderly and Other Medicare Consumers

A recent poll of more than 100 elderly Medicare enrollees asked to prioritize the importance of insurance coverage for specific services revealed that mental healthcare coverage was a very low priority (Danis, 1997). Therefore, the elderly do not have a strong commitment to mental health advocacy. Nevertheless, the Medicare/elderly population, especially patients who already suffer from another chronic illness, is a particularly vulnerable group for depression and other forms of mental illness. Providers should therefore screen these patients regularly for any mental illness. During this screening process, providers should identify what medications patients are currently taking. This will rule out possible drug-related causes of the mental illness and will also help identify any possible drug interactions that may occur if patients are prescribed a particular medication. In addition, it is important for prescribers to stay up to date on the latest treatment recommendations for the elderly because this population is often unable to do this on their own.

Children

Treating children who suffer from any mental illness is also difficult. Too often, many children are not receiving treatment for their problems (Rogers, 1998). Why are these children not being treated? Perhaps because their cries for help (verbal or implied) are ignored by parents (and providers) who may be either embarrassed or ashamed to learn the truth or believe it is a "phase" that their child can and/or will "snap out of." Although teachers and school administrators can sometimes identify problematic children, they often rely on the families to take responsibility for helping children with emotional disorders. Sometimes, teachers and even family members fail to identify a child with emotional disorders when they are not around this child enough (a child may skip school often) or if the child is quiet and keeps to himself or herself.

Obtaining information from children with psychiatric conditions can be particularly complex because the psychiatric problems may be related to the family dynamics, including physical and sexual abuse. In some cases, these situations or parental persuasion may influence a child's ability to provide unbiased information and may prevent the child from receiving proper treatment. Some children may believe that they are or will be punished or blamed for their problem. These children may lie to people in order to protect themselves from their parents. In difficult cases, methods such as drawing pictures, playing with puppets, and using activity books may be used to help understand the nature of the problem (Hart & Chesson, 1998).

Most of these patients have the capacity to make their own decisions about their treatment plan (Stagno & Agioch, 1997). Specific tests of cognitive maturity should determine the child's ability to understand his or her condition and whether the child is capable of making an informed decision. If such tests suggest that the child is mature enough to understand this information, physicians should review all of the treatment options, explaining both the benefits and side effects of treatment as they would with any other patient. It is especially important to provide accurate information when prescribing antipsychotic medications, which may cause acute and long-term side effects.

THE DEMAND FOR QUALITY OUTCOMES AND PATIENT SATISFACTION

Since the rise in managed care many years ago, consumers and providers have been concerned that cost-control efforts have led to a decline in the quality of care patients receive. Traditional measures of quality include examination of structure, process, and outcomes (Srebnik et al., 1997). Most of the time, however, the structure and processes are measured, and little attention is given to outcomes assessment. Yet in mental health, outcomes assessment is a better indicator of quality of care than structure or process. Consumers are now demanding evidence of the effectiveness of these cost-savings programs through outcomes assessments that measure not only clinical endpoints but patient-oriented outcomes such as quality of life and patient satisfaction as well (Srebnik et al., 1997).

What are the quality outcomes that would satisfy mental health consumers? In general, most healthcare consumers are interested in satisfaction, quality of life, and the receipt of effective treatment (clinical and functional status). In addition to these outcomes, mental health consumers are concerned with their ability to make decisions without being influenced by the clinicians' judgments about what is best. The reality is that the quality of mental healthcare is far from ideal in many cases. Although this may be the result of insurance limitations, consumers are still demanding quality outcomes (Lehman, 1996). In fact, the schizophrenia Patient Outcomes Research Team (PORT) study concluded that the actual treatment received by hundreds of schizophrenic patients fell far short of the recommended treatment plan (Lehman & Steinwachs, 1998). Therefore, it is no surprise that many schizophrenics misuse their medication and that treatment for these consumers becomes ineffective. The results of this study have empowered consumers and family members to demand appropriate treatment from scientifically developed guidelines.

TABLE 20-3

Desired Quality Outcomes for Patients with Mental Illnesses

Satisfaction	Functioning/ Rehabilitation	Quality of Life	Clinical Status
Involvement with treatment	Physical	Housing	Treatment outcomes
Appropriateness of treatment	Mental	Safety within the community	Side effects
Safety at treatment center	Social functioning (including basic community living skills)	Ability to perform activities of daily living	Compliance
Understanding of treatment plan	Stress and anger-coping skills	Employment/financial independence. Adequate social support from provider, family, and community	

For psychiatric consumers, satisfactory outcomes and quality of care include the ability to be involved and influence service decisions, and the ability to reintegrate into the community. Important outcome variables that measure the quality of psychiatric treatment and patient satisfaction are shown in Table 20–3 (Lehman, 1996; Srebnik et al., 1997).

In addition to the factors listed in Table 20–3, a study by Rogers et al. (1997) determined that consumer empowerment was related to quality of life, income, and community activism, not related to demographic variables, and inversely related to the use of traditional mental health services. In addition, five different scales determine the individual's feeling of "consumer empowerment":

1. Self-efficacy–self-esteem
2. Power–powerlessness
3. Community activism
4. Righteous anger
5. Optimism–control over the future

CONCLUSIONS: WHAT HAVE WE LEARNED AND WHAT OPPORTUNITIES STILL EXIST?

Although many challenges and obstacles remain for both mental health consumers and their providers, significant developments in medicine and a more united mental health advocacy movement have resulted in a number of positive changes. The impact of these suggestions has been enormous: mental health consumers are now being treated in the community instead of in a hospital and more consumers are seeking treatment (new drugs have and continue to encourage more consumers to seek treatment than ever before). This has resulted in more successful outcomes for consumers who had previously failed to respond to traditional therapy. It has also helped advocacy groups increase in size and become more influential. These influences have helped countless numbers of people live full, productive lives.

The literature suggesting a strong biological basis for mental health disorders, the "Decade of the Brain," and the development of Prozac and new pharmacological treatment became the building blocks of the mental health consumer movement. The language used to describe mental illnesses and persons suffering from a mental disorder can shape public perception. Fortunately, through the media, the prevailing stereotype that people with mental illnesses were to blame for their own conditions has subsided somewhat. As the public begins to accept mental illnesses as a biologically based condition, more and more people are seeking help for their condition. In addition, general practitioners are becoming more familiar with the signs and symptoms associated with many of these conditions and are now able to treat these patients.

The size and strength of the mental health consumer advocacy movement is becoming increasingly important for two main reasons. By demonstrating the positive benefits and cost-effectiveness associated with mental health treatment, a strong advocacy group can lobby politicians and others who influence healthcare financing to provide coverage for mental healthcare. This group can also argue for equal physical and mental healthcare coverage by demonstrating that both components have a biological basis.

Despite the evidence of the commonalties between mental and physical illness, consumerism in mental health is still lagging compared with other areas of healthcare because of limited data on scientific outcomes and the public's limited understanding of neurobiological disorders (Peschel & Peschel, 1996). Although scientific developments and the media have positively impacted the public's perceptions, psychiatric patients are still disliked by many, even doctors in primary care (Byrne, 1999). The vast amount of publicity has influenced public opinion about mental health. Despite several changes in both the treatment for and the public's perception of mental health consumers, some consumers still refuse a psychiatric referral, fearing the resulting stigma attached to psychiatric assessment and treatment. The general public and many primary care providers continue to stereotype these persons as different (Byrne, 1999). To the public, persons with psychiatric conditions are considered patients, not consumers. These "patients" are considered different (Gallo, 1994), aggressive (Wolff et al., 1996), and perhaps even incurable, and they are therefore often feared and excluded (Penn, 1994; Sayce, 1998). The stigma has professional implications as well. Funding for psychiatric research remains scarce, and psychiatry remains one of the first and hardest hit areas for budget cuts (Byrne, 1999).

Until this understanding turns into action, patients will continue to suffer emotionally, and employers, who bear more than 50% of costs related to depression in terms of increased absenteeism and decreased productivity, will continue to suffer economically (Russell, Patterson, & Baker, 1998). Providers, together with other advocates, can then demand effective and equitable treatment programs based on documented evidence of the physical nature of mental illness and the positive outcomes associate with appropriate treatment (Peschel & Peschel, 1996).

Like those with other illnesses, mental health consumers can live full and productive lives with proper treatment and support. Proper treatment includes not only medical treatment but also social and educational treatment. Properly treating these individuals will allow them to understand their illness and integrate with society. While these consumers recover, they will need ongoing support from local community organizations and family members. As they rebuild their lives, they may need help finding residence and obtaining a job. Most important, they need to feel love, support, and normal—like any other person. In fact, for many mental health consumers in both the public and private sector, true "empowerment" means having self-control, the ability to make their own choices, and an end to discrimination in the public and healthcare sectors (Fisher, 1994; McLean, 1995).

REFERENCES

Andreasen NC. Clients, consumers, providers, and products: where will it end? *Am J Psychiatr* 1995; 152(8):1107–1109.

Burns J. Providing care for the mind, body, and soul. *Managed Healthcare* 1997; 7:20–25.

Burns J. Massachusetts suicide points out a critical need. *Managed Healthcare* 1998; 8(8):50.

Byrne P. Stigma of mental illness: changing minds, changing behavior. *Br J Psychiatr* 1999; 174:1–2.

Carlin PA. Depressed mind, sick body. *Hippocrates* 1998; 12(12):36–42.

Chamberlin J. *On our own: patient controlled alternatives to the mental health system.* New York: Hawthorne, 1978.

Corrigan PW, Garman AN. Considerations for research on consumer empowerment and psychosocial interventions. *Psychiatr Serv* 1997; 48(3):347–352.

Danis M, et al. Older Medicare enrollees' choices for insured services. *J Am Geriatr Soc* 1997; 45(6):688–694.

Dinan TG. The physical consequences of depressive illness. *Br J Psychiatr* 1999; 318:826.

Emmanuel NP, Jones CB, Lydiard RB. Use of herbal products and symptoms of bipolar disorder. *Am J Psychiatr* 1998; 155(11):1627.

Fisher DB. Health care reform based on an empowerment model of recovery by people with psychiatric disabilities. *Hosp Commun Psychiatr* 1994; 45(9):913–915.

Frese FJ. Advocacy, recovery, and the challenges of consumerism for schizophrenia. *Psychiatr Clin North Am* 1998; 21(1):233–249.

Gallo K. First person account: self-stigmatisation. *Schizophrenia Bulletin* 1994; 20:407–410.

Gask L. Listening to patients. *Br J Psychiatr* 1997; 171:301–302.

Grinfield MJ. A showdown over medical records privacy looms—or does it? *Psychiatr Times* 1999; 16(5):20–21.

Guralnik O. Psychiatry and managed care: reports from the 149th annual meeting of the American Psychiatric Association. *Drug Benefit Trends* 1996; 8(6):27, 31–32, 51.

Hart C, Chesson R. Children as consumers (see comments). *BMJ* 1998; 316(7144):1600–1603.

Helmchen H. Research with patients incompetent to give informed consent. *Curr Opin Psychiatr* 1998; 11(3):295–297.

Jamison KR. *An unquiet mind: a memoir of moods and madness*. New York: Knopf, 1995.

Kettl PA. Major depression: the forgotten illness. *Hosp Med* 1998; 34(8):41–50.

Kohl M. Shelby Amendment creates concerns about confidentiality, privacy in medical records. *Psychiatr Times* 1999; 16(5):22.

Kramer PD. *Listening to Prozac*. New York: Penguin Books, 1994.

Lehman AF. Evaluating outcomes of treatments for persons with psychotic disorders. *J Clin Psychiatr* 1996; 57(11S):61–67.

Lehman AF. Public health policy, community services, and outcomes for patients with schizophrenia (review). *Psychiatr Clin North Am* 1998; 21(1):221–231.

Lehman AF, Steinwachs DM. Translating research into practice: the schizophrenia Patient Outcomes Research Team (PORT) treatment recommendations. *Schizophrenia Bulletin* 1998; 24(1):1–10.

McLean A. Empowerment and the psychiatric consumer/ex-patient movement in the United States: contradictions, crisis and changes. *Soc Sci Med* 1995; 40(8):1053–1071.

Penn DL, et al. Dispelling the stigma of schizophrenia: what sort of information is best? *Schizophrenia Bulletin* 1994; 20(3):567–578.

Peschel RE, Peschel E. Consumerism for neurobiological disorders. An assessment. *Int J Tech Assess Health Care* 1996; 12(4):644–656.

Petrila J. Medical records confidentiality: issues affecting the mental health and substance abuse systems. *Drug Benefit Trends* 1999; 11(3):6–10.

Pomerantz JM. Behavioral health matters—SSRI dilemmas: a psychiatrist's perspective. *Drug Benefit Trends* 1999a; 11(3):5, 12.

Pomerantz JM. Behavioral health matters—the behavioral health war zone. *Drug Benefit Trends* 1999b; 11(1), 2,5.

Rogers ES, et al. A consumer-constructed scale to measure empowerment among users of mental health services. *Psychiatr Serv* 1997; 48(8):1042–1047.

Rogers JA. Too many people are overlooked. *Philadelphia Inquirer,* December 3, 1998.

Rupp A, Gause EM, Regier DA. Research policy implications of cost-of-illness studies for mental disorders. *Br J Psychiatr* 1998; 173(36S):19–25.

Russell JM, Patterson J, Baker AM. Depression in the workplace: epidemiology, economics and effects of treatment. *Dis Manage Health Outcomes* 1998; 4(3):135–142.

Sayce L. Stigma, discrimination, and social exclusion: what's in a word? *J Mental Health* 1998; 7:331–343.

Scallet LJ. Managing care for mental illness: paradox and pitfalls. *Managed Care Q* 1996; 4(3):93–99.

Scheffler R. The economic implications of managed behavioral health care. *Drug Benefit Trends* 1999; 11(1):6–8.

Shamoo AE, Keay TJ. Ethical concerns about relapse studies. *Cambridge Q Healthcare Ethics* 1996; 5:373–386.

Slater L. *Prozac diaries*. New York: Random House, 1998.

Srebnik D, et al. Development of outcome indicators for monitoring the quality of public mental health care. *Psychiatr Serv* 1997; 48(7):903–909.

Stagno SJ, Agioch GJ. Consent in patients with mental illness. *Curr Opin Psychiatr* 1997; 10(5):423–426.

Tischler GL, Astrachan BM. (1996). A funny thing happened on the way to reform. (review). *Arch Gen Psychiatr* 1996; 53(10):959–963.

Tyrer P. (1998). Whither community care? (editorial; comment). *Br J Psychiatr* 1998; 173:359–360. Published erratum appears in *Br J Psychiatr* 1998; 173:539 (see comments).

Wolff G, et al. Community knowledge of mental illness and reaction to mentally ill people. *Br J Psychiatr* 1996; 168(2):191–198.

Wong AH, Smith M, Boon HS. Herbal remedies in psychiatric practice (review). *Arch Gen Psychiatr* 1998; 55(11):1033–1044.

Wurtzel E. *Prozac nation: young and depressed in America*. Boston: Houghton Mifflin, 1994.

21

CHAPTER

Examining Alternative Medicine: What Consumers Want from Physicians and What Physicians Should Tell Them

John La Puma, M.D., F.A.C.P.

INTRODUCTION

Alternative medicine has become a steamy thicket of medical uncertainty, patient-driven passion, costly hope and hype, and quality hazards left and right. Just when medical pharmaceuticals can be programmed to enter your mitochondria and surgical laser beams can be focused on impossibly small blood vessels, *alternative* medicine has emerged. Is it meaningful, or is it the millennium? What does it mean? And where is it going?

This chapter aims to assess the popularity of alternative medicine, identify what consumers seek from alternative medicine, acknowledge the ethical and product labeling issues that it raises, and analyze several bottom-line financial issues that alternative medicine illuminates.

To accomplish these goals, seven core questions about alternative medicine are proposed. The questions are derived from the author's hand review and computer searching of the peer-reviewed literature, using the PubMed database, as well as personal clinical study and assessment of several hundred patients undergoing an intensive, individualized clinical and educational program to control a chronic medical problem or to optimize their health.

1. What drives the trend in the popularity of alternative medicine?
2. What do consumers really want to know about alternative medicine?
3. What data are available to answer consumers' questions?
4. What do physicians think about alternative medicine?
5. What ethical issues do physicians face as alternative medicine grows more popular?
6. Will payors and employers step into alternative medicine delivery and finance, and what about multilevel marketing?
7. What take-home messages can consumers and physicians walk away with?

WHAT DRIVES THE POPULARITY OF ALTERNATIVE MEDICINE?

Alternative medicine is popular and growing. Published data in 1998 from Harvard Medical School indicate that more than 40% of patients use alternative medicine and more than 70% do not inform their physicians (Eisenberg et al., 1998). In 1997, out-of-pocket expenses for visits to physicians totaled roughly $29.3 billion (Eisenberg et al., 1998); estimated out-of-pocket expenses for visits to alternative practitioners (exclusive of naturopaths, aroma therapists, and chelation therapists) are estimated between $27 billion and $34.4 billion (Eisenberg et al., 1998).

However, conventional medicine is catching up. Nearly 80 medical schools now offer an elective or required course in alternative medicine (Wetzel et al., 1998). In fact, "alternative medicine" was listed as the subject about which physicians want to know more than any other by the American Medical

Association, which, using its family of medical journals, devoted a series to the subject in October and November 1998.

Eisenberg et al. (1998) estimate that visits to alternative medical practitioners exceeded visits to physicians by an estimated 243 million in 1997. In 1990, 19.9% of patients who saw a physician also saw a practitioner of alternative therapy for that same condition during the same year (Eisenberg et al., 1993). In 1997, this percentage jumped to 31.8% (Eisenberg et al., 1998). Chiropractic, relaxation techniques, and massage therapies were among the alternative therapies used most commonly to treat principal medical conditions.

Why are consumers so hungry for alternative medicine? One likely reason is that patient preferences have changed. Consumer interest has accelerated as patients "find health care alternatives to be more congruent with their own values, beliefs and philosophical orientations toward health and life" (Astin, 1998). A second reason is the backlash against well-intended but misguided healthcare reform efforts. Wennberg (1992) categorized healthcare reform's genesis as stemming in part from "weaknesses in the ethical basis for clinical decision making that allow the physician's preferences for outcomes and treatments to dominate the choice of treatment when the right of choice properly belongs to the patient."

With this heady new consumerism, it is perhaps unexpected that the federal government would have been so important in the development of a new field in medicine. In 1993, the Office of Alternative Medicine (OAM) was established at the NIH, with a $2 million budget. In just 5 years, the Office was elevated to an NIH National Center for Complementary and Alternative Medicine with a budget of $50 million in fiscal year 1999. The OAM funded at least 13 research centers, conducting 50 different projects, and has attracted rigorously trained scientific researchers eager to test alternative approaches.

The NIH has devised six categories of alternative medicine:

1. Diet/nutrition/lifestyle changes
2. Mind–body control (e.g., biofeedback, music therapy, relaxation)

3. Traditional/ethnomedicine (e.g., ayurveda, homeopathy, herbal medicine)
4. Structural/energetic therapies (e.g., acupressure, chiropractic, massage)
5. Pharmacological/biological treatments (e.g., chelation, antioxidizing agents)
6. Bioelectromagnetic applications (e.g., magnets, devices that emit low level radiation)

Another force serving to foster alternative medicine's growth and visibility was the passing of the 1994 Dietary Supplement Health and Education Act (DSHEA) by the FDA. Dietary supplements, defined as vitamins, minerals, herbs, other botanicals, amino acids, and any concentrate, metabolite, constituent, extract or combination of these agents, are considered alternative medicine. Until 1994, herbs were considered to be food by the FDA (in fact, most cooks still think of herbs as a leafy garnish). In creating a separate category for supplements, the Act effectively helped get herbs "out of the kitchen," into the pharmacy, and from the pharmacy into superstores. The Act allows supplements to be marketed without testing for efficacy or proof of safety in return for marketers not claiming to diagnose, treat, cure, or prevent disease.

How did the DSHEA come about? Analysts suggest that old-fashioned grassroots campaigning, fueled with industry support, contributed to its enactment. What lawmakers may not have counted on (physicians certainly did not) is that people generally seem to care less about medical terms of proof than an anecdotal favorable story about the effectiveness of, for example, traditional Native-American faith healing. People want a sense of control and choice in their healthcare and a chance to optimize their own health. Alternative medicine gives them both in spades.

WHAT DO CONSUMERS REALLY WANT TO KNOW ABOUT ALTERNATIVE MEDICINE?

In 1998, *Consumers Reports* surveyed a sample of its readers regarding what consumer issues they wanted to know more about. Alternative medicine, especially in regard to supplements, emerged as the number one issue. The questions fell along these lines:

- What is it really for?
- What is the evidence that it works?
- What are the risks?
- Does it contain what it is supposed to?

These questions could be asked about any medication and, with a little modification, any medical device or intervention. Proposed answers are considered in the following section.

WHAT IS IT FOR? WHAT ARE THE SPECIFIC INDICATIONS FOR THIS THERAPY?

As opposed to pharmaceuticals manufactured with specific indications and that are bound by specific FDA regulations, many alternative medical therapies are not specific to any disease or indication. Alternative therapies, at their best, emerge from different value systems, cultures, and beliefs about what causes disease and what improves it. The relationship between the healer and the patient is as important—and in many cases more important—as the chemical complexities of the substances or behaviors given, offered, or prescribed.

Nevertheless, there are specific indications and contraindications in alternative medicine, especially with dietary supplements (discussed later in this chapter). These indications and contraindications are not well known among physicians, and reliable, credible sources for these data have been slow in emerging. Although some of this lag is likely because physicians are generally a conservative lot, suspicious of anything new, the reality is that precious little information fits the Western paradigm for scientific excellence—or even for scientific publication. Specific indications are largely unknown because the data are not published or available or because those data that are published and available seem more like hype than fact.

Those indications for alternative medicine that are known have become or are becoming indications for allopathic medicine. For example, many physicians now recommend low-fat, high-fiber diets and antioxidants to reduce the risk of colorectal and prostate cancers. Chiropractic manipulation is sometimes recommended for spinal problems, especially lower-back problems. Surely, this is not news to consumers, who paid more visits to alternative practitioners in the 1990s than to conventional practitioners.

However, using specific therapies for other indications—not those for which there is scientific evidence, but those that are simply popular—is where alternative medicine remains alternative. For example, even though chiropractic is not "medically indicated" for intestinal, cardiac, infectious, or menstrual problems, or for anything that is not musculoskeletal, patients still see chiropractors, and chiropractors still try to help with these problems. It matters not that the data supporting the use of chiropractic for these reasons is severely wanting.

Similarly, acupuncture is indicated for pain relief and anesthesia. Many clinicians who do acupuncture offer it for this reason, as well as for other reasons. There are lines of people out acupuncturists' office doors, generally speaking, and the lines consist of customers who will pay out of pocket for what their managed care organization may or may not cover. Again, it matters not that acupuncture is not indicated—for the moment, in the United States, anyway—for intestinal, cardiac, infectious, or menstrual problems. In addition, consumers seem unconcerned that the 1998 NIH Consensus conference on the use of acupuncture did not place any of these uses in the "adequate evidence" category.

Any physician with the time to read the research literature in alternative medicine (i.e., in an attempt to learn more about its indications and efficaciousness) would likely find it to be chaotic, wild, unpredictable, and inconsistent. It exists in many languages and comes from many nontraditional sources. Biases are evident from top to bottom, from funding to formulation. Although the papers published in English are generally more reliable than those published in other languages (German, Chinese, and Indian, in descending order), physicians are likely to read only the bottom line and, often, only the bottom line of the abstract.

Assessing research in alternative medicine is actually no different than assessing research in conventional medicine.

Much of alternative medicine's laboratory testing falls into the same category. What do intracellular vitamin levels really mean? How are we to interpret *Candida* counts in the intestine (in which the yeast normally lives)? What relationship does the laboratory evidence of the biochemistry of digestion, absorption, and excretion have to the cramps and diarrhea of irritable bowel syndrome, or the often symptomless colon cancer? No one knows the answers to these questions, and anyone who insists that he or she does has a lot of proving (and probably not homeopathic proving) to do.

So, although physicians will generally want some scientific evidence before offering advice or alternative procedures to their patients, they have different standards than consumers. Consumers see it differently than physicians: if it works for them, and it is unlikely to be very unsafe, most consumers will and have tried alternative medicine—for what ails them, along with whatever their regular allopathic doctor might offer.

WHAT IS THE EVIDENCE? WHAT VALID, RELIABLE DATA EXIST TO SUPPORT ITS USE?

For physicians, payors, and most employers, evidence means Western biomedical proof. However, as noted previously, the triumph of individual experience and personal belief over the generalizations of science and the media are all the evidence that many people need. Also, as noted earlier, these people pay out of pocket.

Convergence and conflict about what counts as evidence are core philosophical issues about which conventional and alternative medicine disagree. It is easy to say that conventional medicine counts well-constructed, double-blinded, randomized controlled clinical trials; accepts cohort studies; and regards case reports as anecdotal, "interesting" observations of little generalizable clinical significance. It is equally easy to say that alternative medicine has little or no history of systematic biomedical analysis and regards peer-reviewed medical journals as emblematic of their own (not in the least objective) biased cultural norms; that alternative medicine individualizes treatment and resists standard protocols because patients are individuals requiring unique herb composition, examination, interview and study; and that alternative medicine regards exceptional cases as worthy of careful reflection and generalization.

What matters to most patients is not whether these truisms about conventional and alternative medicine research are true. Scientific medicine had most patients' rapt attention as little as 10 years ago, and now it is nightly news. Yet educated, successful, thoughtful people will and do take nearly anything, see nearly anyone, try nearly any new substance in the name of optimum health. What happened?

While conventional medicine was worrying about CPT coding and DRG identification and reacting to managed care, quality initiatives, and report cards, it cut time spent with patients to just a few minutes. Patients began to feel even more rushed and less well when they left conventional physicians than they did when they came in. Physicians appeared more knowledgeable about cellular phone service than about cellular mechanisms of disease, not that patients wanted to know the theory of scientific medicine, necessarily. It is just that they wanted to know that their physician knew and, more important, that he or she cared—not just about the evidence and the diagnosis, but about patient values.

Here then is the tension between alternative medicine and "traditional" or allopathic medicine; the belief in self-healing, versus the power of medicine to heal. It is the imbalance of the mind, body, and spirit, versus the dysfunction of an organ; the uniqueness of the individual and his or her illness, versus the generalizability of medical knowledge and conditions; the reliance on special cases, ancient texts, and stories of illness and treatment as a research base, versus randomized, controlled clinical trials.

What *is* the theory behind alternative medicine? Nature, observational science, vitalism, and spirituality are the major themes. Most of the 10,000 acupuncturists in the United States, for example, are taught that illness is caused by blockages in "qi" (pronounced "chee" in Chinese), which means "life energy." Everyone has qi; disease results when qi flow is disturbed or out of balance. Qi runs through the body in 12 (or in one tradition, 59) meridians, and the acupuncturist selects from the 365 (one for each day) available points to unblock qi. The selection of points is influenced by the five elements: wood, water, fire, metal, and earth.

To most Western physicians, this is gobbledygook. To someone with fibromyalgia who is open minded and who has little or no relief from the analgesics and muscle relaxants and steroids and antidepressants prescribed by his or her internist, unblocking energy and using the power of the elements sounds pretty good, and sometimes, it works.

WHAT ARE THE RISKS? WHAT SIDE EFFECTS, ADVERSE EFFECTS, AND INTERACTIONS MIGHT BE ENGENDERED?

Although supplements are not regulated as drugs, the risks of some therapies are significant. The risks fall in two primary categories: (1) adverse effects and interactions of herbs and supplements and (2) opportunity risk with their use.

Adverse Effects

Supplements are supposedly "natural," and by implication, they are conceived as being safer and gentler than pharmaceuticals. They are also less costly, readily available, and completely controlled by the user. "Safer" depends on the compared substance, but many herbs have interactions and effects that are anything but benign.

Among those with well-known counterindications and/or adverse effects: Ma Huang (also known as ephedra), for example, is a deadly ephedrine-packing substance that has killed at least 39 people and spawned hundreds of reports of heart attacks and strokes. Ma Huang should be taken only under a doctor's supervision and not by anyone with high blood pressure or cardiac disease.

And gentler? Coffee enemas for colonic "irrigation" have resulted in an outbreak of amebiasis in Colorado and sodium depletion, resulting in death. Chelation therapy has meant renal failure in several patients. Ginger, Gingko biloba, feverfew, and garlic interfere with platelet function and should not be taken (medicinally) by people taking anticoagulants or blood-thinning medication. St. John's Wort should not be taken with other photosensitizing medications or with many other antidepressants or certain decongestants. Valerian depresses the central nervous system and should not be combined with alcohol, tranquilizers, or other centrally acting drugs. DHEA (dehydroepiandrosterone) and androstenedione should not be taken at all because they may reset endocrine axes and cause glucocorticoid effects. Pennyroyal, a sweet-tasting herb prescribed as an abortifacient tea, has been reported to cause renal failure and death.

Many adverse effects are less well known, but there are now better places to discover them. Web sites (www.quackwatch.com) and the FDA's own MedWatch both list adverse effects of common supplements. Newsletters and journals for clinicians (e.g., *Alternative Medicine Alert, The Scientific Review of Alternative Medicine*) report up-to-date and thorough analyses.

Opportunity Risk

The opportunity risk for using alternative medicine is simply this: if a patient has a chronic medical condition and is taking conventional steps to control it, there is generally little added risk if he or she adds an alternative therapy. However, if a patient has an acute medical condition that is readily curable or controllable with conventional medicine, he or she may do personal harm by trying alternative therapy first—and this, practically speaking, is where the most serious harm is likely to be done. If alternative medicine does not work (e.g., for newly developed diabetes or leukemia), the conventional treatment involved is often more extensive, costly, and intensive than it would have been otherwise. Also, the treatment may be less effective.

DOES IT CONTAIN WHAT IT IS SUPPOSED TO? WHAT ASSURANCES OF PRODUCT QUALITY, FORMULATION, PURITY, AND COMPOSITION ARE EXTANT?

None of the dietary supplement manufacturers appear to test their products as comprehensively as do the pharmaceutical manufacturers—even when one manufacturer produces both products. Few marketers actually manufacture their own products, and most manufacturers do not have in-house analytical capabilities. The 1994 DSHEA notes that a company must know what is in their products and should test for validation. However, there is no penalty for noncompliance because the FDA is not equipped to police and enforce adherence to "recommendations." Furthermore, to seize a product, the FDA must prove it is unsafe. Note that the FDA has banned no supplement since the DSHEA went into effect.

Supplements of everything from saw palmetto (an extract of berries from an Atlantic coast palm tree effective in the treatment of symptoms of benign prostatic hyperplasia) to DHEA (a steroid hormone available over the counter and used for symptoms of fatigue, low libido, and for bodybuilding) are still unregulated. A recent *New England Journal of Medicine* report (Ko, 1998) noted that 24 of 260 Asian patent medicines collected contained a median of 30 parts per million (ppm) of lead, 36 contained a median of 180 ppm of arsenic, and 35 contained a median of 329 ppm of mercury. The U.S. Pharmacopeia "limits heavy metals in most oral pharmaceuticals to 30 ppm, with lower limits for lead, arsenic and mercury."

"WHAT'S IN A LABEL?"

New labels appear on supplements manufactured after March 1999. They resemble the FDA's required labels on packaged foods. Like those labels, however, which omit "trans fat" (every bit as potent in raising low-density lipoprotein [LDL] cholesterol as the required "saturated fat" on the label), much is left unspoken on the labels of dietary supplements. Unlike food labels, there is no guarantee that what is printed is actually inside the bottle. First and foremost, supplement labels market the product. Marketing has been based on ingredients, structure/function claims, and company name and image—not based on science.

Labels do not typically offer the origin of ingredients, unless it offers a perceived sales advantage to the manufacturer. Most vitamin C sold in the United States, for example, comes from corn. Most gelatin in vitamins comes from animal sources.

Paradoxically, the most "natural" formulations can also be the most toxic—oyster shell calcium tablets are much more likely to contain lead than plain calcium carbonate, and they are much more expensive.

Manufacturers can make structure/function claims with little fear of penalty or reprisal. Supplement manufacturers cannot make cause–effect claims and cannot give dosages. However, they can submit label information and label change information to the FDA just 30 days before the product hits the market. To the best of the author's knowledge, no penalty exists for not submitting supporting literature for the claims. Thus, an herb can "promote prostate health" or "enhance circulation" or "elevate mood," and it can show a dropper full of lovely elixir right next to two handfuls of antibiotics and let the reader and viewer draw their own conclusions.

Thus, it is little wonder that there have been countless examples of violations in labeling, but minimalist FDA response. Why? Because the FDA is hard pressed to acknowledge, inspect, analyze, and approve anything within 30 days, much less new product labeling.

Manufacturers are not accountable to the FDA—or to anyone else—unless the product has "a significant or unreasonable risk of illness or injury." Only then can the FDA withdraw the supplement from public harm (although again, it has never done so). A recent federal court decision (Pearson v. Shalala) made it even tougher on the FDA. The FDA can now ban claims that are "inherently misleading" but not those that are "potentially misleading." From a practical perspective, however, the FDA does neither.

Finally, company name and image in alternative medicine carry the weight that scientific evidence should. Johnson & Johnson and American Home Products are strong household names (despite their past fiascos—Tylenol, Fenfluramine, and Dexfenfluramine, among them), and Bayer (One-a-day products) and Whitehall-Robins (Centrum Herbals) are entering the market as well. Large pharmaceutical companies have not entered this market previously because plants could not be patented: even with the market's growth, supplements are barely 3% of all pharmaceuticals sold in the United States.

Improving quality, quality control, and safety will be their first order of business, and big companies will likely improve industry credibility because they have much to lose if they do not.

The problem is that there are no incentives for even a trustworthy, honorable company to go public with test results because there are no national standards for purity, dissolution, or safety and because competitor company B is unwilling to release their test results, if it has bothered to collect them. Moreover, it is not clear that consumers care—a recent Kaiser/NPR poll showed that 73% of consumers would continue to take supplements "if it worked for them," even if government research found the supplements to be ineffective (NPR/Kaiser, 1999).

The evidence, such as we are able to measure and assess it, continues to accrue, and it lands on both sides. Since 1997, high-dose beta carotene has been shown to increase the incidence of lung cancer in smokers, and the beta carotene arm of the Women's Health Initiative has been discontinued. Vitamin E supplementation appears to reduce the incidence of myocardial infarction, much like aspirin, but not mortality. And the link between vitamin C and heart disease remains as murky as ever.

So, unfortunately for consumers, messages from the supplement industry are truly mixed. Responsibility for the safety and effectiveness of dietary supplements resides with their manufacturer. There is no nationally accepted, mandatory standard for purity, dissolution, safety, or consistency of supplements. Most scientists are uncertain whether the ingredient that is isolated and purified and standardized (by the company, without external review) is even the active ingredient that has the promoted effect. In short, buying supplements without standards is like eating food that someone tells you is transitional between organically produced and conventionally produced: what this means to one person is not what it means to another.

WHAT DO DOCTORS THINK OF ALTERNATIVE MEDICINE?

Most physicians have encouraged at least one form of alternative medicine—usually diet or exercise. Many want to learn about alternative medicine, and those with the greatest enthusiasm tend to be younger and female. Because many patients believe their doctors to have a negative attitude about alternative medicine—patients fear being judged, embarrassed, and laughed at—physicians who put their skepticism in their pocket and try to earn their patients' trust differentiate themselves from their peers.

Doctors seem to fall into three camps about alternative medicine: true believers, prudent skeptics, and committed skeptics. Only a few are in the first category—maybe 5% to 10%; most are in the second category—maybe 60% to 70%. More than a few are in the latter category.

Among the believers, there are some avid ones and some salespeople. Alternative medicine has become an entrepreneur's delight. Retail markups of more than 50% are not uncommon for supplements sold in or nearby the office, and some physicians (after running the numbers) have supplements made under their own name to be marketed out of the office and in fitness centers. Buyouts and mergers of chiropractic practices with allopathic ones is the most recent wave of business activity, soon to be superseded by something else.

Some of these physicians truly believe that their patients deserve better choices, and they want to spend 45 to 60 minutes per patient to recapture the joy of medicine and to learn a patient's biography. Some are just tired of being told what, where, how, and when to practice by physician-managers who not uncommonly fled full-time clinical practice themselves for the comfort of a PC and no windows but a 6 o'clock dinner most nights at home without call. And some always wanted the rewards of the business world, the excitement of entrepreneurship, the challenge of creating and honing a brand, the riddles of the PR game. However, all of them believe, and they want their patients to believe too, and for the most part, they do.

Among prudent skeptics, there may not be a lot of financial remuneration in alternative medicine, but there is interest. A survey by Mehta (1997) found that as early as 1995, cardiologists were practicing as much as they preached. Mehta surveyed cardiologists listed in the American College of Cardiology. Almost half (44%) of all respondents took prophylactic antioxidants themselves. Vitamin E was the most commonly used antioxidant vitamin (39%), followed by vitamin C (33%) and beta carotene (19%). The most common dosage of aspirin taken was 325 mg daily; of vitamin E, 400 IU daily; vitamin C, 500 mg daily; and beta carotene, 20,000 units daily. Many took aspirin routinely (42%). Thirty-seven percent reported routinely prescribing antioxidants to their patients with coronary artery disease (response rate, 40%; mean age of respondents, 46).

On a similar note, Daaleman et al. (1999) mailed a questionnaire about personal and spiritual beliefs to a random national sample of active members of the American Academy of Family Physicians who had the self-designated professional activity of direct patient care (response rate, 58%). Survey results suggest that family physicians believe and practice as their patients do, especially in nonurban settings. There appears to be common, unexpected ground for spirituality in the office (La Puma, 1999). Of the surveyed physicians, 74% reported at least weekly or monthly religious service attendance. Seventy-nine percent reported a strong religious or spiritual orientation. Thirty-five percent reported daily time in private religious or spiritual practices. Although there are limitations to the study (e.g., significant regional variations in reported religiosity; differences between spirituality [conceptual and personal] and religion [doctrine, ritual and practice], biased toward nonurban family physicians [already more religious than their brethren in the city]), the data may be useful.

Finally, there are the committed skeptics, who will always regard all of alternative medicine as demonstration of the placebo effect (and may discount its usefulness and propriety as well). They may be right, but at bottom, medicine is consequentialist and pragmatic—physicians do what works. In many cases, the placebo effect works well enough to use as an actual clinical intervention. In fact, some physicians actively use the placebo effect with their enthusiasm, creation of the expectation of improvement, and warm, caring, attentive and positive attitude, especially about minor illnesses. Why? Because it often makes the patient feel better.

ETHICAL ISSUES: HELPING PROVIDERS AND PRACTITIONERS BALANCE ALLOPATHIC AND ALTERNATIVE THERAPIES

Allopathic physicians still have the opportunity to do good for most Americans. Only 3% of Americans have never seen an allopathic physician; for physicians, that is the first, perhaps most important, fact. Yet faced with consumers who do not want to wait until doctors have accumulated a library full of studies to test what they should already know, with which ethical voice should a physician speak?

- Should I try to do good by learning more about and then using alternative remedies with my patients?
- Or, should I just try to prevent patients from harm by warning of alternatives' dangers and interactions?

For many physicians, other major questions arise in daily practice, and first among them is informed consent. Can adequate information, reasonable understanding, and complete volition be satisfied if 300 mg of St. John's Wort "standardized" to contain 0.3% hypericin actually contains 0.1% or 0.9%? Or, what if some ginseng extracts contain up to 40% alcohol and are available at gas station check-out counters, next to the sunglasses?

Second is the issue of dual loyalty—especially economic dual loyalty. This issue deserves separate, more detailed treatment, as does the issue of managed care coverage. Some physicians believe it is unethical not to sell their formulation of skin cream (perhaps with calendula, perhaps with lavender essence) because it is the best available, in their opinion. Others believe that the medical office should not be a storefront because patients cannot know what they are getting any more than doctors can know what they are giving.

Third is the issue of professionalism and standards. An age-old turf battle if there ever was one is who qualifies: who can actually be termed a conventional provider and who an alternative provider is key to plans and providers alike. Do physicians need just a short course on the evidence for herbal therapies, on the indications for bodywork to call themselves integrated? Can patients tell the difference between an in-plan registered dietitian, harried and seldom paid-for, and a fee-for-service "nutritionist," paid for out of pocket? You bet they can.

Fourth is the issue of respect for persons—patients and providers—with non-Western beliefs and traditions. Staying with a young Hodgkin's patient who takes astragalus when chemotherapy and low-dose irradiation will likely cure him is much better than signing off his case. Keeping open communication lines, demonstrating openness to values and choices, and encouraging and providing information will be more successful than discharging the patient from your care.

Finally, language matters. Some say that the term *alternative medicine* legitimizes it as alternatives used to be options physicians offered as a second choice: for example, medical versus surgical treatment for triple vessel disease. Others say that the term *alternative medicine* derides what colleagues have to offer, despite the fact that theirs is a multibillion dollar industry and growing.

WILL PAYORS AND EMPLOYERS STEP IN? AND WHAT ABOUT MULTILEVEL MARKETING?

Despite dense discussions about the integration of complementary and allopathic medicine, the facts are that few organizations or practitioners know how to do it effectively or cost-effectively. The facts also are that saw palmetto's cost for treatment of benign prostatic hyperplasia (BPH) is a fraction of finasteride's for the same indication. Formulary costs are next on the list of expenses for which primary care physicians may be held responsible. Thus, price pressure is beginning to force consideration of effectiveness and cost-effectiveness, where popular considerations have not.

Plans have moved cautiously to cover the services of providers they cannot credential or assess qualitatively, much less empirically. Who is qualified to deliver herbalist services has become no more clear than the occasional lawsuit. Whether suits are occasional because little money is to be gained from an alternative provider's insurance (if it exists) or because the harm done is often minor is unknown.

Alternative medicine is still paid for largely out of pocket. However, more insurance companies, health plans, and employers are picking and choosing alternative therapies to cover. In every state in the country, chiropractors are licensed, and in 46 states, as of this writing, reimbursement for their services is mandated. Acupuncturists are licensed in 33 states, and 43 states recognize acupuncture as within the scope of physician practice (Leake & Broderick, 1999). The numbers are fewer for naturopaths and massage therapists, but they are also rising.

The opportunity for financial innovation is unlimited. HMO Illinois, a Blue Cross company, recently contracted with an alternative medicine independent practice association (IPA), using chiropractors as primary care physicians. American Whole Health, a privately held aggressive national chain of holistic health centers, which hires allopathic physicians to captain teams of nonallopathic providers, has raised $39 million in venture capital and owns eight centers at the time of this writing, with plans to buy and build more.

Will managed care kill what patients like about alternative medicine? Saddle it with credentialing, quality checking, and accountability mechanisms? Dictate when referrals to consultants are indicated? Decide whether the primary allopathic physician is responsible for the nonallopathic consultant's recommendations? Create and test algorithms and gauge cost-effectiveness? Rank coverage for alternative medicine next to hypertension screening and prenatal vitamins, for members to debate? These are questions for executives and, ultimately, patients to answer.

CREDENTIALING AND LICENSURE HURDLES

Employers and payors will be keenly interested in licensure hurdles. In some states, any licensed physician can practice acupuncture (or surgery, for that matter). In others, extensive training and examination are required. Naturopaths are licensed in only a few states, and homeopaths in even fewer. However, licensing is one of the few absolute standards for quality that conventional structures have, and consumers are learning that to have a chance of having alternative care paid for, licensed practitioners are the way to go.

WHAT ARE THE TAKE-HOME MESSAGES?
Suggestions/Rules of Thumb for Patients

- Look at quality in manufacturing. Is the manufacturer licensed to produce prescription pharmaceuticals and over-the-counter supplements/drugs, or just the latter? Both is better because they likely have higher internal standards, having had to deal with the FDA on a bit stricter level, and have more to lose if they falter.

- Are there good manufacturing practices/inspection violations that are public record? These are published on the FDA's Web site, at www.fda.gov.
- Is the product kosher? Stricter manufacturing regulations are required than what ordinary dietary supplements meet.
- If you are bent on knowing how good your supplement company really is, show up for a surprise facility visit. Sourcing, raw material handling, cataloging, air quality, and potential for cross-contamination are all ways in which companies do actually surprise consumers.
- Caveat emptor.

Suggestions for Executives and Physicians

Because the best techniques and sharpest insights for alternative medicine will likely be subsumed by allopathic medicine does not mean that alternative medicine can guarantee success. However, patients are not asking for guarantees. They are asking for effort, openness, interest, time, and a more personal, natural approach to everyday living.

We are aiming toward food as medicine, and the myriad ways in which people can prevent the diseases that clinicians spend so much time trying to treat once developed. Can you imagine prescribed meals on the formulary? Nutraceuticals next to beta-blockers? A reduced fat soybean with improved flavor characteristics? HCFA or NCQA grading plans and physicians on percentage of patients with a body mass index of less than 25 or 30?

It's not that far off. However, most of health policy and managed care are nowhere close to this—most patients depend on their next-door neighbor and on Oprah for their everyday, preventive medical advice.

CONCLUSION

Many doctors in managed care view alternative medicine as another procedure to add, or medication with which to become familiar, instead of a set of modalities that may be especially or differently useful or that may be culturally or socially linked to a different set of personal values. Physicians are, under most circumstances, so pressed by the day-to-day struggles of making a living that the movement toward alternative medicine has more chance to catch their fancy if it has immediate, real, and practical application. Physicians feel plainly impotent in creating their relationship with patients, and alternative medicine to most seems not so much like a way out as something else to be wary of, like capitation rates or managed care formalities. Unfortunately, most physicians have been "caught with their pants down by alternative medicine," like they were by managed care. As with managed care, they feel as if they have been ambushed.

On the upside, medical schools are just starting to teach alternative medicine. Many physician-centered newsletters and medical journals have arisen to educate physicians in practice, and postgraduate fellowships (e.g., at the University of Minnesota, the University of Arizona, and Cedars-Sinai Medical Center in Los Angeles) have been created to help physicians who want to take leadership. It is the dream of many ambitious academics (e.g., in the alternative medicine arena, no differently than in internal medicine or surgery) to foster a young cadre of researchers and clinicians who will some day head academic departments in their field. In this way, legacies are built, and former trainees model what they have learned for trainees in their own specialties.

However, it is unlikely that alternative medicine fellowships and residencies will allow graduates to march down this path and carve out new space within medical school walls or teaching program rotations. Alternative medicine seems unlikely to become a stand-alone, board-certified, CPT-coding specialty within medicine any more than lifestyle modification or medical ethics. Instead, the new available research monies and the tremendous popular interest in optimal health will foster the growth of alternative medicine within traditional allopathic medicine and will likely set the stage for the gradual integration of "alternative" techniques as part of allopathic medicine.

Consumers are the real driver of the interest in alternative medicine. Dissatisfied with the limits that managed care has placed on them, their healthcare, and their doctors, patients want to be regarded as human beings with personal needs, not as a number in a bed or a diagnosis on a billing slip. Patients do not care that alternative medicine's assumptions are not based in Western medical science or that its methods appear unorthodox or are used in other cultures. Patients want fewer medications, not more prescriptions, and fewer side effects from the medications that they have to take. Patients have come to expect wellness and are not finding it from physicians who are used to making decisions *for* patients.

What should be done is this: turn managed care from a health insurance program into a health program, especially for the Medicare population. What does this mean? Not a change from vaccinations, Pap smears, mammography, and colorectal cancer screening. *It means an addition to it.*

Employers should require exercise, nutrition, and smoking-cessation programs, delivered in the communities in which people live, and they should offer financial incentives for enrollment. People with low-risk profiles should have to pay less, both for the programs and for their premiums.

Is this feasible? Is it cost-effective? These are the questions of the managed care age. They have to be answered. However, they are not the questions patients are asking. Also, patients are using alternative medicine as a complement to allopathic medicine. Physicians should find out what patients find so compelling. (See Table 21–1 for more resources.)

TABLE 21-1

Key Credible Resources

Alternative Medicine on the Web

Acupuncture and Oriental Medicine National Certification Commission. www.nccaom.org.

Acupuncture/NIH Consensus Statement. http://odp.od.nih.gov/consensus/statements/cdc/107/107_stmt.htm.

American Botanical Council (translators of the German Commission E monographs—package inserts). www.herbalgram.org.

American Health Consultants (publishers of *Alternative Medicine Alert* and *Alternative Medicine Watch*). www.pubmed.com.

Cochrane Database of Systematic Reviews (an international network of reviews of randomized controlled clinical trials). http://hiru.mcmaster.ca/cochrane/default.htm.

Cranial Osteopathy (osteopathic manipulation how to site). http://users.dircon.co.uk/~med-man.

European Agency for Evaluation of Medical Products (part of the European Union overseeing drugs/medical devices). www.eucra.org/emea.html.

FDA List of Unsafe Herbs (updated periodically). http://lep.cl.msu.edu/msueimp/htdoc/mod03/03900066.html.

Herb Gardens, Medicinal. http://nnlm.nlm.nih.gov/pnr/uwmhg.

Herb Research Foundation (nonprofit educational agency—publisher of Herbalgram). www.herbs.org.

National Center for Complementary and Alternative Medicine (links to funded research, and the Citation Index, with more than 90,000 bibliographic citations, culled from Medline). http://altmed.od.nih.gov/nccam.

Prescriber's Letter (excellent, detailed documents on new drug developments, including conventional ones). www.prescribersletter.com.

United States Pharmacopeia (some botanical monographs now available). www.usp.org.

University of Texas Center for Alternative Medicine Research (cancer research). www.sph.uth.tmc.edu/utcam.

Alternative Medicine on the Web   Continued

Website on Ineffective Complementary Medicine Practices (a very skeptical, very careful physician compiles data here). www.quackwatch.com.

Selected General Articles

Angell M, Kassirer JP. Alternative medicine—the risks of untested and unregulated remedies. *N Engl J Med* 1998; 339:839–841.

Carroll RJ. When patients want alternative care. *ACP-ASIM Observer* 1998; 18–21.

Eisenberg D. Advising patients who seek alternative medical therapies. *Ann Intern Med* 1997; 127:61–69.

Eliason BC, et al. Dietary supplement users: demographics, product use and medical system interaction. *J Amer Board Fam Prac* 1997; 10:265–271.

Ernst E. Harmless herbs? A review of the recent literature. *Am J Med* 1998; 104:170.

Furnham A, Vincent C, Wood R. The health beliefs and behaviors of three groups of complementary medicine and general practice group of patients. *J Alt Med Comp Med* 1995; 1:347–359.

Moxos DA. Science, alternative care and third party payors. *Mt Sinai J Med* 1995; 62(2):159–162.

Core Texts

Blumenthal M (ed). German Commission E Monographs. IntegrativMedicine.

Robbers JE, Tyler VE. *Tyler's herbs of choice.* Haworth Press, 1999.

Rosenfeld I. *Dr. Rosenfeld's guide to alternative medicine.* Random House, 1997.

Schulz V, Hänsel R, Tyler VE. *Rational phytotherapy: a physician's guide to herbal medicine.* New York: Springer-Verlag, 1998.

Herbal PDR—Medical Economics, 1999.

REFERENCES

Astin JA. Why patients use alternative medicine: results of a national study. *JAMA* 1998; 279:1548–1553.

Daaleman TP, et al. Spiritual and religious beliefs and practices of family physicians—a national survey. *J Fam Pract* 1999; 48:98–104.

Eisenberg DM, et al. Unconventional medicine in the United States: prevalence, costs, and patterns of use. *N Engl J Med* 1993; 328:246–252.

Eisenberg DM, et al. Trends in alternative medicine use in the United States, 1990-1997: results of a follow-up national survey. *JAMA* 1998; 280:1569–1575.

Ko RJ. Adulterants in Asian patent medicines (Correspondence). *N Engl J Med* 1998; 339(12):847.

La Puma J. Why patients use alternative medicine. *Alternative Medicine Alert* 1999; 2(4):48.

Leake R, Broderick JE. Current licensure for acupuncture in the United States. *Alter Ther Health Med* 1999; 5(4):94–96.

Mehta J. Intake of antioxidants among American cardiologists. *Am J Cardiology* 1997; 79(11):1558–1560.

NPR/Kaiser Family Foundation/Kennedy School of Government. Survey on Americans and Dietary Supplements, February 1999. Web site: http://www.npr.org/programs/specials/survey/front.html.

Wennberg JE. AHCPR and the Strategy for Health Care Reform. *Perspective* 1992; 67–71.

Wetzel MS, Eisenberg DM, Kaptchuk TJ. Courses involving complementary and alternative medicine at US medical schools. *JAMA* 1998; 280(9):784–787.

ABOUT THE AUTHORS

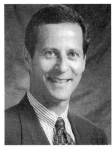 **David B. Nash,** M.D., M.B.A., is the founding Director of the Office of Health Policy and Clinical Outcomes at Thomas Jefferson University Hospital and the Associate Professor of Medicine at Jefferson Medical College in Philadelphia, positions he has held since 1990. In December 1996, Dr. Nash assumed additional responsibilities as the first Associate Dean for Health Policy at Jefferson Medical College. Nationally recognized for his work in outcomes management, medical staff development, and quality-of-care improvement, his publications have appeared in four dozen articles in major journals and in 10 edited books, including *The Physician's Guide to Managed Care* by Aspen Publishers and *A Systems Approach to Disease Management* by the American Hospital Publishing Company. In 1995, he was awarded the Clifton Latiolais Prize by the American Managed Care Pharmacy Association for his leadership in disease management, formulary design, and pharmacoeconomics. He also received the Philadelphia Business Journal Healthcare Heroes Award in October 1997.

Repeatedly named by Faulkner & Gray as one of the most influential policy makers in academic medicine, his national activities include appointment to the JCAHO National Performance Council, Vice Chair of the AMA Physician Measurement Advisory Committee, and the Foundation for Accountability (FACCT) Board. Recently, Dr. Nash completed his tenure as the Chairman of both the Center for Clinical Quality Evaluation and the Clinical Evaluative Sciences Council of the University HealthSystems Consortium (UHC) in Chicago, Illinois. He continues as one of the principal faculty members for quality-of-care issues of the American College of Physician Executives in Tampa, Florida, and the developer of the ACPE Capstone Course on Quality. He also directs the Physician's Track of the National Managed Health Care Congress. Dr. Nash recently was appointed as the Associate Director of the Pew Charitable Trusts-Managed Care Education Program, responsible for liaison activities with all interested outside parties. He is also a member of the board of trustees of Catholic Healthcare Partners in Cincinnati, Ohio.

Dr. Nash is a consultant to organizations in both the public and private sectors, including the Technical Advisory Group of the Pennsylvania Health Care Cost Containment Council, The Hartford Foundation, the Federal Agency for Health Care Policy and Research, and numerous corporations within the pharmaceutical industry. He is on the board of directors and advisory board of several national biotechnology and patient diagnostic firms. He is on the editorial board of three major peer-reviewed journals on medical quality management and three additional journals concerned with the cost-effectiveness of pharmaceuticals. From 1984 to 1989, Dr. Nash was Deputy Editor of *Annals of Internal Medicine* at the American College of Physicians. Currently, he is the Editor of *New Medicine* and a member of the *Medical Economics* editorial board.

Dr. Nash received his BA in economics (Phi Beta Kappa) from Vassar College, Poughkeepsie, New York; his M.D. from the University of Rochester School of Medicine and Dentistry; and his M.B.A. in Health Administration (with honors) from the Wharton School at the University of Pennsylvania. While at Penn, Dr. Nash was a former Robert Wood Johnson Foundation Clinical Scholar and Medical Director of a nine-physician faculty group practice in general internal medicine.

Dr. Nash lives in Lafayette Hill, Pennsylvania, with his wife, Esther J. Nash, M.D., twin daughters, and a son.

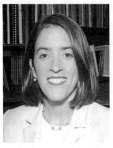 **Mary Pat Manfredi,** MPH, is the Project Director and assists in the development and coordination of educational programs for pharmaceutical industry clients. She also spearheads the Office's communications and publishing projects and is Managing Editor of the *Office of Health Policy Newsletter.* Among Ms. Manfredi's topical areas of interest and expertise are self-care, consumerism, and the impact of the switch of prescription drugs to over-the-counter status in the managed care setting. She received her dual BA degree in Health and Exercise Science and French from Furman University in Greenville, South Carolina, and her Master of Public Health degree, with focus on Health Promotion and Education, from the University of South Carolina in Columbia, South Carolina. Before joining the Office, Ms. Manfredi was a health and welfare analyst for a healthcare consulting firm in Atlanta, Georgia, which is also her hometown.

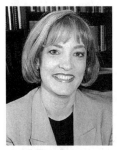 **Barbara L. Bozarth,** MSEd, as Program Director for the Office of Health Policy's educational programs, is responsible for the development and implementation of more than 25 new programs a year. In this capacity, she serves as primary liaison for Office clients, who comprise diverse sectors, including the public, academic, and nonprofit sectors. Ms. Bozarth works closely with clients to assess their educational objectives and to ensure that Office programs meet their unique needs. To this end, Ms. Bozarth is responsible for enlisting and coordinating the necessary resources, both within the Office and within the Jefferson Health System and Jefferson's CME partners. Ms. Bozarth received her BS in Zoology from Iowa State University, her BS in Diagnostic Imaging from Thomas Jefferson University, and her MS in Education from the University of Pennsylvania. Her prior experience includes having been a clinical research associate for a contract research organization and an education coordinator for the Department of Radiology at Thomas Jefferson University.

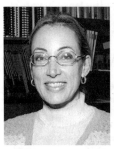 **Susan Howell,** MSS, is an editor and writer for the Office. In addition to serving as a developmental editor for Office publications, she is former managing editor for the *Office of Health Policy Newsletter.* Her responsibilities also include development and implementation of Office public events that promote the knowledge of health policy issues, such as the annual Grandon Lecture and the Health Policy Forum. Before joining the Office full time in 1995, Ms. Howell was a project coordinator and research assistant for Jefferson's Center for Research in Medical Education and Health Care, where her primary responsibilities were writing grant proposals, reports, and grants monitoring, including project budgets. While at the Center, Susan was a contributing author on a number of articles in health services research. The former Managing Editor of the *Journal of Outcomes Management,* she has also contributed to and/or served as editor on *The Physician's Guide to Managed Care, The Managed Care Manual: Future Practice Alternatives in Medicine,* and *Accountability and Quality in Health Care: The New Responsibility.* Ms. Howell has a background in marketing and healthcare program planning and development. She received her MSS from Bryn Mawr College, with a concentration in Advocacy, Planning and Program Development. She received her BS in Business Studies from SUNY College at Buffalo.

INDEX

ABOUT THE CONTRIBUTORS

Diane Bechel, Dr.P.H., received her doctorate in health policy in 1998 from the University of Michigan, as a Pew Charitable Trust Fellow. She currently serves as National Director of Hospital Profiling for a joint Big Three Automakers/American Hospital Association effort to distribute comparative hospital technical quality, cost, and patient reports of care results to active and retired workers in six U.S. regions. From 1996 to 1998, she was the Senior Health Policy Advisor for Ford Motor Company, where she created risk-adjusted quality measurement methodologies to inform employees and retirees about health plan and hospital performance and coordinated national Ford health policy efforts, including projects to increase safety belt use and projects to decrease workplace violence and tobacco use. Before that, she worked at Blue Cross and Blue Shield of Michigan in corporate strategy and quality management and managed two urgent care centers for the Daughters of Charity's first joint venture with physicians.

Dr. Bechel serves on the National Advisory Committee for the Consumer Assessment of Health Plans (CAHPS) National Benchmarking Data Base, and on the Advisory Committee for the Report on Scorecards project from the Midwest Business Group on Health. Her applied research interests focus on consumer healthcare informatics, and she is involved in local community hunger coalition and adult literary programs.

J. Marvin Bentley, Ph.D., is an Associate Professor of Health Economics at Penn State University. He teaches graduate courses in health administration at Penn State's School of Public Affairs. He earned a Ph.D. in economics from Tulane University. Dr. Bentley's research centers on state-sponsored medical outcome report cards. He is especially interested in how the information in these reports is used by health providers and ultimately shapes markets for healthcare in the United States. His studies on these topics have been published in *Health Services Research, The Joint Commission Journal on Quality Improvement,* and *American Journal of Medical Quality.*

Christina Bethell, Ph.D., M.B.A., M.P.H., is the Director of Research for FACCT—The Foundation for Accountability. FACCT is a not-for-profit organization dedicated to helping consumers make better healthcare decisions. Dr. Bethell has more than 15 years of experience in both healthcare policy and administration and public health at the state, local, and federal levels. She is a former senior policy analyst with VHA Inc. in Washington, D.C.; senior research associate with Chicago's Rush Primary Care Institute; and health policy analyst with both the American Association of Retired Persons and California's Health Access Foundation. In each of these roles, her primary focus has been on shaping a healthcare system that is organized, financed, and evaluated in ways that meet the health needs of the public.

Dr. Bethell has extensive experience working with communities to assess health needs and develop partnerships to improve health. She holds a Ph.D. in health services and policy research from the University of California at Berkeley. Her research has focused on both the role of the healthcare system in improving community health and the development and testing of indicators of performance for the healthcare system in the area of prevention and primary care. At FACCT, Dr. Bethell is responsible for the development of quality performance measures and consumer research. She is director of the Children and Adolescent Health Measurement Initiative, a national collaborative between FACCT and the National Committee for Quality Assurance.

John B. Coombs, M.D., is Associate Vice President for Medical Affairs (Clinical Systems & Networks) and the Associate Dean for Regional Affairs & Rural Health at the University of Washington School of Medicine in Seattle, Washington. In 1996–1997, he served as Acting Dean and Vice President for Medical Affairs for the University of Washington Academic Medical Center. Dr. Coombs is the T. J. Phillips Professor of Family Medicine and adjunct professor of pediatrics at the University of Washington. He has had 10 years experience in rural family practice, 8 years of which were spent as chief of staff in two under-fifty-bed rural hospitals. Before coming to the University of Washington, Dr. Coombs served as vice president for medical affairs at MultiCare Health Systems in Tacoma, Washington.

At the University of Washington, Dr. Coombs is responsible for the day-to-day operations of the Academic Medical Center (the hospitals, faculty practice plan, and medical school clinical activity) and oversees the School's Regional Medical Education Program—WWAMI, providing medical school activities for the States of Washington, Alaska, Montana, Idaho, and Wyoming. He is also responsible for graduate medical education programs at the University of Washington, with more than 1,500 residents and fellows in 57 programs.

After completing a master's degree in Nutritional Science from Cornell University, Dr. Coombs has pursued a career of linking sound nutritional care with primary care practice. He has lectured extensively on the topic and written many articles in this area as well. In addition to nutrition, he has published numerous articles on rural healthcare, healthcare public policy, and quality, and he is a frequent speaker nationally on these topics. He received his medical degree from Cornell University Medical College, New York City.

Tim R. Covington, M.S., Pharm.D., currently serves as Bruno Professor of Pharmacy and Executive Director of the Managed Care Institute of Samford University in Birmingham, Alabama. Dr. Covington has authored five books, edited the APhA *Handbook of Nonprescription Drugs* and the Facts and Comparisons book titled *Nonprescription Drug Therapy: Guiding Patient Self Care*, contributed to nine other books, published more than 160 professional and scientific articles, and presented more than 300 invited lectures and presentations.

Dr. Covington has been principal or co-principal investigator on a variety of research and service projects, generating more than $4 million in extramural support from 1973–1998. Dr. Covington has held elected and appointed offices in several state and national pharmacy organizations, including the American Pharmaceutical Association and American Society of Hospital Pharmacists. He currently serves on the Board of Directors and is Treasurer of the Pharmacy and Therapeutics Society. Dr. Covington is the recipient of seven national professional recognition awards and currently serves on advisory boards of seven national organizations and corporations. Dr. Covington serves as a consultant to numerous national healthcare corporations, governmental agencies, and managed care organizations.

Ann Danish, M.S.W., is the Director of Social Work and Chaplaincy Services at the Main Line Health Hospitals of the Jefferson Health System in suburban Philadelphia, Pennsylvania. She has many years of experience in providing, developing, and managing services and programs for patients and the community, including geriatric initiatives. She has also directed a hospice program and presently coordinates Main Line Health's domestic violence project.

Ms. Danish has served on numerous boards and advisory committees of organizations for the elderly, such as The Philadelphia Corporation for Aging, Main Line Adult Day Center, CARIE (Coalition of Advocates for the Rights of the Infirm Elderly), and Montgomery County Eldercare, as well as on the local Board of Health.

Felicia Gevirtz, M.S.P.H., has more than four years of research experience in health policy and outcomes research, having received her Master of Science of Public Health in 1996 from the University of North Carolina—Chapel Hill. Currently, she is attending the School of Policy, Planning and Development at the University of Southern California, where she plans to graduate in 2003 with a Ph.D. in Public Policy. She is also a consultant and works part-time at the RAND Corporation. Before this, she was an Assistant Project Director in the Office of Health Policy and Clinical Outcomes at Thomas Jefferson University.

Ms. Gevirtz's research interests include examining healthcare quality through provider report cards and patient satisfaction surveys, pharmacoeconomics, disease management, and mental health policy. Ms. Gevirtz was a Research Analyst in the Outcomes Research Department at PCS HealthSystems. She received her bachelor's degree from the State University of New York (SUNY) at Binghamton in 1994.

Stuart Gitlow, M.D., M.P.H., is the Chair of the American Medical Association's Young Physician Section. He is responsible for the one-third of the nation's physicians who are younger than 40 or in their first 5 years of practice. Dr. Gitlow is currently a member of the AMA's Online Oversight Panel, the American Psychiatric Association's Telemedical Services Committee, the Pennsylvania Medical Society's Physician Technology Education Committee, and chairman of the American Society of Addiction Medicine's Telemedicine Committee. He has been active in organized medicine since 1985 and is past-chair of the Pennsylvania Medical Society's Young Physician Section. He has provided consultation for the U.S. Public Health Service, the New York Board of Medicine, the New Hampshire Public Defender Office, the Pennsylvania Bureau of Disability Determination, and the Massachusetts Disability Determination Services. He provides peer review services for Core, Inc.'s Behavioral Management section in Boston and is a Medical Expert for the Social Security Administration's Office of Hearings and Appeals. He currently is medical director of the Family and Children's Service of Nantucket, where he sees patients in the outpatient and residential settings.

Dr. Gitlow is board certified by the American Board of Psychiatry and Neurology in general, addiction, and forensic psychiatry. He has presented internationally on topics of substance dependence, depressive disorders, and the integration of computers with the field of medicine. Dr. Gitlow's training in both addiction and forensic psychiatry took place at Massachusetts General Hospital and Harvard Medical School. His general psychiatric training and psychiatric epidemiology work were both at the University of Pittsburgh following his basic medical training at Mount Sinai in New York.

Since 1985, Dr. Gitlow has been involved in the field of telecommunications. In April of that year, he founded Laser-Board, New York's full-time bulletin board system dedicated to the Macintosh computer. After three years, LaserBoard was taken national as Mac Symposium and PC Symposium, the successful computing forums of the Connect Business Information Network. He and many of his staff then helped build the computing forums of Quantum Computing's online service, which would later be named America Online. By 1995, he had been brought in as Coordinator of America Online's Mac Computing Forums, where he was responsible for a staff of more than 200 and for a site receiving tens of millions of hits each month. Dr. Gitlow is now Chief Medical Officer of Healant, Inc., the online health communities company based in Greensboro, North Carolina.

Julianna S. Gonen, Ph.D., serves as Director of Family Health at the Washington Business Group on Health (WBGH). WBGH represents employers in promoting performance-driven health-care systems and competitive markets that improve the health and productivity of companies and communities. The business group's family health programs include initiatives relating to maternal and child health, women's health, and work-life issues. These programs foster partnerships and corporate best practices in areas such as prenatal care, breast-feeding support, domestic violence, preventative care and screening, and family-friendly workplace policies.

Before joining WBGH, Dr. Gonen served as Research Associate with the Jacobs Institute of Women's Health in Washington, D.C., an independent, nonprofit, multidisciplinary membership organization that studies and disseminates infor-mation to advance the knowledge, understanding, and practice of women's healthcare. There she worked primarily on issues re-lating to women's health and managed care, authoring a briefing paper series titled *Insights* and planning related symposia.

Before her work at the Jacobs Institute, Dr. Gonen was Senior Research Associate in the Medical Affairs Department at the American Association of Health Plans (AAHP), the principal national trade association representing managed healthcare or-ganizations. At AAHP, Dr. Gonen worked on issues relating to women's health, accreditation and performance measurement, technology assessment, electronic data interchange, medical ed-ucation, and childhood immunization. Previous to her position at AAHP, she was Director of Industry Research at the American Managed Care and Review Association (AMCRA), another man-aged care association that merged with the former Group Health Association of America (GHAA) to form AAHP.

Dr. Gonen received her Bachelor of Arts degree in govern-ment from Cornell University and holds a doctorate in political science from the American University in Washington, D.C. Her dissertation examined public policy litigation around employ-ment discrimination against women based on reproductive haz-ards in the workplace.

In addition to her work with the Jacobs Institute, Dr. Gonen is an adjunct professor at American University in the Depart-ment of Government and serves on the Long Range Planning Committee of Washington's Whitman-Walker Clinic. She also does independent consulting research on women's health services.

Steven Haimowitz, M.D., has devoted his full time energies to the field of health communication for the past 10 years and is a co-founder of Healthology.com, a leading online health media company. He has extensive experience in effectively delivering health information to both the consumer and healthcare professional audiences. He has a reputation as a forward-thinking leader in developing unique educational programs that embrace emerging trends, with a focus on health consumerism and physician–patient communication.

Dr. Haimowitz served as a senior level consultant to leading international healthcare communications companies. He has worked with companies from virtually all sectors of the healthcare marketplace, with a roster including academic associations, Fortune 100 pharmaceutical companies, biotechnology companies, hospitals and health systems, managed care organizations, physician practice management companies, and nutritional and consumer product companies.

Dr. Haimowitz was a participant in the seven-year accelerated B.A./M.D. program of the City and State University of New York. After receiving his B.A. degree in three years from the City University of New York in 1984, he went on to Downstate Medical Center of the State University of New York, receiving his M.D. in 1988. He did his postgraduate training at the Albert Einstein College of Medicine in New York.

James Hereford, M.S., is currently the Executive Director of Customer Services for Group Health Cooperative, one of the nation's oldest and most prestigious HMOs. Mr. Hereford's duties at Group Health include strategy development for customer services, assessment of service quality, customer service operations, and leading major process and systems improvement projects.

Before taking this position, Mr. Hereford was a Senior Quality Consultant and Quality Education Manager at Group Health. Before coming to Group Health Cooperative in 1991, Mr. Hereford was an independent consultant in statistical process control for manufacturing companies in the Puget Sound region, including the Boeing Commercial Airplane Group. Mr. Hereford began his professional career as a mathematics teacher and basketball coach in 1982 in Lewistown, Montana.

Mr. Hereford also serves on the faculty of the Institute for Healthcare Improvement in Boston, Massachusetts, where he teaches courses on improvement methods in healthcare and the use of quantitative approaches to improvement. Mr. Hereford has a master's degree in Mathematics from Montana State University.

Naomi R. Klayman, Ph.D., has been consulting for health insurance, pharmaceutical, and medical education institutions for well over a decade. Her academic training is in social communication and qualitative research methods, with a focus on physician–patient communication and gender. She has taught medical interviewing skills and biopsychosocial medicine for residents and faculty. She has worked extensively in the fields of managed care, having spent nine years conducting research for major health insurers. Dr. Klayman is continuing to explore how consumers, health professionals, and health-related industries respond to health policy.

David J. Lansky, Ph.D., is the president of FACCT—The Foundation for Accountability. FACCT is a not-for-profit organization dedicated to helping consumers make better healthcare decisions. FACCT's board of trustees is made up of consumer organizations, corporate healthcare purchasers, and government purchasers representing 80 million Americans.

FACCT believes that America's ability to create a more responsive healthcare system depends on informed, empowered consumers who help shape the system, hold it accountable for quality, and act as partners in improving their health. To achieve this goal, FACCT creates tools that help people understand and use quality information, develops consumer-focused quality measures, supports public education about healthcare quality, supports efforts to gather and provide quality information, and encourages health policy to empower and inform consumers.

Before joining FACCT, Dr. Lansky was regional director of clinical information for Oregon-based Providence Health System, a statewide integrated system that includes six hospitals, primary care groups, home health services, and both HMO and PPO insurance services. At Providence, he led the Center for Outcomes Research and Education, which helps members, patients, doctors, and managers measure and understand the quality of healthcare delivery. Dr. Lansky's team was responsible for outcomes research, measurement of consumer satisfaction, health risk and health status assessment, development of electronic member and patient records, and communications with purchasers and the larger community about healthcare quality.

During 1993 and 1994, Dr. Lansky provided support to the Jackson Hole Group, with responsibility for national accountability measures under the "managed competition" model. He holds a Doctor of Philosophy degree from the University of California in Berkeley.

John La Puma, M.D., F.A.C.P., was the first physician in the United States to enter a postgraduate fellowship in medical ethics, at the University of Chicago. Dr. La Puma was also the first physician in this country to graduate from the Cooking and Hospitality Institute of Chicago. Since 1995, he has cooked regularly at Rick Bayless' Frontera Grill/Topolobampo in Chicago, and he has represented the Society for General Internal Medicine to the Healthy People 2000 Consortium.

Formerly a Clinical Associate Professor of Medicine at the University of Chicago, Dr. La Puma has been invited to speak at the Brookings Institution and has testified before the U.S. Senate. His work has been published by the *New England Journal of Medicine,* the *Encyclopedia Britannica, The Wall Street Journal, USA Today,* and *Prevention Magazine.* Dr. La Puma has written 3 scholarly books and more than 250 articles, published in scientific, culinary, and popular journals and newspapers.

Dr. La Puma is currently a Professor of Nutrition at Kendall College in Evanston, Illinois, and Founding and Executive Editor of *Alternative Medicine Alert,* the leading evidence-based clinical newsletter for physicians. He is the national spokesperson for the D.A.S.H. (Dietary Approaches to Stop Hypertension) Eating Plan. He directs *C.H.E.F.* (Cooking, Healthy Eating and Fitness) *Clinic* and *C.H.E.F. Research,* which teach and study the hands-on lifestyle management of food-related medical problems.

Marnie LaVigne, Ph.D., is the Executive Director of Consumer Editorial for Medscape, Inc., a healthcare Web site that provides comprehensive, authoritative, and timely medical information and interactive programs to physicians; allied healthcare professionals, such as pharmacists and nurses; and consumers at www.Medscape.com. Previously she co-founded Patient Info-systems, Inc., where she was responsible for interactive, behavior-

and outcomes-based services, including disease management, demand management, Internet, surveys, and other healthcare support programs.

Dr. LaVigne has 15 years of experience in health psychology and behavioral medicine, with nearly 10 of those years in research, development, and operation of disease management programs and outcomes studies in multiple therapeutic areas. She has authored numerous conference presentations and publications regarding disease management. In addition, she has taught psychology courses at several universities. Dr. LaVigne has a doctorate in clinical psychology from the University of Rochester.

Paul C. LePore, Ph.D., as Assistant Professor at the University of Washington, specializes in social psychology, social structure and personality, and the sociology of education, with focus on adolescents. In addition to his work on the adolescent self-concept, Dr. LePore has written on the social psychological processes associated with blood donation and other forms of medical volunteerism. In addition, he has worked on a number of projects analyzing the role of schools and classroom organization on student achievement.

Dr. LePore's current projects include studies on the impact of employment during high school on academic outcomes, the development of "home schooling" as a recent educational reform effort in Washington state and throughout the nation, and a long-term project on the processes of family educational decision making. In particular, Dr. LePore is analyzing the individual-, family-, and school-level variables that affect school choice decisions.

Mike Magee, M.D., is Senior Medical Advisor of Pfizer Inc. and director of the Pfizer Medical Humanities Initiative. In this capacity, he is called on to speak for Pfizer worldwide, and for the pharmaceutical industry, on a wide range of clinical and public policy issues that impact quality of life.

Dr. Magee is Professor of Surgery at Jefferson Medical College and has consulted for Congress, the American Medical Association, the American Association of Medical Colleges, and the American Hospital Association. His work on creating positive and productive relationships among doctors, nurses, health managers, trustees, health suppliers, payors, and patients is well known, often quoted, and has placed him at the center of health-care reform.

Dr. Magee is past president of the National Association of Physician Broadcasters and a former radio and television columnist, titled by the *Boston Globe,* "the most optimistic physician in America—Medicine's own Norman Vincent Peale." He is an accomplished public speaker and prolific writer with more than 100 titles to his name.

Dr. Magee is the son of a house-call-making doctor and one of 12 children. He attended medical school in Syracuse, New York, and did his surgical residency at the University of North Carolina. He spent 13 years as a country doctor in rural New England before assuming progressive academic and leadership posts, including Senior Vice President of Pennsylvania Hospital in Philadelphia, our nation's first hospital. He and his wife, Trish, have four children and live in New York City.

Suzanne Mercure's experience is from the perspective of the employer as a purchaser of health and healthcare services for employees, retirees, unions, and family members. Ms. Mercure has work experience in all areas of benefits, including work/family programs, health promotion and prevention, behavioral health, lost work time, pension and savings, and health plans. Ms. Mercure's work for employers and as a consultant has included strategic planning, program value assessment, marketplace and policy change, quality improvement and measurement, consumer information, consumer input processes, consumer information, and problem resolution for consumers.

Ms. Mercure worked for Southern California Edison in the Los Angeles area. Before this California experience, she worked on the East Coast. She has developed collaborative projects with employers, health plans, providers, academia, and government. Currently, she works as an independent consultant on purchaser issues with Centers for Disease Control and Prevention, National Committee for Quality Assurance, Institute for Health Policy Solutions, Managed Health Care Association, and National Business Coalition on Health.

In these roles, Ms. Mercure has had numerous opportunities to speak at conferences, provide testimony for congressional committees, as well as work directly with purchasers, providers, and plans. She has served on the boards of Washington Business Group on Health, Employers Managed Health Care Association, Health Action Committee for Greater Boston, Visiting Nurse Association of Boston, California Health Information Reporting Initiative, California Primary Care Consortium, and California Health Decisions.

Molly Mettler, M.S.W., is Senior Vice President of Healthwise, Inc., a not-for-profit consumer health information group located in Boise, Idaho. In 1995, Ms. Mettler began directing the Healthwise Communities Project, a community-based health education project.

Ms. Mettler is known nationally as an expert in medical self-care program design, medical consumer issues, and patient empowerment. She devotes most of her time speaking to national audiences and writing about how to empower patients, improve doctor–patient partnerships, and the concept of shared medical decision making.

Ms. Mettler serves on the advisory boards of many organizations and is a Fellow of the Health Forum's Creating Healthier Communities Fellowship. She has co-authored four books on medical self-care and health promotion, including *Healthwise for Life: Medical Self-Care for Healthy Aging* and *It's About Time: Better Health Care in a Minute (or two)*, and has written numerous articles for national publications. She holds a Master of Social Work degree from the University of Washington.

Joel E. Miller is Director of Policy for the National Coalition on Health Care, a broad-based alliance composed of employers, unions, consumer and religious organizations, payors, and medical organizations. In this capacity, he provides technical expertise on a wide range of healthcare issues to Coalition members, policy makers, and the media and provides analyses on proposed legislation that affects the Coalition and its principles. He oversees the Coalition's commissioned studies and has authored several reports on cost, coverage, and quality issues. In 1998, Mr. Miller conducted for the Coalition a meta-analysis of 22 healthcare public opinion surveys published in 1997 and 1998.

Mr. Miller served as Director of Professional Relations at the Health Insurance Association of America (HIAA), where he organized and managed HIAA's Medical Practice Assessment

Unit. That body provided technical assistance to health insurers on healthcare technology assessment and quality assessment issues affecting third-party payors.

Mr. Miller has also served as Director of the Illinois Health Care Coalition, which served as a forum for employers, unions, insurers, and provider groups to advance cost containment and quality assurance initiatives. He has consulted for many pharmaceutical companies and several healthcare organizations such as the American Medical Association (AMA) and the American Hospital Association (AHA).

Mr. Miller has also served on advisory committees on quality of care issues to the Health Care Financing Administration, American College of Cardiology, Institute of Medicine, the AMA, and the AHA. He has written articles on medical practice assessment issues, physician reimbursement, continuous quality improvement in healthcare, and managed mental healthcare.

Woodrow A. Myers, Jr., M.D., M.B.A., is Director of Healthcare Management for the Ford Motor Company in Dearborn, Michigan. In that role, he has management responsibility for the Ford healthcare benefit for active and retired Ford employees and their dependents, as well as for workplace safety, occupational health, worker's compensation, and disability benefit issues. Before taking his current position, he was Senior Vice President and Corporate Medical Director of The Associated Group, a corporation with major interests in managed healthcare and health insurance, whose national headquarters are in Indianapolis, Indiana. Dr. Myers also served as the New York City Health Commissioner under former New York City Mayor David Dinkins.

In the 5 years before joining the New York City Department of Health, Dr. Myers served as Indiana State Health Commissioner and Secretary to the Indiana State Board of Health. From 1982 to 1984, he was an Associate Director of the medical-surgical intensive care unit and chairman of the quality assurance program at the San Francisco General Hospital, as well as an Assistant Professor of Medicine at the University of California-San Francisco.

A past president of the Association of State and Territorial Health Officials and former advisor to the U.S. Senate Committee on Labor and Human Resources, Dr. Myers has held faculty positions at the Cornell University Medical College and the Institute of Health Policy Studies at the University of California-San Francisco and at the Indiana University School of Medicine.

He received a B.S. from Stanford University, his M.D. from Harvard Medical School, and his M.B.A. from Stanford University Graduate School of Business. He currently holds an appointment as Clinical Associate Professor of Medicine, Wayne State University School of Medicine, and Adjunct Associate Professor of Internal Medicine, University of Michigan School of Medicine.

Dr. Myers is a member of the Institute of Medicine, the Medicare Payment Advisory Commission, and the national advisory councils for the Centers for Disease Control and Prevention and the Agency for Health Care Policy and Research. He is also a member of the Board of Overseers of Harvard University and the Board of Directors of UCSF (University of California-San Francisco)-Stanford University Health Care. He is a Master of the American College of Physicians and a Fellow of the American College of Physician Executives.

Ira S. Nash, M.D., F.A.C.C., is Associate Director of the Zena and Michael A. Wiener Cardiovascular Institute of the Mount Sinai Medical Center in New York and an Assistant Professor of Medicine of the Mount Sinai School of Medicine. He is a summa cum laude graduate of Harvard College and received his M.D. degree cum laude from the Harvard-MIT Program in Health Sciences and Technology at Harvard Medical School. He completed his residency in internal medicine and his fellowship in both clinical and interventional cardiology at Boston's Beth Israel Hospital. Before taking his current position, he was on the full-time academic staff of the Cardiac Unit at the Massachusetts General Hospital and on the faculty of Harvard Medical School.

In addition to being an active clinician and teacher, Dr. Nash directs the quality assessment and improvement activities of the Cardiovascular Institute. His interests include the exploration of the role of generalists and specialists in the changing healthcare environment, the application of computer technology to clinical practice, and the assessment and improvement of clinical outcomes in cardiology. He has edited two books and been published in a variety of journals about these and other issues in cardiology.

Since 1998, Dr. Nash has also served as the on-air spokesman for the Mount Sinai Hospital in the "2 Your Health" series of television public service announcements and promotions produced by WCBS-TV in New York. He is married and has two daughters.

Philip A. Newbold, President/CEO of Memorial Health System and Memorial Hospital of South Bend, Indiana, has been with Memorial since 1987. Before taking his position at Memorial, he was the President/CEO of Baptist Medical Center in Oklahoma City. In 1992, Newbold was awarded the Philip Kotler Award for Excellence in Healthcare Marketing and, in 1991, he was awarded the THF-3M 21st Century Innovators Award. He has received the THF-Korn/Ferry International Emerging Leaders Award and is a Fellow in the American Academy of Medical Administrators and the American College of Healthcare Executives. He also serves as Past Board Chairman of The Healthcare Forum. Mr. Newbold has authored numerous articles on healthcare issues and is the co-author of two books on healthcare sales and acquiring physician practices.

Diane Serbin Stover joined Memorial Health System in 1990 and is currently Vice President, Market Communications. Before her arrival in South Bend, Indiana, she served as Director of Marketing for AMI Alabama and was responsible for market communications, public affairs, and physician relations at AMI Brookwood Medical Center in Birmingham. She also served as a corporate marketing consultant for AMI hospitals in Tuscaloosa, Denver, Baton Rouge, and Tarzana. Ms. Stover is a native of Philadelphia, Pennsylvania, and has held market communications positions with the U.S. Department of Health & Human Services, Northwestern Institute of Psychiatry and the Medical College of Pennsylvania.

Ms. Stover has been recognized with numerous local and national healthcare marketing awards, including recognition as the Young Marketer of the Year—1996 from the Alliance for Healthcare Strategy and Marketing. She is a life-time volunteer with the YMCA and is active in various school and church committees in South Bend.

Linda M. Stutz, R.N., M.B.A., is now the Manager of Health Management Development for Roche Diagnostics Corporation, Indianapolis, Indiana, with more than 15 years of progressive hospital and healthcare experience and 5 years developing new companies. In this capacity, she is responsible for the conceptual design, development, implementation, and evaluation of disease management and health management initiatives for the diabetes patient care division. Ms. Stutz is the past CEO for the National Institute for Managed Care Education, a training company that educates healthcare providers and consumers about the changing healthcare environment. In addition, she has served as a senior consultant for Health Evolutions, Inc., a health management consulting firm, and as Vice President of Operations for Summex Corporation, an employer-focused health promotion and demand management consulting company.

Ms. Stutz is currently authoring the book *Nurses in Managed Care: New Roles in a Changing System.* She has an M.B.A. from Indiana Weslyan University and a B.S. in Nursing from the University of Evansville. Ms. Stutz is a member of the American Nurses Association, the Indiana State Nurses Association, the American Organization for Nurse Executives, the National Nurses in Business Association, and the Executive Women in Healthcare organization. She also serves as faculty at the University of Southern Indiana, where she is a member of the Advisory Board for Healthier Communities.

Elizabeth White, M.D., is currently Medical Director, Senior Health for the Jefferson Health System in Philadelphia, where she is involved in developing integrated long-term care services for seniors. She studied medicine in Hamburg, Germany; completed a Family Medicine Residency in Portland, Maine; and a Fellowship in geriatrics at the University of Pennsylvania. Since residency, she has focused on caring for the elderly and has served as Medical Director in a variety of settings, including nursing homes, home health care, and hospice.